Current Controversies in Perinatology

Editors

ROBERT H. LANE
ROBERT M. KLIEGMAN

CLINICS IN PERINATOLOGY

www.perinatology.theclinics.com

Consulting Editor
LUCKY JAIN

December 2014 • Volume 41 • Number 4

ELSEVIER

1600 John F. Kennedy Boulevard • Suite 1800 • Philadelphia, Pennsylvania, 19103-2899

http://www.theclinics.com

CLINICS IN PERINATOLOGY Volume 41, Number 4
December 2014 ISSN 0095-5108, ISBN-13: 978-0-323-32672-8

Editor: Kerry Holland
Developmental Editor: Casey Jackson

Clinics in Perinatology (ISSN 0095-5108) is published quarterly by Elsevier Inc., 360 Park Avenue South, New York, NY 10010-1710. Months of issue are March, June, September, and December. Business and Editorial Offices: 1600 John F. Kennedy Blvd., Ste. 1800, Philadelphia, PA 19103-2899. Customer Service Office: 3251 Riverport Lane, Maryland Heights, MO 63043. Periodicals postage paid at New York, NY and additional mailing offices. Subscription prices are $285.00 per year (US individuals), $445.00 per year (US institutions), $340.00 per year (Canadian individuals), $545.00 per year (Canadian institutions), $420.00 per year (foreign individuals), $545.00 per year (foreign institutions), $135.00 per year (US students), and $195.00 per year (Canadian and foreign students). Foreign air speed delivery is included in all Clinics subscription prices. All prices are subject to change without notice. **POSTMASTER:** Send address changes to *Clinics in Perinatology*, Elsevier Health Sciences Division, Subscription Customer Service, 3251 Riverport Lane, Maryland Heights, MO 63043. **Customer Service: Telephone: 1-800-654-2452** (U.S. and Canada); **1-314-447-8871** (outside U.S. and Canada). **Fax: 1-314-447-8029. E-mail: journalscustomerservice-usa@elsevier.com** (for print support); **journalsonlinesupport-usa@elsevier.com** (for online support).

Reprints. For copies of 100 or more, of articles in this publication, please contact the Commercial Reprints Department, Elsevier Inc., 360 Park Avenue South, New York, NY 10010-1710. Tel. 212-633-3874; Fax: 212-633-3820; E-mail: reprints@elsevier.com.

Clinics in Perinatology is also publlshed in Spanish by McGraw-Hill Interamericana Editores S.A., P.O. Box 5-237, 06500 Mexico D.F., Mexico.

Clinics in Perinatology is covered in *MEDLINE/PubMed (Index Medicus) Current Contents, Excepta Medica, BIOSIS and ISI/BIOMED.*

Contributors

CONSULTING EDITOR

LUCKY JAIN, MD, MBA
Richard W. Blumberg Professor and Executive Vice Chairman, Department of Pediatrics, Emory University School of Medicine; Executive Medical Director, Children's Healthcare of Atlanta Faculty Practices, Atlanta, Georgia

EDITORS

ROBERT H. LANE, MD, MS
The Barri L. and David J. Drury Chair in Pediatrics; Pediatrician in Chief, Children's Hospital of Wisconsin; Chair, Department of Pediatrics, Medical College of Wisconsin, Milwaukee, Wisconsin

ROBERT M. KLIEGMAN, MD
Professor and Chair Emeritus, Department of Pediatrics, Children's Hospital of Wisconsin, Medical College of Wisconsin, Milwaukee, Wisconsin

AUTHORS

KANWALJEET J. S. ANAND, MBBS, D.Phil., FAAP, FCCM, FRCPCH
Professor of Pediatrics, Anesthesiology, Anatomy & Neurobiology, Department of Pediatrics/Critical Care Medicine, Le Bonheur Children's Hospital & University of Tennessee Health Science Center, Memphis, Tennessee

MIR A. BASIR, MD, MS
Associate Professor of Pediatrics, Section of Neonatology, Department of Pediatrics, Children's Corporate Center, Medical College of Wisconsin, Milwaukee, Wisconsin

DAVID A. BATEMAN, MD
Professor of Pediatrics, Division of Neonatal-Perinatal Medicine, Department of Pediatrics, College of Physicians and Surgeons, Columbia University, New York, New York

MANEESH BATRA, MD, MPH, FAAP
Associate Professor of Pediatrics, Division of Neonatology, Department of Pediatrics, University of Washington School of Medicine, Seattle, Washington

MARYLOU BEHNKE, MD
Professor Emeritus, Department of Pediatrics, University of Florida, Gainesville, Florida

DAVID P. BICK, MD
Professor and Chief of Genetics, Department of Pediatrics, Medical College of Wisconsin, Milwaukee, Wisconsin

DAVID P. DIMMOCK, MD
Associate Professor, Department of Pediatrics, Medical College of Wisconsin, Milwaukee, Wisconsin

MICHELE A. FROMMELT, MD
Professor, Pediatric Cardiology, Division of Cardiology, Children's Hospital of Wisconsin, Milwaukee, Wisconsin

RICHARD W. HALL, MD, FAAP
Professor of Pediatrics, Obstetrics & Gynecology, University of Arkansas for Medical Sciences, Little Rock, Arkansas

M. ELIZABETH HARTNETT, MD, FACS, FARVO
Professor of Ophthalmology, Adjunct Professor of Pediatrics, Neurobiology and Anatomy, Department of Ophthalmology and Visual Sciences, John A. Moran Eye Center, University of Utah, Salt Lake City, Utah

SHERI JOHNSON, PhD
Assistant Professor, Department of Pediatrics, Center for the Advancement of Underserved Children, Medical College of Wisconsin, Milwaukee, Wisconsin

U. OLIVIA KIM, MD
Assistant Professor of Pediatrics, Section of Neonatology, Department of Pediatrics, Children's Corporate Center, Medical College of Wisconsin, Milwaukee, Wisconsin

DAVID W. KIMBERLIN, MD
Professor of Pediatrics, Division of Pediatric Infectious Diseases, The University of Alabama at Birmingham, Birmingham, Alabama

MARK KLEBANOFF, MD
Professor, Departments of Pediatrics and Obstetrics and Gynecology, The Ohio State University; Professor, Division of Epidemiology, The Ohio State University College of Public Health; Principal Investigator, The Research Institute, Nationwide Children's Hospital, Columbus, Ohio

JACQUELYN KUZMINSKI, MD, FAAP
Assistant Professor of Pediatrics, Department of Pediatrics Global Health Program, Medical College of Wisconsin, Milwaukee, Wisconsin

JOANNE LAGATTA, MD, MS
Assistant Professor, Department of Pediatrics, Medical College of Wisconsin, Milwaukee, Wisconsin

ROBERT H. LANE, MD, MS
The Barri L. and David J. Drury Chair in Pediatrics; Pediatrician in Chief, Children's Hospital of Wisconsin; Chair, Department of Pediatrics, Medical College of Wisconsin, Milwaukee, Wisconsin

ANNE CC LEE, MD, MPH, FAAP
Assistant Professor of Pediatrics, Department of Pediatric Newborn Medicine, Brigham and Women's Hospital, Harvard Medical School, Boston, Massachusetts

STEVEN R. LEUTHNER, MD, MA
Professor of Pediatrics and Bioethics, Medical College of Wisconsin, Wauwatosa, Wisconsin

NORMA MAGALLANES, BSc
Department of Pediatrics, Center for the Advancement of Underserved Children, Medical College of Wisconsin, Milwaukee, Wisconsin

AMBER MAJNIK, PhD
Department of Pediatrics, Division of Neonatology, Medical College of Wisconsin, Milwaukee, Wisconsin

KARA B. MARKHAM, MD
Assistant Professor, Maternal Fetal Medicine Division, Department of Obstetrics & Gynecology, The Ohio State University College of Medicine, Columbus, Ohio

PATRICIA McMANUS, PhD, RN
President/CEO Black Health Coalition of Wisconsin, Inc, Milwaukee, Wisconsin

MICHAEL E. MITCHELL, MD
Division of Cardiothoracic Surgery, Department of Surgery, Medical College of Wisconsin, Milwaukee, Wisconsin

JOSEF NEU, MD
Professor of Pediatrics, Department of Pediatrics, Division of Neonatology, University of Florida, Gainesville, Florida

CLIFF O'CALLAHAN, MD, PhD, FAAP
Assistant Professor of Pediatrics, University of Connecticut, Mansfield, Connecticut; Director of Nurseries and Faculty FM Residency, Middlesex Hospital, Middletown, Connecticut

JULIE PANEPINTO, MD, MSPH
Professor, Department of Pediatrics; Director, Center for Clinical Effectiveness Research, Medical College of Wisconsin, Milwaukee, Wisconsin

SWETHA G. PINNINTI, MD
Instructor, Division of Pediatric Infectious Diseases, The University of Alabama at Birmingham, Birmingham, Alabama

RICHARD A. POLIN, MD
William T. Speck Professor of Pediatrics; Vice Chair Academic and Clinical Affairs; Director, Division of Neonatal-Perinatal Medicine, Department of Pediatrics, College of Physicians and Surgeons, Columbia University, New York, New York

DIKEA ROUSSOS-ROSS, MD
Assistant Professor, Department of Obstetrics and Gynecology and Department of Psychiatry, University of Florida, Gainesville, Florida

JOHN ROUTES, MD
Professor of Pediatrics and Microbiology, Division of Allergy/Immunology, Department of Pediatrics, Medical College of Wisconsin, Milwaukee, Wisconsin

RAKESH SAHNI, MD
Professor of Pediatrics, Division of Neonatal-Perinatal Medicine, Department of Pediatrics, College of Physicians and Surgeons, Columbia University, New York, New York

NICOLE E. ST CLAIR, MD, FAAP
Assistant Professor of Pediatrics, Department of Pediatrics Global Health Program, Medical College of Wisconsin, Milwaukee, Wisconsin

AOY TOMITA-MITCHELL, PhD
Division of Cardiothoracic Surgery, Department of Surgery, Medical College of Wisconsin, Milwaukee, Wisconsin

MICHAEL UHING, MD
Professor, Department of Pediatrics, Medical College of Wisconsin, Milwaukee, Wisconsin

JAMES VERBSKY, MD, PhD
Associate Professor of Pediatrics and Microbiology, Division of Rheumatology, Department of Pediatrics, Medical College of Wisconsin, Milwaukee, Wisconsin

AMY J. WAGNER, MD
Division of Pediatric Surgery, Department of Surgery, Medical College of Wisconsin, Milwaukee, Wisconsin

TAMARA D. WARNER, PhD
Research Assistant Professor, Department of Pediatrics, University of Florida, Gainesville, Florida

EARNESTINE WILLIS, MD, MPH
Kellner Professor in Pediatrics, Department of Pediatrics; Director, Center for the Advancement of Underserved Children, Medical College of Wisconsin, Milwaukee, Wisconsin

Contents

> Simple low-cost, evidence-based interventions such as clean delivery
> practices, immediate warming, umbilical cord care, and neonatal resusci-
> tation could prevent 40% to 70% of newborn deaths globally, but many
> obstacles preclude the provision of those basic interventions for all
> newborns, particularly in low-resource regions. Global efforts have led to
> widespread development of neonatal clinical practice guidelines, training
> programs, and policies. Because of a shortage of health care resources,
> standards of care have been redefined to meet the needs of underserved
> populations. This article provides an overview of the challenges, efforts,
> and controversies surrounding neonatal health in low-resource settings.

> Spontaneous preterm labor is a complex process characterized by the
> interplay of multiple different pathways. Prevention of preterm labor and
> delivery is also complicated. The most effective interventions for preven-
> tion of preterm birth (PTB) are progestin prophylaxis and lifestyle modifica-
> tions, with cerclage placement also playing a role in selected populations.
> Interventions such as activity modification, home tocometry, and routine
> antibiotic use have fallen out of favor because of lack of effectiveness
> and possibility of harm. The solution to the problem of PTB remains
> elusive, and researchers and clinicians must collaborate to find a cure
> for preterm labor.

> Today, almost 70% of babies with hypoplastic left heart syndrome (HLHS)
> will survive into adulthood, although significant long-term morbidity and
> mortality still exists. Prenatal diagnosis of HLHS is increasingly common,
> allowing improved counseling, and the potential for fetal intervention if
> indicated. Exciting progress continues to be made in the area of fetal diag-
> nosis and intervention, specifically catheter intervention for intact atrial
> septum or severe aortic stenosis. Pediatric cardiologists should be keenly

neonatal HSV infections remain uncommon, due to the significant morbidity and mortality associated with the infection, HSV infection in the newborn is often considered in the differential diagnosis of ill neonates. This review summarizes the epidemiology and management of neonatal HSV infections and discusses strategies to prevent HSV infection in the newborn.

Noninvasive prenatal testing (NIPT) using cell-free fetal (cfDNA) offers potential as a screening tool for fetal anomalies. All pregnant women should be offered prenatal screening and diagnostic testing based on current guidelines. Adoption of NIPT in high-risk pregnancies suggests a change in the standard of care for genetic screening; there are advantages to an accurate test with results available early in pregnancy. This accuracy decreases the overall number of invasive tests needed for diagnosis, subjecting fewer pregnancies to the risks of invasive procedures. Women undergoing NIPT need informed consent before testing and accurate, sensitive counseling after results are available.

One of the most controversial areas in neonatology is whether probiotics should be provided routinely to preterm infants to prevent necrotizing enterocolitis (NEC). This review provides the reader with a brief overview of NEC and current concepts of its pathophysiology, discusses the microbial ecology of the intestine in preterm infants and factors that may lead to a "dysbiosis", summarizes studies of probiotics in preterm infants, elaborates on the need for regulation in this area, and discusses alternatives to probiotics and what is the future for the prevention of NEC.

The current process of educating and informing parents of the concerns and outcomes of premature infants is suboptimal, mostly because of modifiable factors. Proven methods to improve the transference of information are underused. In most institutions, the task to inform and educate parents is left to individual providers. Effective parent-clinician communication depends collectively on parents, clinicians, and the health care systems. Efforts must focus on improving communication and not on decreasing information provided to parents. If done successfully, we might find new and worthy allies in the trenches of the NICU.

With the recognition of genetic disorders in the newborn, there is the potential to offer new lifesaving therapies. For other conditions such as hypothyroidism in Down syndrome or hypercalemia in the 22q11 microdeletion syndrome, the early identification of an untreatable condition permits prompt screening for potential comorbid conditions. DNA testing for disorders and DNA-based screening are rapidly evolving. With new more powerful tests, there is an increasing ability to see into a potential future and change the outcome for newborns. However, there remain significant ethical and structural issues to be considered before routine implementation of DNA testing.

PROGRAM OBJECTIVE
The goal of *Clinics in Perinatology* is to keep practicing perinatologists, neonatologists, obstetricians, practicing physicians and residents up to date with current clinical practice in perinatology by providing timely articles reviewing the state of the art in patient care.

TARGET AUDIENCE
Perinatologists, neonatologists, obstetricians, practicing physicians, residents and healthcare professionals who provide patient care utilizing findings from *Clinics in Perinatology*.

LEARNING OBJECTIVES
Upon completion of this activity, participants will be able to:
1. Review prematurity prevention.
2. Discuss pain management in the newborn.
3. Recognize methods to inform and educate parents about the risk and outcome of prematurity.

ACCREDITATION
The Elsevier Office of Continuing Medical Education (EOCME) is accredited by the Accreditation Council for Continuing Medical Education (ACCME) to provide continuing medical education for physicians.

The EOCME designates this enduring material for a maximum of 15 *AMA PRA Category 1 Credit*(s)™. Physicians should claim only the credit commensurate with the extent of their participation in the activity.

All other health care professionals requesting continuing education credit for this enduring material will be issued a certificate of participation.

DISCLOSURE OF CONFLICTS OF INTEREST
The EOCME assesses conflict of interest with its instructors, faculty, planners, and other individuals who are in a position to control the content of CME activities. All relevant conflicts of interest that are identified are thoroughly vetted by EOCME for fair balance, scientific objectivity, and patient care recommendations. EOCME is committed to providing its learners with CME activities that promote improvements or quality in healthcare and not a specific proprietary business or a commercial interest.

The planning committee, staff, authors and editors listed below have identified no financial relationships or relationships to products or devices they or their spouse/life partner have with commercial interest related to the content of this CME activity:
Mir A. Basir, MD, MS; David A. Bateman, MD; Maneesh Batra, MD, MPH, FAAP; Mary Lou Behnke, MD; David P. Bick, MD; Michele A. Frommelt, MD; Richard W. Hall, MD, FAAP; M. Elizabeth Hartnett, MD; Kristen Helm; Kerry Holland; Brynne Hunter; Lucky Jain, MD, MBA; Sheri Johnson, PhD; U. Olivia Kim, MD; David Kimberlin, MD; Mark Klebanoff, MD; Robert M. Kliegman, MD; Jacquelyn Kuzminski, MD, FAAP; Joanne Lagatta, MD, MS; Robert H. Lane, MD, MS; Sandy Lavery; Anne CC Lee, MD, MPH, FAAP; Steven R. Leuthner, MD, MA; Norma Magallanes; Amber Majnik, PhD; Kara B. Markham, MD; Patricia McManus, PhD, RN; Jill McNair; Palani Murugesan; Cliff O'Callahan, MD, PhD, FAAP; Julie Panepinto, MD, MSPH; Lindsay Parnell; Swetha G. Pinniti, MD; Richard A. Polin, MD; Dikea Roussos-Ross, MD; John Routes, MD; Rakesh Sahni, MD; Nicole E. St. Clair, MD, FAAP; Megan Suermann; Michael Uhing, MD; James Verbsky, MD, PhD; Amy J. Wagner, MD; Tamara D. Warner, PhD; Earnestine Willis, MD, MPH.

The planning committee, staff, authors and editors listed below have identified financial relationships or relationships to products or devices they or their spouse/life partner have with commercial interest related to the content of this CME activity:
Kanwaljeet J. S. Anand, MBBS, D. Phil., FAAP, FCCM, FRCPCH has royalties/patents with Elsevier Science Publishers, Inc., and Up-To-Date, Inc.
David P. Dimmock, MD is a consultant/advisor for Illumina, Inc. and Complete Genomics Incorporated; has stock ownership in Global Health Incorporated; and has an employment affiliation with Medical College of Wisconsin
Aoy Tomita-Mitchell, PhD along with spouse/partner, has the following financial relationships with Ariosa Diagnostics: has stock ownership, research grants and royalties/patents.
Michael E. Mitchell, MD along with spouse/partner, has the following financial relationships with Ariosa Diagnostics: has stock ownership, research grants and royalties/patents.
Josef Neu, MD is a consultant/advisor for Medela and BioGaia/Infant Microbial Therapeutics.

UNAPPROVED/OFF-LABEL USE DISCLOSURE
The EOCME requires CME faculty to disclose to the participants:
1. When products or procedures being discussed are off-label, unlabelled, experimental, and/or investigational (not US Food and Drug Administration [FDA] approved); and

2. Any limitations on the information presented, such as data that are preliminary or that represent ongoing research, interim analyses, and/or unsupported opinions. Faculty may discuss information about pharmaceutical agents that is outside of FDA-approved labelling. This information is intended solely for CME and is not intended to promote off-label use of these medications. If you have any questions, contact the medical affairs department of the manufacturer for the most recent prescribing information.

TO ENROLL

To enroll in the *Clinics in Perinatology* Continuing Medical Education program, call customer service at 1-800-654-2452 or sign up online at http://www.theclinics.com/home/cme. The CME program is available to subscribers for an additional annual fee of $235 USD.

METHOD OF PARTICIPATION

In order to claim credit, participants must complete the following:
1. Complete enrolment as indicated above.
2. Read the activity.
3. Complete the CME Test and Evaluation. Participants must achieve a score of 70% on the test. All CME Tests and Evaluations must be completed online.

CME INQUIRIES/SPECIAL NEEDS

For all CME inquiries or special needs, please contact elsevierCME@elsevier.com.

CLINICS IN PERINATOLOGY

Foreword

Current Controversies in Perinatology: Why They Don't Go Away

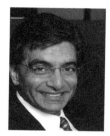

Lucky Jain, MD, MBA
Consulting Editor

Controversies are not new to neonatal perinatal medicine. They are an inevitable consequence of the rapid progress witnessed in this field, progress that is reflected in an across-the-board improvement in neonatal outcomes. A *New York Times* Op-Ed[1] from 2012 summarizes it well: "NICUs are the triumph of modern medicine's investment in technology, pharmacy and know-how. They exist to finish nature's work because more than 500,000 times a year—more than anywhere else in the industrialized world—an American baby is born prematurely. The most precarious are born at the margin of life: somewhere between 23 and 26 weeks of gestation, or what is called the limit of viability. Now we face a difficult choice: whom we fight for and whom we let go."

Indeed, this problem is emblematic of the price we must pay for the progress. It is not just babies with extreme prematurity; those with severe birth defects face similar challenges, leaving parents and providers with difficult choices to make. And the issue is not just cost of care; it is the overwhelming uncertainty in predicting bad outcomes, particularly the ones that can persist an entire lifetime.

Scientists and clinicians are united in finding answers to vexing questions and furthering the field. Yet, there is much work to be done. As you will see from this issue of the *Clinics in Perinatology*, many fairly simple and common interventions in neonatology deserve urgent attention. What oxygen concentrations do we use for resuscitating newborns?[2] What saturations do we accept that minimize morbidity and mortality? Which probiotic and how much? How do we manage pain?[3] How expansive should our neonatal screening programs be? The list goes on and on.

New challenges have also emerged that threaten to severely impede the pace of progress. Legal and societal challenges to the "SUPPORT" trial have shaken the

Clin Perinatol 41 (2014) xv–xvii
http://dx.doi.org/10.1016/j.clp.2014.09.002
0095-5108/14/$ – see front matter

Table 1
Examples of current clinical trials in the field of neonatal-perinatal medicine

Trial	Sponsor	Sponsor Type	Clinical Trials Gov Identified
A Randomized Trial of Induction Versus Expectant Management	NICHD NIH	Government	NCT01990612
Triple Dye Plus Alcohol Versus Triple Dye Alone for Newborn Umbilical Cord Care	Penn State University	Public university	NCT00127699
Pentavalent DTaP-Hep B-IPV	NIAID NIH	Government	NCT00133445
Antenatal Micronutrient Supplementation and Infant Survival (JiVitA-3)	Johns Hopkins Bloomberg School of Public Health	Multiple sponsors, including The Gates Foundation	NCT00860470
Umbilical Cord Blood Use for Admission Blood Tests of VLBW Preterm Infants	Captain Alicia Prescott	Government-military	NCT02103296
Lung Injury Prediction Study	Mayo Clinic	Private university	NCT00889772

Data from Ref.[6]

very foundation on which research and innovation is based.[4,5] Clinical trials like the SUPPORT trial are needed to bridge gaps in our knowledge and to reduce the unacceptably high levels of variation in care. This will require the unwavering commitment of funding and regulatory agencies, public and private institutions, along with individuals engaged in research. **Table 1** shows a sampling of clinical trials that are currently being undertaken along with their official sponsors.[6] Clinical controversies will continue, but there is no cause more worthy of attention at the moment than preserving clinical research.

Drs Kliegman and Lane are to be congratulated for addressing many burning controversies in clinical care in this issue. As always, I am grateful to the dedicated publishing team at Elsevier led by Kerry Holland.

Lucky Jain, MD, MBA
Department of Pediatrics
Emory University School of Medicine &
Children's Healthcare of Atlanta
2015 Uppergate Drive
Atlanta, GA 30322, USA

E-mail address:
ljain@emory.edu

REFERENCES

1. Parikh RK. Preemies, better care also means hard choices. The New York Times. August 13, 2012; section-Health.

2. Chalkias A, Xanthos T, Syggelou A, et al. Controversies in neonatal resuscitation. J Matern Fetal Neonatal Med 2013;26:50–4.
3. Nemergut ME, Yaster M, Colby C. Sedation and analgesia to facilitate mechanical ventilation. Clin Perinatol 2013;40:539–58.
4. SUPPORT Study Group. Target ranges of oxygen saturation in extremely premature infants. N Engl J Med 2010;362:1959–69.
5. Drazen JM, Solomon CG, Greene MF. Informed consent and SUPPORT. N Engl J Med 2013;368:1929–31.
6. Clinical Trials.gov is a registry and results database of publicly and privately supported clinical studies of human participants conducted around the world. Available at: https://clinicaltrials.gov/.

Preface

Current Controversies in Perinatology

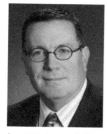 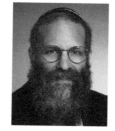

Robert H. Lane, MD, MS   Robert M. Kliegman, MD
Editors

As participants in and observers of the "new perinatology," we have become increasingly aware of the need for continued critical evaluations of innovative approaches to the care of the pregnant woman and her child. Such evaluations have always been important and have taught us the potential dangers of introducing untested or unquestioned innovations in fetal or premature care. New interventions should not be introduced without the benefit of properly controlled trials or other appropriate assessments of the risks and benefits, if we are to avoid the possibility of unanticipated adverse side effects for the mother, fetus, neonate, and later, child. Without the benefit of such critical analysis, well-intended clinicians may unintentionally do harm. Social or medical diagnostic or therapeutic interventions that are not always easily amendable to randomized controlled trials require special attention and critical review.

Although this issue of *Clinics in Perinatology* is entitled "Controversies in Perinatology," we have included some topics that at first appearance may not seem controversial; however, when examined in closer detail, these problems warrant a fresh re-examination of their public health implications as well as their epidemiology, treatment, or ethics.

In addition to a continuing critical analysis of our current care practices for individual patients, there is a need to re-evaluate what is known about significant perinatal health trends, such as the differences in infant mortality between black and white infants and the challenges of global approaches to infant mortality. Furthermore, as new diseases or syndromes are identified, there is a need to integrate these observations with past knowledge and update our understanding of underlying mechanisms. For example, as new, diagnostic advances develop and are applied to newborn screening or prenatal or neonatal diagnosis, we need to assess their accuracy and the ethical implications involved.

We have selected contributors to this volume of *Clinics in Perinatology* who have been working actively on the problems they discuss. We greatly appreciate their efforts

Clin Perinatol 41 (2014) xix–xx
http://dx.doi.org/10.1016/j.clp.2014.09.001
0095-5108/14/$ – see front matter © 2014 Published by Elsevier Inc.

perinatology.theclinics.com

to analyze these important matters critically. It is hoped that the issues raised in these articles will initiate further discussions in perinatal obstetric units, neonatal intensive care centers, and related research laboratories, all of which will lead to improved outcomes of pregnancy and newborn care.

This is the sixth edition of "Controversies in Perinatology" for Dr Kliegman and the first for Dr Lane. As the baton gets passed to the next generation of academic pediatric and neonatal leaders, we look forward to a continued tradition of examining, questioning, and validating new practices in the NICU by outstanding clinician-scientists.

We would also like to express our appreciation to Carolyn Redman for her outstanding editorial assistance and dedication to this edition.

Robert H. Lane, MD, MS
Department of Pediatrics
Children's Hospital of Wisconsin
Medical College of Wisconsin
Children's Corporate Center
999 North 92nd Street
Suite 450
Milwaukee, WI 53201, USA

Robert M. Kliegman, MD
Department of Pediatrics
Children's Hospital of Wisconsin
Medical College of Wisconsin
Children's Corporate Center
999 North 92nd Street
Suite 450
Milwaukee, WI 53222, USA

E-mail addresses:
rlane@mcw.edu (R.H. Lane)
rkliegma@mcw.edu (R.M. Kliegman)

Global Challenges, Efforts, and Controversies in Neonatal Care

Nicole E. St Clair, MD[a],*, Maneesh Batra, MD, MPH[b],
Jacquelyn Kuzminski, MD[a], Anne CC Lee, MD, MPH[c],
Cliff O'Callahan, MD, PhD[d]

KEYWORDS

- Global health • Millennium Development Goals • Neonatal mortality • Low-resource
- Low-income • Community health worker • Traditional birth attendant
- Essential newborn care

KEY POINTS

- Despite impressive advancements for the care of preterm infants in high-income countries, the greatest reduction in global neonatal mortality can be achieved by ensuring universal access to essential newborn care, such as clean delivery, cord care, and immediate warmth of infants, both for facility-based and in-home births.
- Low-income countries suffer from a significant shortage of resources and health care professionals amidst burgeoning needs. Global mobilization and innovative solutions are required to address this gap.
- Intervention packages are being implemented to achieve Millennium Development Goals 4 and 5, combining health care system improvements along a continuum of care (preconception, antenatal, childbirth, and postnatal) and also involving actions from the community, primary care, referral, and governmental levels.
- High-resource institutions can play a vital role in improving the care of newborns globally, particularly through engaging in twinning initiatives, which help to build health care infrastructure with global partners in low-resource settings.
- As global neonatal mortality is reduced, outcomes need to be measured, including tracking for incremental increase in childhood rates of disability.

Disclosures: the authors have no financial relationships to disclose.
[a] Global Health Program, Department of Pediatrics, Children's Corporate Center, Medical College of Wisconsin, Suite C560, PO Box 1997, Milwaukee, WI 53201-1997, USA; [b] Division of Neonatology, Department of Pediatrics, University of Washington School of Medicine, 4800 Sand Point Way Northeast Mailstop M1-12, Seattle, WA 98105, USA; [c] Department of Pediatric Newborn Medicine, Brigham and Women's Hospital, Harvard Medical School, 75 Francis Street, Boston, MA 02115, USA; [d] FM Residency, Middlesex Hospital, 90 South Main Street, Middletown, CT 06457, USA
* Corresponding author.
E-mail address: nstclair@mcw.edu

Clin Perinatol 41 (2014) 749–772
http://dx.doi.org/10.1016/j.clp.2014.08.002
0095-5108/14/$ – see front matter © 2014 Elsevier Inc. All rights reserved.

INTRODUCTION

The fourth Millennium Development Goal (MDG) targets a two-thirds reduction of the under-5-year mortality (U5MR) between 1990 and 2015 (from 90 deaths per 1000 live births to 30). Although progress has been made, the rate of U5MR reduction has averaged 2.6% annually worldwide (2000–2010), less than the 4.4% rate that is required to reach the MDG goal. Neonatal deaths account for approximately 3 million of the total 7.6 million under-5 deaths annually, primarily related to preterm birth complications (14% of under-5 deaths), intrapartum-related complications (9%), and neonatal sepsis or meningitis (5%) (**Fig. 1**).[1] Approximately 99% of neonatal deaths occur in low-income and middle-income countries, up to two-thirds of which are preventable.[2] More than half the total neonatal deaths occur in 5 countries: India, Nigeria, Pakistan, China, and the Democratic Republic of the Congo.

The reduction in U5MR has been faster among children aged 1 to 59 months than neonates (2.9% reduction per year compared with 2.1%, respectively). This disparity has resulted in an increase in the proportion of under-5 child deaths occurring among newborns, from 37% to 44% (1990–2012).[3] These numbers do not capture the huge and equal burden of third-trimester stillbirths, which are not tracked in the MDGs, thereby underestimating the childbirth-related deaths by almost half.

Given these statistics, the issue of newborn deaths has gained attention on the world's agenda over the past decade, coupled with increased awareness of

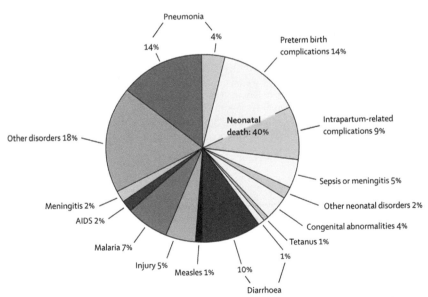

Fig. 1. Global causes of childhood deaths in 2010. Note that more than 60% of neonatal deaths are associated with low birth weight (causes that led to <1% of deaths are not shown). (*From* Liu L, Johnson HL, Cousens S, et al. Global, regional, and national causes of child mortality: an updated systematic analysis for 2010 with time trends since 2000. Lancet 2012;379(9832):2155; with permission.)

maternal health and the continuum of care (**Fig. 2**).[4] The *Lancet Neonatal Survival Series* first brought newborns into the global spotlight in 2005. More recently, stakeholders drafted the Global Newborn Action Plan (2013–14), a roadmap outlining specific objectives and goals to reduce preventable neonatal deaths, and the *Lancet* released the *Every Newborn Series*, outlining the status of global neonatal health (2014). Global leaders are also now determining how to prioritize neonatal health issues in the post-2015 United Nations (UN) development agenda.

The authors of this article recognize that the majority of its readers are employed in tertiary care, high-technology centers, and work under the assumption that the necessary resources to care for acutely ill mothers and newborns will be available. The purpose of this article is to provide an overview of health care for newborns who are born outside that setting, in low-income and

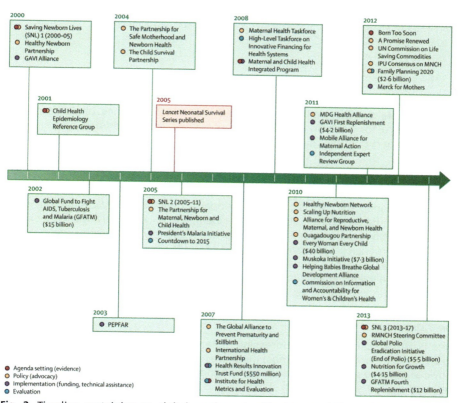

Fig. 2. Timeline pertaining to global newborn health, January 2000 to December 2013. GAVI, Global Alliance for Vaccines and Immunisation; IPU, Inter-Parliamentary Union; MNCH, maternal, newborn, and child health; PEPFAR, President's Emergency Plan for AIDS Relief; RMNCH, reproductive, maternal, newborn, and child health and nutrition. (*From* Darmstadt GL, Kinney MV, Chopra M, et al. Who has been caring for the baby? Lancet 2014;384(9938):179; with permission.)

Table 1
Example of a referral facility in a low-income country

Demographics	Sole facility serving a rural population of 500,000 people MMR 545/100,000 live births (US rate is 24/100,000) NMR 52/1000 live births (US rate is 4/1000)

Facility/resources	Total bed capacity for ≤300 patients
	Intermittent access to electricity
	No access to ambulances nor adequate roads for patient transport
	Newborn unit has limited supplies, including:
	  2 functioning isolettes
	  Cup and nasogastric tube feedings
	  Limited phototherapy equipment
	  Limited number of oxygen concentrators for use with nasal cannula
	  (no ventilators)

Staffing	Physician/patient ratio is 1:75 (trained to level of a general practitioner; no pediatricians) Nurse/patient ratio is 1:30–70, depending on shift There are no neonatal specialists available for patient consultations

Abbreviations: MMR, maternal mortality rate; NMR, neonatal mortality rate.

middle-income countries. To best enter that paradigm, envision the setting outlined in **Table 1**. With that reality in mind, this article outlines challenges surrounding care for newborns under resource limitations, efforts to address the challenges, and controversies therein.

CHALLENGES

When considering the world's least developed countries, approximately 46% of deliveries are attended by a skilled birth attendant, and only 43% of births occur in facilities that may or may not have appropriate equipment to handle maternal or neonatal emergencies.[5] In addition, in most of South Asia and sub-Saharan Africa, fewer than 5% of facility-based births are estimated to have access to neonatal intensive care.[6] The following sections describe a few of the many challenges in delivering effective care in those settings.

The 3 Delays

Time is of the essence when addressing maternal and newborn medical emergencies, and in low-resource countries, there are pervasive issues that result in gaps in provider coverage and delays at critical periods (**Fig. 3**). Approximately 46% of all maternal deaths and 40% of all stillbirths and neonatal deaths occur in a 48-hour window: at the time of labor and the day of birth.[7] In countries most affected by neonatal mortality, there is approximately 60% coverage for skilled attendance at birth,[8] but often there is only 1 provider to attend to both newborn and maternal emergencies. Investigators frequently cite the 3-delay classification scheme to describe causes related to delays in health care delivery for mothers and newborns: (1) delay in recognition of the problem and the decision to seek care; (2) delay in reaching a health facility; and (3) delay in receiving quality care at the

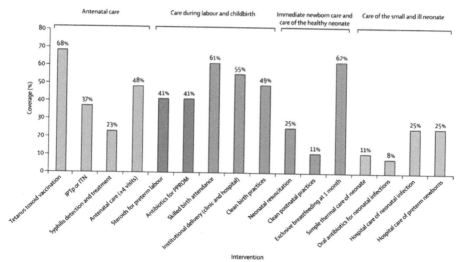

Fig. 3. Coverage of selected interventions (interventions modeled and not shown on graph have estimated coverage <10% in the 75 Countdown countries) to improve neonatal health in Countdown countries (weighted average). Countdown countries include 75 low-resource countries where greater than 95% of global maternal and child deaths occur. IPTp, intermittent preventive treatment in pregnancy; ITN, insecticide-treated bed nets; PPROM, preterm premature rupture of membranes. (*From* Bhutta ZA, Das JK, Bahl R, et al. Can available interventions end preventable deaths in mothers, newborn babies, and stillbirths, and at what cost? Lancet 2014;384(9940):361; with permission.)

facility.[9] Examples of infrastructural issues in low-income countries that contribute to these 3 categories of delays are outlined in **Table 2**.

The severity and the number of barriers leading to delays in care in low-income countries are difficult to fathom if one's career is nested in a tertiary-care center in

Table 2
Examples of issues that contribute to delays in health care delivery for mothers and newborns in low-resource countries

(1) Delay in recognition of the problem and the decision to seek care	Insufficient health literacy of the mother Maternal cultural factors influencing choice of medical care or decision for home birth Paucity or undertraining of CHWs or TBAs Lack of community mobilization
(2) Delay in reaching a health facility	Geographic barriers (eg, mountains, rivers, distance, difficult terrain) Communication barriers Inability to pay for transport Lack of transportation (public or private; non-existent or suboptimal emergency medical system)
(3) Delay in receiving quality care at the facility	Shortage of health care personnel Insufficient training of clinicians Lack of supplies Financial barriers for patient (ie, pay before service model)

> **Box 1**
> **Clinical case scenario in a low-resource setting**
>
> A 16-year-old G2P1 woman is 33 weeks pregnant. She lives in Lesotho, in a hut in a rural moun-
> tainous region. She has not received antenatal care, does not know the danger signs for when
> she should seek care, and there is no community health worker in that region to recognize
> that she has preeclampsia (delay 1). After several days of worsening edema and severe head-
> aches, she decides to seek medical advice, necessitating a 2-hour walk down the mountainside,
> a 3-hour walk on the road, a 4-hour wait for the bus, and an additional 3-hour drive to the near-
> est health facility (delay 2). Once at the hospital, she is admitted, is noted to be hypertensive, but
> is not evaluated by a physician until 10 hours later, because of overnight staffing issues. Further-
> more, she is not treated for her preeclampsia until her family members gather enough money to
> purchase intravenous magnesium sulfate. She and the baby are not monitored overnight, and a
> cesarean section is not performed until she tells the nurse she has not felt fetal movement for
> several hours (delay 3). The infant emerges apneic and bradycardic. The nurse in attendance stim-
> ulates and dries the infant without a response, but she does not have the appropriate training or
> supplies to perform bag-and-mask ventilation. She asks a security officer to notify another physi-
> cian that the infant is in distress; response time requires 15 additional minutes, during which the
> infant dies (delay 3). The infant's cause of death is erroneously classified as a stillbirth.

a high-income country. Consider the case example in **Box 1**. Variations of that scenario regularly occur in low-resource settings, necessitating interventions as microscopic as modifying individual care-seeking behaviors and as macroscopic as
implementing maternal and newborn health policy changes.

Health Worker Migration

Even if physical barriers were improved, such as transportation infrastructure,
there remains a paucity of trained personnel to deliver care. In general, regions
that have high maternal and neonatal mortality also have the fewest physicians
per capita (**Fig. 4**),[10] complicated by significant urban-rural disparities within
many of those regions. The long-standing issue of brain drain, pertaining to

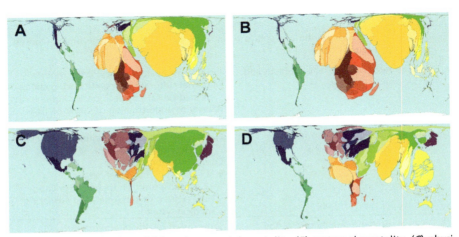

Fig. 4. Global distribution of (*A*) early neonatal mortality, (*B*) maternal mortality, (*C*) physician workforce, and (*D*) midwife workforce (territories are resized according to the subject
of interest). (*From* worldmapper.org. © Copyright Sasi Group (University of Sheffield) and
Mark Newman (University of Michigan).)

international migration of skilled health care workers from low-resource areas (particularly sub-Saharan Africa, Asia, and Pacific countries) to high-resource areas, has contributed to a strikingly disproportionate allocation of health care personnel. Although high-income countries have only one-third of the world's population, they contain three-fourths of the world's physicians. High-income countries have also secured 89% of the world's migrating physicians, two-thirds of whom originated from low-income or low-middle–income countries. Similar statistics exist for the nursing workforce. Africa carries approximately 24% of the global burden of disease but has only 3% of the health care workforce and 1% of the world's financial resources to tackle the issues.[11] The motivation for health care personnel to migrate is multifactorial, often beginning with a lack of local training infrastructure to gain expertise, and sustained by better economic and lifestyle prospects elsewhere. In addition, there are no universal codes of practice on international recruitment of health personnel, although some high-income countries have implemented policies to mitigate targeted recruitment from low-income countries.[12] Approximately 25% of US accredited postgraduate medical training positions are filled by foreign medical graduates annually, many of whom remain stateside for their careers.

Insufficient Supplies

Health service provision assessments (facility-based audits) in 6 countries in sub-Saharan Africa showed that only 15% of hospitals were equipped to provide basic neonatal resuscitation.[13] Similar supply shortages permeate other low-resource regions. In 2012, the UN Commission on Life-Saving Commodities for Women's and Children's Health identified 13 life-saving commodities, which, if more widely accessed and properly used, could cumulatively save the lives of more than 6 million women and children at a cost of $2.6 billion over 5 years.[14] Suggested newborn supplies were injectable antibiotics, antenatal corticosteroids, chlorhexidine, and resuscitation equipment.

Scalability and Sustainability

Despite evidence to support many low-cost, high-impact interventions for newborns (**Table 3**), many barriers exist that inhibit implementation at local and national levels. In addition, effectiveness of an intervention in one context may not equate to similar outcomes in a different region or community. Kangaroo mother care (KMC) is a prime example. Although KMC has been successful in many settings in Latin America, it has had slow uptake in South Asia, and implementation research is being conducted to understand why. Building on preexisting infrastructure helps promote longer-term sustainability in settings with severe resource limitations.[15] Local champions, engagement of key stakeholders, and ownership are required to promote both scalability and sustainability of neonatal interventions.

Lack of Effective Prevention Strategies for Preterm Birth

Preterm births are globally the second most common cause of death for children under 5 years, and are a significant risk factor for long-term morbidity. Rates of preterm births are rising in both low-income and high-income settings, and there are few effective public health prevention strategies. Additional investigation is required to understand the physiology of preterm births, to elicit the cause of increasing rates, and to identify prevention strategies.[16]

Table 3
Overview of interventions showing effect on selected neonatal outcomes (relative risk [95% confidence interval])

	Stillbirth	Preterm Birth	Perinatal Mortality	Small for Gestational Age	Neonatal Mortality
PRECONCEPTION AND ANTENATAL INTERVENTIONS					
Iron supplementation	—	0.88 (0.77–1.01)	—	—	0.90 (0.68–1.19)
Iron and folic acid supplementation	—	1.55 (0.40–6.00)	—	—	0.81 (0.51–1.30)
Multiple micronutrient supplementation	0.95 (0.85–1.06)	0.99 (0.97–1.02)	0.96 (0.84–1.10)	**0.87 (0.83–0.92)**	1.01 (0.89–1.16)
Calcium supplementation	—	**0.76 (0.60–0.97)**	0.90 (0.74–1.09)	1.01 (0.84–1.21)	1.07 (0.39–2.95)
Balanced energy protein supplementation	**0.62 (0.40–0.98)**	0.96 (0.80–1.15)	—	**0.68 (0.49–0.89)**	0.63 (0.37–1.06)
Tetanus toxoid immunization	—	—	—	—	**0.06 (0.02–0.2)**
Haemophilus influenzae type b vaccine	1.69 (0.41–6.94)	1.37 (0.20–9.16)	—	—	—
Influenza virus vaccine	—	0.77 (0.36–1.64)	—	—	—
Syphilis screening and treatment	**0.18 (0.10–0.33)**	**0.36 (0.27–0.47)**	—	—	**0.20 (0.13–0.32)**
Intermittent preventive treatment of malaria in pregnancy	0.96 (0.72–1.27)	0.86 (0.62–1.21)	0.83 (0.66–1.05)	**0.65 (0.55–0.77)**	**0.69 (0.49–0.98)**
Insecticide-treated bed nets	—	—	—	**0.65 (0.55–0.77)**	—
Maternal anthelminthic treatment	—	0.88 (0.43–1.78)	0.97 (0.68–1.40)	—	—
Lower genital infection screening and management	—	**0.55 (0.41–0.75)**	—	—	—
Prophylactic antibiotics	—	0.96 (0.70–1.33)	0.80 (0.31–2.06)	1.29 (0.42–3.96)	0.19 (0.01–3.82)
Antibiotic prophylaxis for group b *Streptococcus* colonization	—	—	—	—	—
Antibiotics for bacterial vaginosis	—	0.88 (0.71–1.09)	0.71 (0.36–1.39)	—	—
Asymptomatic bacteriuria treatment	—	0.37 (0.10–1.36)	—	—	—
Periodontal disease management	**0.49 (0.26–0.94)**	—	0.96 (0.60–1.54)	1.04 (0.84–1.27)	0.79 (0.14–4.34)
Antihypertensive for mild to moderate hypertension	1.14 (0.60–2.17)	1.02 (0.89–1.16)	0.98 (0.88–1.10)	—	1.16 (0.94–1.42)
Magnesium sulfate for prevention of preeclampsia	0.99 (0.87–1.12)	—	0.86 (0.70–1.07)	1.05 (0.86–1.29)	—
Calcium supplementation for hypertension	0.90 (0.74–1.09)	**0.76 (0.60–0.97)**	0.89 (0.74–1.08)	—	—
Antiplatelets for preeclampsia	1.15 (0.88–1.49)	**0.92 (0.88–0.97)**	—	**0.90 (0.83–0.98)**	0.89 (0.64–1.22)

Intervention				
Preconception diabetes education	—	0.83 (0.62–1.12)	0.31 (0.19–0.53)	—
Optimum vs suboptimum glucose control	0.51 (0.14–1.88)	—	0.40 (0.25–0.63)	—
Education/psychotherapy to quit smoking	—	0.79 (0.52–1.21)	—	—
Nicotine replacement therapy	—	0.77 (0.61–0.97)	—	—
Incentives to quit smoking	—	0.49 (0.22–1.08)	—	—
Prenatal antidepressants	—	1.55 (1.38–1.74)	—	—
Doppler velocimetry	—	—	—	0.81 (0.53–1.24)
Fetal movement monitoring	0.65 (0.41–1.04)	0.71 (0.52–0.98)	—	—
Cesarean section for breech	—	1.12 (0.72–1.75)	—	—
Postterm labor induction	0.28 (0.05–1.67)	—	0.33 (0.19–0.56)	—
Antibiotics for preterm premature rupture of membrane	—	—	0.30 (0.09–0.99)	0.88 (0.80–0.97)
Steroids for preterm labor	—	—	0.96 (0.63–1.44)	0.47 (0.35–0.64)
Basic emergency obstetric care	—	—	—	0.60 (0.48–0.60)
Comprehensive emergency obstetric care	—	—	—	0.15 (0.12–0.32)
Skilled birth care	—	—	—	0.75 (0.70–0.85)
Clean birth practices at home	—	—	—	0.85 (0.80–0.90)
Clean birth practices at facility	—	—	—	0.73 (0.64–0.76)
NEWBORN AND NEONATAL INTERVENTIONS				
Delayed cord clamping in full-term neonates	—	—	—	0.37 (0.04–3.41)
Umbilical cord antiseptics	—	—	—	0.77 (0.63–0.94)
Neonatal resuscitation at home	—	—	—	0.80 (0.75–0.85)
Neonatal resuscitation at facility	—	—	—	0.70 (0.59–0.84)
Anticonvulsants for asphyxia	—	—	—	0.87 (0.54–1.40)
Hypothermia for hypoxic ischemic encephalopathy	—	—	—	—
Continuous positive airway pressure for respiratory distress syndrome	—	0.52 (0.32–0.87)	—	0.75 (0.64–0.88)

(continued on next page)

Table 3
(continued)

	Stillbirth	Preterm Birth	Perinatal Mortality	Small for Gestational Age	Neonatal Mortality
Surfactant therapy for respiratory distress syndrome	—	—	—	—	**0.68 (0.57–0.82)**
Preventive surfactant therapy for preterm neonates	—	—	—	—	**0.60 (0.47–0.77)**
Antibiotics for meconium aspiration syndrome	—	—	—	—	1.29 (0.36–4.54)
Systemic steroids for meconium aspiration syndrome	—	—	—	—	0.61 (0.22–1.71)
Inhaled steroids for meconium aspiration syndrome	—	—	—	—	0.39 (0.08–1.94)
Surfactant lung lavage for meconium aspiration syndrome	—	—	—	—	0.38 (0.09–1.57)
Bolus surfactant for meconium aspiration syndrome	—	—	—	—	0.80 (0.39–1.66)
Topical emollient therapy	—	—	—	—	**0.73 (0.56–0.94)**
Hypothermia prevention for preterm infants	—	—	—	—	**0.80 (0.55–0.92)**
Kangaroo mother care in preterm infants	—	—	—	—	**0.60 (0.39–0.93)**
Oral antibiotics for pneumonia	—	—	—	—	**0.58 (0.41–0.82)**
Injectable antibiotics for pneumonia	—	—	—	—	**0.25 (0.19–0.30)**
Antibiotics for sepsis	—	—	—	—	**0.35 (0.30–0.50)**

Numbers in bold indicate a significant effect, whereas nonbold data indicate no significant effect. — indicates no evidence.
From Bhutta ZA, Das JK, Bahl R, et al. Can available interventions end preventable deaths in mothers, newborn babies, and stillbirths, and at what cost? Lancet 2014;384(9940):349–50; with permission.

Minimal Infrastructure to Track Progress

Although there are clear actions to reduce maternal and newborn morbidity and mortality globally, there is insufficient infrastructure to evaluate and show measurable outcomes. Most births (and deaths) in low-income countries may never be counted. Data collection is hindered at many levels, including invisible deaths from unregistered home births, poor vital registration in rural areas and in facility-based health information systems, and misclassification of deaths as stillbirths.

CURRENT EFFORTS

"It always seems impossible until it's done." Although the world is by no means "done" in achieving health equity for all newborns, Nelson Mandela's words embrace the striking improvements that have occurred globally to achieve the MDGs over the past decade. This section outlines a few of those efforts to improve global neonatal health.

Educational Initiatives

In 2009, the World Health Organization (WHO) estimated that it would take an additional 2.4 million physicians, nurses, and midwives to meet the world's health needs, along with an extra 1.9 million pharmacists, health aides, technicians, and other auxiliary personnel.[11] To mitigate brain drain and promote sustainability, governmental and non-governmental organizations (NGOs) are allocating more resources toward educational initiatives for local providers. Clinical practice guidelines, such as those provided in Integrated Management of Childhood Illnesses (IMCI)[17] and Integrated Management of Pregnancy and Childbirth, have been developed for community health workers (CHWs) and rural providers and tailored to various health literacy levels to promote recognition, stabilization, and referral of ill mothers and newborns. Considered a major step forward in addressing newborn issues, IMCI incorporated young infant (<2 months) guidelines in 2005. Examples of curriculum designed for low-resource settings include *Helping Babies Breathe* (HBB) (neonatal resuscitation) and the WHO essential newborn care course. Some countries offer perinatal diploma programs for general practitioners. Twinning programs are growing worldwide, involving partnerships between institutions from high-income countries and low-income or low-middle–income countries to improve clinical, educational, and research capacity in the low-resource regions. The Human Resources for Health Program in Rwanda is one such example.[18]

Task Shifting

Keeping in line with the "use what you have" mentality, many countries have adopted task shifting strategies by training cadres of workers to perform tasks that would normally be performed only by clinicians with higher levels of training. For example, cesarean surgical training programs have been developed for non-physician clinicians[19] (midlevel providers) in low-resource settings with favorable outcomes. A 2011 systematic analysis of 6 nonrandomized controlled trials[20] reported that rates of maternal and perinatal deaths did not differ between physician and trained non-physician groups, although postoperative complications were higher in the non-physician group. In 2012, WHO issued a maternal and newborn task shifting guide, outlining interventions that could safely and effectively be delivered by different levels of trained providers.[21]

Clinical Care

Recognizing that newborn health is heavily intertwined with maternal health, global efforts are moving toward packaged approaches to clinical system improvements to achieve MDGs 4 and 5. Such approaches ideally combine interventions along a continuum of care (preconception, antenatal, childbirth, and postnatal) and also involve actions from the community, primary care, referral, and governmental levels (**Fig. 5**).

Essential care for all newborns

In referring to the care of healthy newborns, there is a bundle of provisions dubbed by WHO as "essential newborn care," including thermal care (drying, warming, skin-to-skin, and delayed bathing), hygienic cord and skin care (hand washing, delayed cord care, chlorhexidine), early and exclusive breastfeeding, and neonatal resuscitation if not breathing at birth.[22] Efforts are being made to ensure that all newborns receive these services at birth, although coverage globally varies significantly.

Special care for small or sick newborns

The care of sick and preterm newborns becomes more complicated in low-resource settings. Approximately 15 million babies are born preterm annually, and two-thirds

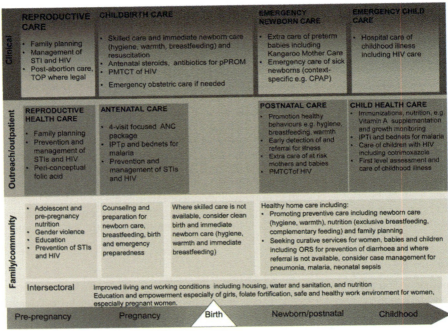

Fig. 5. Integrated maternal, newborn, and child health service delivery packages. ANC, antenatal care; CPAP, continuous positive airway pressure; HIV, human immunodeficiency virus; IPTi, intermittent preventive treatment in infants; IPTp, intermittent preventive treatment during pregnancy for malaria; ORS, oral rehydration solution; PMTCT, prevention of maternal to child transmission of HIV; pPROM, prelabor premature rupture of membranes; STI, sexually transmitted infection; TOP, termination of pregnancy. (*From* Lawn JE, Kinney MV, Black RE, et al. Newborn survival: a multi-country analysis of a decade of change. Health Policy Plan 2012;27(Suppl 3):iii9; with permission.)

of them are born in low-income countries. More than 85% are between 32 and 37 weeks of gestation; 10% are between 28 and less than 32 weeks gestation, and 5% less than 28 weeks. South Asia and sub-Saharan Africa account for more than three-quarters of the world's newborn deaths caused by preterm complications.[22] An additional 10.6 million babies are born with low birth weight and are growth restricted at term[23] and carry higher risk of mortality and other neonatal morbidities.[24] It is unrealistic to envision neonatal intensive care unit (NICU)-level care for these newborns globally, particularly when many of them are not even receiving essential care. However, apart from ventilation, there are many low-cost measures that are feasible and could save lives, especially for infants more than 28 weeks gestation. **Table 4** outlines the tools and technology required to implement those measures in low-resource facilities.

Noteworthy examples of low-cost, high-impact interventions for preterm infants include kangaroo mother care (KMC) and low-cost bubble continuous positive airway pressure (CPAP). KMC was developed in 1978 by a Colombian pediatrician. Originally introduced out of necessity because of limited hospital resources, mothers were asked to provide continuous skin-to-skin contact with their low birth weight infants to promote warmth and breastfeeding. Over time, this methodology has demonstrated positive impacts for both newborns and mothers, with particular importance in improving neurocognitive outcomes and decreasing mortality in preterm infants (**Table 5**). In contrast to many medical advancements that eventually trickle down to low-resource regions, this approach was developed and used first in low- and middle-income countries, and is now gaining popularity in high-income countries, although global implementation has faced many barriers.

Over the past several years, NICUs in high-income countries have increased their utilization of non-invasive respiratory support for newborns with respiratory distress, with evidence that it is superior to intubation, surfactant, and ventilation.[25] Non-invasive respiratory support, such as CPAP, is a reasonable intervention for low-income regions with medical centers that are staffed with pediatricians but are insufficiently resourced to provide mechanical ventilation. Bubble CPAP, widely used in high-income countries, can cost approximately $6000 for a device stateside. Alternative low-cost bubble CPAP systems have been designed, costing approximately $350, with maintenance costs of less than $1 every 2 years.[26] A Malawi-based study recently reported a 27% absolute improvement in survival for neonates with respiratory distress syndrome treated with CPAP when compared with standard therapy (nasal oxygen), with the greatest beneficial effect observed in neonates with very low birth weight, respiratory distress syndrome, or sepsis.[27]

Research and Quality Improvement

Collaborations have formed to promote capacity building for research to effectively measure outcomes of health initiatives in various settings. One example is the African Newborn Network, a network of research studies funded in whole or part by the Bill and Melinda Gates Foundation through the Saving Newborn Lives Program of Save the Children. This collaboration, involving researchers, ministries of health, UN agencies, and technical assistance partners across Africa, is testing various community-based initiatives for newborn health to determine which interventions are effective and scalable in African settings. Participating countries include Ethiopia, Ghana, Malawi, Mali, Mozambique, South Africa, Tanzania, and Uganda, most of which are also measuring costs of interventions through the Cost of Integrated Newborn care tool.

Quality improvement methodologies have also yielded a decrease in perinatal mortality in low-income countries. Perinatal mortality audits, or systematic inquiries into

Table 4
Tools, technologies, and innovations required for the care of preterm babies

Priority Packages and Interventions	Current Technology/Tools	Technological Innovations Required
All Babies		
Essential newborn care and extra care for preterm babies	Protocols for care, training materials, and job aids	Generic communications and counseling toolkit for local adaptation
Thermal care (drying, warming, skin-to-skin, and delayed bathing)	Materials for counseling, health education, and health promotion	Generic, modular training kit for adaptation, novel methods (eg cell phone prompts)
Early initiation, exclusive breastfeeding	Weighing scales	Birth kits for frontline workers
Hygienic cord and skin care	Cord clamp and scissors, clean birth kit if appropriate	Chlorhexidine preparations for application to the umbilical cord
	Vitamin K for LBW babies	Simplified approaches to identifying preterm babies such as foot size
Neonatal resuscitation for babies who do not breathe at birth	Materials for training and job aids	Wide-scale novel logistics systems to increase availability of devices for basic resuscitation and training manikins
	Training manikins	Additional innovation for resuscitation devices (eg, upright bag-and-mask, adaptable, lower-cost resuscitation stations)
	Newborn resuscitation devices (bag-and-mask)	
	Suction devices	
	Resuscitation stations with overhead heater	
	Clock with large face and second hand	
Preterm Babies		
KMC for small babies (birthweight <2000 g)	Cloth or wrap for KMC	Generic communications and counseling toolkit for local adaptation, Innovation to address cultural, professional barriers
	Baby hats	Generic, modular training kit and job aids for local adaptation

		Lower-cost and more robust versions of:
Care of preterm babies with complications, including:	Nasogastric tubes, feeding cups, breast milk pumps	
Extra support for feeding preterm and small babies	Blood sugar testing sticks	Blood sugar testing for babies on low volume samples, heel pricks
	Intravenous fluids including glucose and more accurate giving sets	
Case management of babies with signs of infection	Syringe drivers	Oxygen condensers, including portable options
	Injection antibiotics, 1-mL syringes/27-G needles, preloaded syringes	Pulse oximeters and robust probes, including with alternative power options
Safe oxygen management and supportive care for RDS	Oxygen supply/concentrators	Syringe drivers able to take a range of syringes
	Nasal prongs, head boxes, other O_2 delivery systems	Bilirubin testing devices, including lower-cost transcutaneous devices
Case management of babies with significant jaundice	Pulse oximeters to assess blood oxygen levels with reusable cleanable neonatal probes	Hemoglobin and blood grouping, rhesus point of care
Managing seizures	Bilirubinometers (table top and transcutaneous)	Point of care for C-reactive protein/procalcitonin
	Phototherapy lamps and eye shades	Apnea alarm
	Exchange transfusion kits	Phototherapy devices such as portable Bilibed (Medela, Switzerland) to provide both phototherapy treatment and heat
	Hot cots, overhead heaters	
Neonatal intensive care	CPAP devices with standardized safety features	Lower-cost robust CPAP equipment with standardized settings
		Neonatal intensive care context specific kits (eg, district hospital) with ongoing support for quality use and for equipment maintenance
		Surfactant as more stable, lower-cost preparations

Note: this table refers to care after birth, so does not include interventions for the mother, such as antenatal steroids.

Abbreviations: CPAP, continuous positive airway pressure; LBW, low birth weight; RDS, respiratory distress syndrome.

From Howson CP, Kinney MV, Lawn JE, editors. Born too soon: the global action report on preterm birth. Geneva (Switzerland): March of Dimes, PMNCH, Save the Children, World Health Organization; 2012. p. 73; with permission.

Table 5
Documented benefits of KMC when compared with conventional neonatal care in (1) low birth weight infants and (2) healthy newborns

Low Birth Weight Infants[51,52]

Reduction in	Risk of mortality (RR 0.6, 95% CI 0.39–0.93)
	Hypothermia (RR 0.23, 95% CI 0.10–0.55)
	Length of hospital stay (typical MD 2.4 d, 95% CI 0.7–4.1)
Increase in	Infant growth
	Breastfeeding
	Mother-infant attachment
	Psychomotor development

Healthy Newborns[53]

Increase in	Breastfeeding at 1–4 mo after birth (RR 1.27, 95% CI 1.06–1.53)
	Cardiorespiratory stability for late preterm infants (MD 2.88, 95% CI 0.53–5.23)
	Blood glucose 75–90 min after birth (MD 10.56 mg/dL, 95% CI 8.4–12.72)

Abbreviations: CI, confidence interval; MD, mean difference; RR, relative risk.

the cause of maternal and neonatal deaths, have led to a 30% reduction in mortality in low-resource settings in which the audit process is linked to solutions.[28]

For all quality and research efforts, there is continued recognition that the capturing of denominator data (number of births) needs improvement in low-resource countries. According to the United Nations Children's Fund (UNICEF), in 2000, approximately 50 million births went unregistered, accounting for more than 40% of all estimated births that year, with the unregistered rates most prominent in sub-Saharan Africa (70%) and South Asia (63%). Governmental and NGOs are working to optimize birth registration systems through training, advocacy, implementation of protocols, cell phone technology, and provision of resources.

Community Mobilization

Improvement of facility-based health care through clinical, research, and quality improvement will help to address delay 3 (receiving care at the facility), but efforts need to also solve delay 1 (recognition of the problem and the decision to seek care) and delay 2 (reaching a health facility). Organizations are addressing those delays through optimizing community education, increasing coverage with CHWs, improving transport infrastructure, and promoting community mobilization. Community mobilization is defined as "a capacity-building process through which community individuals, groups, or organizations plan, carry out, and evaluate activities on a participatory and sustained basis to improve their health and other needs, either on their own initiative or stimulated by others."[29] Positive benefits have been observed in low-resource settings from community mobilization strategies, including reduction in maternal and neonatal mortality.[30,31] Mobilization efforts vary widely based on a community's needs, but examples that address maternal and newborn health include promoting community education surrounding antenatal care, increasing community demand for skilled birth care, and improving the community's capacity to bring pregnant women closer to health facilities when needed.[32]

Community-Based Interventions

Despite global efforts to improve women's access to facility-based care, the reality is that annually approximately 60 million women give birth outside facilities, primarily at home, 52 million of whom do not have trained birth attendants, particularly in remote settings.[33,34] There are generally 3 categories of community-based resources for these women: (1) skilled birth attendants (accredited health professionals, such as midwives, nurses, or physicians); (2) traditional birth attendants (TBAs, community members who provide childbirth care, with varying levels of experience, non-salaried or fee-for-service, and usually minimally trained); and (3) community health workers (CHWs), employed or volunteer village health workers selected and trained to work in the communities from which they come, sometimes possessing basic skills to ensure clean deliveries, to recognize and treat neonatal infections, and to provide basic neonatal resuscitation.[33] For communities without skilled birth attendants, there is a growing body of evidence highlighting the importance of CHWs and TBAs in providing essential newborn care and in linking patients to health care systems when needed.

Mobile Technology

Seventy-five percent of the world has access to mobile phones (1 in every 6 African owns a cell phone), allowing contact with populations that cannot otherwise be easily reached. Small-scale projects using cell phones in low-resource settings have yielded improvement in health care services, including improved registration of births, increased adherence to IMCI guidelines,[35] improved maintenance of medication inventory, and improved vaccination reminder systems. In addition, compact laboratory equipment such as a quarter-size microscope, designed to plug into cell phones for a mobile laboratory, allow for telemedicine and improved diagnostic techniques in the field.

Global Mobilization

Historically, there has been minimal oversight for organizations and individuals involved in neonatal health initiatives in low-resource settings. Ministries of health and global leaders are attempting to better coordinate the various stakeholders to ensure that initiatives are evidence-based, synergistic, sustainable, and partnered with local infrastructure. Some organizations that have assumed leadership roles in those efforts are listed in **Box 2**.

Box 2

Examples of governmental organizations and NGOs that have assumed instrumental leadership roles in addressing neonatal mortality

American Academy of Pediatrics (AAP)

Bill and Melinda Gates Foundation

The Canadian Neonatal Network

Maternal and Child Health Integrated Program (MCHIP)

Save the Children's Saving Newborn Lives Program

Society for Education Action and Research in Community Health (SEARCH)

The Partnership for Maternal, Newborn and Child Health (PMNCH)

United Nations Children's Fund (UNICEF)

US Agency for International Development (USAID)

World Health Organization (WHO)

A recent large-scale collaborative effort involved the drafting of *Every Newborn: An Action Plan to End Preventable Deaths*. The development of this report was led by WHO and UNICEF, but many additional organizations participated in leadership roles, and consultative input was obtained from various stakeholders. The action plan highlights 5 guiding principles and 5 strategic objectives in **Box 3**. It also sets forth targets for incremental decreases in global neonatal mortality, with a goal reduction in global neonatal mortality from 21 deaths/1000 live births to 7/1000 by 2035.

CONTROVERSIES

Few would debate the importance of essential newborn care and neonatal resuscitation. However, controversy arises with the implementation of these services in low-resource settings with varying degrees of health care coverage, complicated by different cultural paradigms. This section provides examples of controversies that have emerged out of efforts to address newborn health disparities.

Implementation Gaps: We Know What Works, But How Do We Implement and Scale Up?

Despite increasing global consensus around essential maternal and child health interventions, there remain significant gaps in implementation (see **Fig. 3**). Dubbed as the know-do gap (a disconnect between what is known to work and what is done in practice), this gap in some situations is related to lack of resources, but in others, the explanation is more complex and at times controversial.[22] Implementation research in low-income and middle-income countries is necessary to address the gaps in coverage, ensure buy-in and sustainability, and effect change.

Facility Versus Community Births: Where Do We Focus Our Efforts?

Worldwide, only 63% of births occur in facilities, with the rural poor in low-income countries experiencing the highest rates of home births. In 1997, WHO lobbied for countries to promote facility-based births for all women. Many countries successfully made this transition. Latin American countries now on average achieve 90% coverage for facility-based births; however, the average rate in the world's least developed countries remains at only 43%.[5] The controversial question, therefore, is whether to allocate limited training resources and supplies to facilities or to community-based interventions. Darmstadt and colleagues[33] estimated that an average TBA assists 30 births annually: if trained, the TBA could save approximately 1 neonate for every 1000 births, or 1 neonate every 33 years, at a cost of US $3630 per life saved. The

---

Box 3
Summary of guiding principles and strategic objectives in the Every Newborn Action Plan

Guiding principles: country leadership, integration, equity, accountability, innovation

Strategic objectives

1. Strengthen and invest in care during labor, childbirth, and the first day and week of life

2. Improve the quality of maternal and newborn care

3. Reach every woman and every newborn to reduce inequities

4. Harness the power of parents, families, and communities

5. Count every newborn: measurement, program tracking, and accountability

same training interventions in a facility, in which the patient numbers are greater and resources are available to escalate care, would yield a more cost-effective approach to saving lives. Low-income countries are struggling with resource allocation decisions to maximize lives saved yet still maintain health equity for the rural poor.

Lay Providers: How Much Empowerment Is Too Much?

Although countries strive for promoting births in facilities, the reality remains that universal access to clinics or hospitals for all women in labor is not possible now or in the near future. That situation, coupled with the aforementioned critical shortage of health care providers in low-resource areas, has resulted in the development of a growing trend to train lay providers (CHWs and TBAs) in perinatal care practices. The role of such providers, particularly TBAs, has been a source of controversy over the past several decades, with fluctuating degrees of support from WHO. With increasing data to suggest that community-based interventions reduce neonatal and perinatal mortality,[36,37] in 2012 the WHO outlined a list of maternal child health interventions that could be considered for lay workers in the context of clinician shortages (**Box 4**). In considering the top 3 causes of neonatal deaths ([1] preterm birth complications, [2] intrapartum-related complications, and [3] neonatal sepsis or meningitis), there is evidence to support lay providers intervening in each, with the caveat being that training infrastructure, oversight, outcomes tracking, and linkages to health care systems are required components of lay provider clinical programs. Examples are provided below. Controversy remains regarding whether such task shifting compromises appropriate standards of care for the rural poor.

Preterm birth complications

Preterm infants require extra attention for feeding, thermal support, and prevention of infection. TBA and CHW training packages have incorporated some strategies for addressing preterm infant needs, including promoting skin-to-skin contact. However, further data are required to determine whether lay provider interventions for preterm infants are effective in reducing neonatal mortality.

Box 4
WHO maternal and newborn health interventions through task shifting recommendations: summary of interventions that can be considered for lay workers in the appropriate context and training infrastructure

Recommend the option

Promotional interventions for maternal and newborn health

Continuous support during labor

Distribution of oral supplements to pregnant women (with targeted monitoring and evaluation)

Consider the option only in the context of rigorous research

Prevention and treatment of postpartum hemorrhage

Management of puerperal sepsis using parenteral antibiotics before referral

Initiation and maintenance of kangaroo mother care

Delivery of antibiotics for neonatal sepsis

Delivery of neonatal resuscitation

Contraceptive delivery (not including intrauterine devices)

Intrapartum-related complications

Over the last 2 decades, multiple studies have been performed using the modified neonatal resuscitation program (NRP) curriculum for TBAs, with a wide variety of results, including: (1) the SEARCH (Society for Education Action and Research in Community Health) trial, which combined a TBA with a trained CHW, yielding a 60% reduction in asphyxia-specific neonatal mortality[38]; (2) the First Breath Study, which showed no change in neonatal mortality when comparing outcomes for rural TBAs across 6 low-income countries trained with essential newborn care plus modified NRP compared with only essential newborn care[39]; and (3) the Lufwanyama Neonatal Survival Project in Zambia, which reported a 63% reduction (0.37, 0.17–0.81) in deaths caused by birth asphyxia for infants born to TBAs who had been trained in modified NRP.[40] The Helping Babies Breathe (HBB) curriculum, implemented in 2010 (after the aforementioned studies were performed), is targeted specifically toward providers with lower health literacy, including CHWs and TBAs. Reduction in mortality has been noted after HBB facility-based implementation,[41] but further trials are necessary to show mortality reduction from HBB training for TBAs and CHWs. In addition, as asphyxia-related deaths decline, data collection needs to occur longitudinally to follow whether there is an increase in disability rates for newborns who suffered intrapartum hypoxia and survived.[42]

Neonatal infections

Evidence suggests that lay providers can decrease mortality related to neonatal infections with assistance from neonatal-specific tools to guide the assessment, management, and referral process.[17,43] Previously controversial, many programs now use lay providers to administer oral and intramuscular antibiotics for suspected infections. Examples of successful lay provider intervention trials for sepsis include the SEARCH trial in India (sepsis-specific neonatal mortality declined by 90%, $P<.005$),[44] and the Projahnmo Study Group in Bangladesh (neonatal mortality declined by 34%, absolute risk reduction 0.66; 95% confidence interval 0.47–0.93).[45] Data also support the lay provider use of topical chlorhexidine for prevention of omphalitis and reduction of neonatal mortality.[46,47] Ongoing trials are using lay providers to provide oral antibiotic regimens for suspected severe infections, a modality that has the potential to incite controversy in both low-income and high-income countries if found to be effective.[48]

Educational Initiatives: Are We Draining Local Resources?

Although the natural response to international brain drain is to develop educational initiatives from within a low-resource region to promote sustainability, an unexpected consequence is the development of intermittent local brain drain. A common educational intervention involves a train-the-trainer model, in which foreigners train local clinicians to become educators of a specific curriculum. However, during the initial and future training rollouts, the local clinicians often do not have backup to cover their clinical responsibilities, leaving patients without providers. Similar shortages occur when NGOs hire local providers out of local health systems.

Stillbirths: Who Is Keeping Track?

Stillbirths, estimated at 2.65 million annually when referring to the death of a baby at 28 weeks gestation or more,[49] are unaccounted for in the numerators when discussing death statistics, are not counted in the MDGs, and are not tracked in the Global Burden of Disease metrics. Approximately 98% of stillbirths occur in low-income and middle-income countries, about half of which occur during labor and are potentially preventable with quality intrapartum obstetric care. Data collection on stillbirths is hampered by many factors, including misclassifications, differing classification schemes, and non-reporting to avoid culpability. The inability to accurately quantify stillbirth numbers leads to a gross underestimation of neonatal mortality. Experts are advocating for a more universal classification system, improved data collection of stillbirths, and counting of stillbirths in neonatal mortality as programs and policies are developed to improve prioritization of interventions.[49]

Resources: Who Comes First, and Are We Outgrowing Ourselves?

An additional and overarching controversy involves the resources allocated for saving newborn lives amidst a sea of other health care issues in underserved populations. The ethics of resource allocation are beyond the scope of this article, but a pressing issue. Another concern, as our population increases by approximately 74 million people per year, is whether we are contributing to the issue of overpopulation with these efforts to save lives at birth. Although intuitively the answer is yes, data from countries suggest otherwise. Broadly speaking, demographers have shown that a decrease in child death rates is followed by a decrease in birth rates. Such changes are of course multifactorial, and require contraceptive counseling and services while concomitantly saving maternal and newborn lives in the quest for global health equity.

SUMMARY

The MDGs and the Every Newborn Action Plan set high standards and prioritize the care of newborns on the world's agenda. The challenges in optimizing care at birth are immense, yet there are many evidence-based interventions that could save newborn lives if implemented more widely. The Global Investment Framework for Women and Children's Health estimates that an investment of US $5 per person per year could prevent 147 million child deaths (including 60 million newborns), 32 million stillbirths, and 5 million maternal deaths by 2035, yielding an estimated 9-fold return on investment in the form of social and economic benefits over a 23-year period (2012–35).[3,50] As initiatives are developed, it is crucial for organizations and individuals to balance the "something is better than nothing" mentality with a push for optimal standards of care in all regions of the world. Global partnerships, innovative strategies, and ongoing audits of the effectiveness of interventions are required in the attempts to save lives at birth.

REFERENCES

1. Liu L, Johnson HL, Cousens S, et al. Global, regional, and national causes of child mortality: an updated systematic analysis for 2010 with time trends since 2000. Lancet 2012;379(9832):2151–61.
2. Darmstadt GL, Bhutta ZA, Cousens S, et al. Evidence-based, cost-effective interventions: how many newborn babies can we save? Lancet 2005;365(9463): 977–88.
3. World Health Organization/UNICEF. Every newborn: an action plan to end preventable deaths. Available at: http://www.everynewborn.org/. Draft action plan. Available at: http://origin.who.int/maternal_child_adolescent/topics/newborn/every-newborn-action-plan-draft.pdf. Accessed May 1, 2014.
4. The Partnership for Maternal, Newborn and Child Health. 2013. Available at: http://www.who.int/pmnch/en/. Accessed May 1, 2014.
5. UNICEF. State of the world's children report. New York: UNICEF; 2014.

6. Blencowe H, Lee AC, Cousens S, et al. Preterm birth-associated neurodevelopmental impairment estimates at regional and global levels for 2010. Pediatr Res 2013;74(Suppl 1):17–34.

7. Lawn JE, Blencowe H, Olza S, et al. Progress, priorities, and potential beyond survival. Lancet 2014. http://dx.doi.org/10.1016/S0140-6736(14)60496-7.

8. Bhutta ZA, Das JK, Bahl R, et al. Can available interventions end preventable deaths in mothers, newborn babies, and stillbirths, and at what cost? Lancet 2014. http://dx.doi.org/10.1016/S0140-6736(14)60792-3.

9. Rosenfeld A, Maine D. Maternal health in third world. Lancet 1987;1:691.

10. Lawn JE, Kerber K, Enweronu-Laryea C, Cousens S. 3.6 million neonatal deaths–what is progressing and what is not? Semin Perinatol 2010;34(6): 371–86.

11. Serour G. Healthcare workers and the brain drain. Int J Gynaecol Obstet 2009; 106(2):175–8.

12. UK Department of Health. Code of practice for the international recruitment of healthcare professionals. Gateway reference: 4174. 2004. Available at: http://webarchive.nationalarchives.gov.uk/20130107105354/http://dh.gov.uk/prod_consum_dh/groups/dh_digitalassets/@dh/@en/documents/digitalasset/dh_4097734.pdf. Accessed May 1, 2014.

13. Wall SN, Lee AC, Carlo W, et al. Reducing intrapartum-related neonatal deaths in low- and middle-income countries-what works? Semin Perinatol 2010;34(6): 395–407.

14. UN Commission on Life Saving Commodities - report. 2012.

15. Bhutta ZA, Soofi S, Cousens S, et al. Improvement of perinatal and newborn care in rural Pakistan through community-based strategies: a cluster-randomised effectiveness trial. Lancet 2011;377(9763):403–12.

16. Chang HH, Larson J, Blencowe H, et al. Preventing preterm births: analysis of trends and potential reductions with interventions in 39 countries with very high human development index. Lancet 2013;381(9862):223–34.

17. World Health Organization. Handbook IMCI: integrated management of childhood illness. Geneva (Switzerland): World Health Organization; 2005. ISBN 9241546441.

18. Binagwaho A, Kyamanywa P, Farmer PE, et al. The human resources for health program in Rwanda–new partnership. N Engl J Med 2013;369(21): 2054–9.

19. Bergström S. "Non-physician clinicians" in low-income countries. BMJ 2011; 342:d2499.

20. Wilson A, Lissauer D, Thangaratinam S, et al. A comparison of clinical officers with medical doctors on outcomes of caesarean section in the developing world: meta-analysis of controlled studies. BMJ 2011;342:d2600.

21. World Health Organization. Optimizing health worker roles to improve access to key maternal and newborn health interventions through task shifting. Geneva (Switzerland): World Health Organization; 2012. ISBN 978 92 4 1504843.

22. Lawn JE, Kinney MV, Belizan JM, et al. Born too soon: accelerating actions for prevention and care of 15 million newborns born too soon. Reprod Health 2013; 10(Suppl 1):S6.

23. Lee AC, Katz J, Blencowe H, et al, for the CHERG Preterm-SGA Working Group. National and regional estimates of term and preterm babies born small for gestational age in 138 low-income and middle-income countries in 2010. Lancet Glob Health 2013;1:e26–36.

24. Katz J, Lee AC, Kozuki N, et al, for the CHERG Small-for-Gestational-Age-Preterm Birth Working Group. Mortality risk in preterm and small-for-gestational-age infants in low-income and middle-income countries: a pooled country analysis. Lancet 2013;382(9890):417–25.
25. Hillman N, Jobe A. Noninvasive strategies for management of respiratory problems in neonates. Neoreviews 2013;14:e227.
26. Brown J, Machen H, Kawaza K, et al. A high-value, low-cost bubble continuous positive airway pressure system for low-resource settings: technical assessment and initial case reports. PLoS One 2013;8(1):e53622.
27. Kawaza K, Machen HE, Brown J, et al. Efficacy of a low-cost bubble CPAP system in treatment of respiratory distress in a neonatal ward in Malawi. PLoS One 2014;9(1):e86327.
28. Pattinson R, Kerber K, Waiswa P, et al. Perinatal mortality audit: counting, accountability, and overcoming challenges in scaling up in low- and middle-income countries. Int J Gynaecol Obstet 2009;107(Suppl 1):S113–21, S121–2.
29. Howard-Grabman L, Snetro G. How to mobilize communities for health and social change. Baltimore (MD): Health Communication Partnership; 2003.
30. Colbourn T, Nambiar B, Bondo A, et al. Effects of quality improvement in health facilities and community mobilization through women's groups on maternal, neonatal and perinatal mortality in three districts of Malawi: Mai-Khanda, a cluster randomized controlled effectiveness trial. Int Health 2013; 5(3):180–95.
31. Prost A, Colbourn T, Seward N, et al. Women's groups practising participatory learning and action to improve maternal and newborn health in low-resource settings: a systematic review and meta-analysis. Lancet 2013;381(9879):1736–46.
32. Lawn JE, Kinney M, Lee AC, et al. Reducing intrapartum-related deaths and disability: can the health system deliver? Int J Gynaecol Obstet 2009; 107(Suppl 1):S123–40, S140–2.
33. Darmstadt GL, Lee AC, Cousens S, et al. 60 Million non-facility births: who can deliver in community settings to reduce intrapartum-related deaths? Int J Gynaecol Obstet 2009;107(Suppl 1):S89–112.
34. UNICEF. The state of the world's children 2009. New York: UNICEF; 2009.
35. Mitchell M, Getchell M, Nkaka M, et al. Perceived improvement in integrated management of childhood illness implementation through use of mobile technology: qualitative evidence from a pilot study in Tanzania. J Health Commun 2012; 17(Suppl 1):118–27.
36. Lassi ZS, Haider BA, Bhutta ZA. Community-based intervention packages for reducing maternal and neonatal morbidity and mortality and improving neonatal outcomes. Cochrane Database Syst Rev 2010;(11):CD007754.
37. Wilson A, Gallos ID, Plana N, et al. Effectiveness of strategies incorporating training and support of traditional birth attendants on perinatal and maternal mortality: meta-analysis. BMJ 2011;343:d7102.
38. Bang AT, Bang RA, Baitule SB, et al. Management of birth asphyxia in home deliveries in rural Gadchiroli: the effect of two types of birth attendants and of resuscitating with mouth-to-mouth, tube-mask or bag-mask. J Perinatol 2005; 25(Suppl 1):S82–91.
39. Carlo WA, Goudar SS, Jehan I, et al. Newborn-care training and perinatal mortality in developing countries. N Engl J Med 2010;362(7):614–23.
40. Gill CJ, Phiri-Mazala G, Geurina NG, et al. Effect of training traditional birth attendants on neonatal mortality (Lufwanyama Neonatal Survival Project): randomized control study. BMJ 2011;342:346–56.

41. Msemo G, Kidanto HL, Massawe A, et al. Newborn mortality and fresh stillbirth rates in Tanzania after Helping Babies Breathe training. Pediatrics 2013;131: e353–60.
42. Lee AC, Kozuki N, Blencowe H, et al. Intrapartum-related neonatal encephalopathy incidence and impairment at regional and global levels for 2010 with trends from 1990. Pediatr Res 2013;74(Suppl 1):50–72.
43. Young Infants Clinical Signs Study Group. Clinical signs that predict severe illness in children under age 2 months: a multicentre study. Lancet 2008; 371(9607):135–42.
44. Bang AT, Bang RA, Stoll BJ, et al. Is home-based diagnosis and treatment of neonatal sepsis feasible and effective? Seven years of intervention in the Gadchiroli field trial (1996 to 2003). J Perinatol 2005;25(Suppl 1):S62–71.
45. Baqui AH, El-Arifeen S, Darmstadt GL, et al. Effect of community-based newborn-care intervention package implemented through two service-delivery strategies in Sylhet district, Bangladesh: a cluster-randomised controlled trial. Lancet 2008;371(9628):1936–44.
46. Mullany LC, Darmstadt GL, Khatry SK, et al. Topical applications of chlorhexidine to the umbilical cord for prevention of omphalitis and neonatal mortality in southern Nepal: a community-based, cluster-randomised trial. Lancet 2006; 367(9514):910–8.
47. Arifeen SE, Mullany LC, Shah R, et al. The effect of cord cleansing with chlorhexidine on neonatal mortality in rural Bangladesh: a community-based, cluster-randomised trial. Lancet 2012;379(9820):1022–8.
48. Esamai F, Tshefu AK, Ayede AI, et al. Ongoing trials of simplified antibiotic regimens for the treatment of serious infections in young infants in South Asia and sub-Saharan Africa: implications for policy. Pediatr Infect Dis J 2013; 32(Suppl 1):S46–9.
49. Lawn JE, Blencowe H, Pattinson R, et al. Stillbirths: where? when? why? how to make the data count? Lancet 2011;377(9775):1448–63.
50. Stenberg K, Axelson H, Sheehan P, et al. Advancing social and economic development by investing in women's and children's health: a new Global Investment Framework. Lancet 2014;383(9925):1333–54.
51. Conde-Agudelo A, Belizán JM, Diaz-Rossello J. Kangaroo mother care to reduce morbidity and mortality in low birthweight infants. Cochrane Database Syst Rev 2011;(3):CD002771.
52. Tessier R, Cristo MB, Velez S, et al. Kangaroo mother care: a method for protecting high-risk low-birth-weight and premature infants against developmental delay. Infant Behav Dev 2003;26:384–97.
53. Moore ER, Anderson GC, Bergman N, Dowswell T. Early skin-to-skin contact for mothers and their healthy newborn infants. Cochrane Database Syst Rev 2012;(5):CD003519.

Prevention of Preterm Birth in Modern Obstetrics

 CrossMark

Kara B. Markham, MD[a],*, Mark Klebanoff, MD[b,c,d,e]

KEYWORDS

- Preterm birth • Preterm birth prevention • Progestins • Cerclage • Pessary

KEY POINTS

- Tocolytic therapy may be useful for delaying delivery long enough to permit administration of antenatal corticosteroids and/or maternal transport to a tertiary care center, but long-term use does not result in clinically significant pregnancy prolongation.
- Activity restriction has no proven benefit in the prevention of preterm birth and may result in substantial maternal morbidity.
- Cervical pessary usage is a potentially promising intervention, but further research is needed to determine the effectiveness of this device.
- Progestin prophylaxis and, in certain situations, cerclage placement are the most effective interventions in prevention of recurrent spontaneous preterm birth.
- Although there has been progress in recent decades, obstetricians and researchers still have a long way toward preventing preterm birth.

Preterm birth (PTB) continues to be the leading cause of neonatal death, causing more than 1 million deaths worldwide each year. In the United States, 11.72% of all babies were born before 37 weeks of gestation in 2011, representing the lowest PTB rate in more than a decade.[1] Despite this reassuring trend, the United States continues to have the highest PTB rate of any industrialized country. Despite the dedication of billions of dollars and untold hours of work, the solution to the problem of PTB remains elusive worldwide. This article focuses specifically on prevention of spontaneous preterm delivery, processes that account for 70% to 80% of all early births. The

Disclosure: The authors report no conflict of interest.
Disclaimer: No funding was received for this work.
[a] Maternal Fetal Medicine Division, Department of Obstetrics & Gynecology, The Ohio State University College of Medicine, 395 West 12th Avenue, 5th Floor, Columbus, OH 43210, USA; [b] Department of Pediatrics, Nationwide Children's Hospital, 700 Children's Drive, Columbus, OH 43205, USA; [c] Department of Obstetrics and Gynecology, The Ohio State University, 395 West 12th Avenue, 5th Floor, Columbus, OH 43210, USA; [d] Division of Epidemiology, The Ohio State University College of Public Health, 250 Cunz Hall, 1841 Neil Avenue, Columbus, OH 43210, USA; [e] Center for Perinatal Research, The Research Institute, Nationwide Children's Hospital, 700 Children's Drive, WB 5231, Columbus, OH 43205, USA
* Corresponding author.
E-mail address: kara.markham@osumc.edu

Clin Perinatol 41 (2014) 773–785
http://dx.doi.org/10.1016/j.clp.2014.08.003
0095-5108/14/$ – see front matter Published by Elsevier Inc.

perinatology.theclinics.com

interventions that have been attempted to prevent spontaneous PTB are reviewed, some of which have been successful in some populations, whereas others have ultimately fallen out of favor because of lack of effectiveness.

INEFFECTIVE INTERVENTIONS
Home Tocometry

Home uterine activity monitoring has been proposed as a method of identifying women in early preterm labor, potentially allowing intervention to prevent delivery. This type of monitoring may be performed via subjective patient report or, more commonly, via use of home tocometry. Despite being initially heralded as a useful tool, tocometry has since fallen out of favor.

Numerous randomized controlled trials have evaluated the use of home monitors such that an exhaustive review of all of the available literature is beyond the scope of this article. For example, a recent Cochrane Review included 15 randomized controlled trials.[2] This meta-analysis showed no reduction in delivery before 37 weeks of gestation with home uterine monitoring.[2] When low-quality studies were excluded from the analysis, there were also no significant reductions in PTB before 34 weeks of gestation or neonatal intensive care unit admissions.[2]

If there is any benefit to home uterine activity monitoring, it may simply be the increased exposure of high-risk patients to specialized nurses and/or physicians. At present, the American College of Obstetricians and Gynecologists does not recommend use of home tocometry to screen for or prevent spontaneous PTB.[3]

Tocolytics

Several tocolytic agents have been used over the last several decades. These agents vary in mechanisms of action, dosing regimens, and side effects but they all have one thing in common: their lack of efficacy in preventing PTB. As shown in **Table 1**, these agents may be beneficial in the short term, thereby allowing administration of antenatal corticosteroids and/or maternal transport to a level 3 center, but long-term effectiveness has not been shown. These agents are almost destined to fail because they are not initiated until it is too late.[16] By the time a woman presents with symptomatic preterm labor or preterm premature rupture of membranes, the underlying process has been ongoing for weeks if not months.[16] Tocolytic agents thus address the symptoms of preterm labor without affecting the cause of the process.[16]

Activity Restriction

Many women diagnosed with advanced cervical dilatation, advanced cervical effacement, or threatened preterm labor are asked to adhere to activity restrictions. Activity restriction is probably the most commonly prescribed intervention to prevent PTB. These restrictions range from light restriction (1 hour or less of continuous rest during waking hours) to moderate restriction (1–8 hours of continuous rest) or even strict bed rest.

Despite its common use, literature supporting the efficacy of bed rest for prevention of spontaneous PTB is lacking, with randomized controlled trials showing no benefit.[17,18] Furthermore, although the recommendation for bed rest is primarily based on a no-harm-no-foul principle, emerging data indicate that there are potential negative effects to activity restriction. Pregnant women in general are at an increased risk for venous thromboembolic disease, a risk that is only increased in the setting of bed rest. Activity restriction is also associated with a significant decrease in muscle strength and coordination, and there are psychological and socioeconomic impacts that must be considered. Not only can activity restriction result in financial difficulties

Table 1
Effectiveness of tocolytic agents

Class of Tocolytic	Examples	Short-term Benefits	Long-term Effects	Comments
Beta-adrenergic receptor agonists	Terbutaline sulfate Ritodrine hydrochloride	PTB rates reduced within 48 h of administration (RR, 0.68; 95% CI, 0.53–0.88)[4] May postpone delivery long enough to permit antenatal corticosteroid administration	No reduction in either total PTB rates or perinatal mortality[4] Prolonged use not associated with differences in gestational ages at delivery or PTB rates[5,6]	FDA warning against the use of terbutaline for >48–72 h (lack of efficacy and concerns about serious maternal heart problems)[7]
Calcium channel blockers	Nifedipine	PTB rates reduced within 7 d (RR, 0.82; 95% CI, 0.7–0.97)[8] Decreased PTB rates before 34 wk of gestation (RR, 0.77; 95% CI, 0.66–0.91)[8] Reduction in neonatal respiratory distress syndrome (RR, 0.63; 95% CI, 0.46–0.86)[8]	One randomized controlled trial comparing nifedipine with placebo (APOSTEL-II): no difference in adverse perinatal outcomes, gestational age at delivery, or pregnancy prolongation[9]	May be beneficial in the short term or for symptomatic contractions
Cyclooxygenase inhibitors	Indocin	Reduced PTB rates within 48 h of administration[10]	No difference in neonatal outcomes[11]	Use limited by fetal side effects, including premature closure of the ductus arteriosus and oligohydramnios Short courses (48 h) reasonable before 32 wk of gestation
Magnesium sulfate	Not applicable	None identified	No differences in PTB rates or neonatal respiratory distress[12]	Administration recommended for fetal neuroprotection (prevention of cerebral palsy specifically)[13]
Selective oxytocin-vasopressin receptor antagonists	Atosiban	Trend toward increased delivery within 48 h[14]	Trend toward increased risks of PTB at <28 wk and <37 wk of gestation[14]	Not available in the United States
Nitric oxide donors	Transdermal nitroglycerin	None identified	No clear benefit identified[15]	Further research needed

Abbreviations: APOSTEL, assessment of perinatal outcome with sustained tocolysis in early labor; CI, confidence interval; FDA, US Food and Drug Administration; RR, relative risk.

caused by lack of work, this intervention is clearly associated with disruption of family life and increased anxiety and depression.

In the setting of potential harm with no proven benefit, the use of activity restriction should be minimized for the prevention of spontaneous PTB. Per the American College of Obstetricians and Gynecologists, "these measures have not been shown to be effective for the prevention of PTB and should not be routinely recommended."[19]

INTERVENTIONS OF QUESTIONABLE EFFICACY
Treatment of Urogenital Tract Infections

Given the suspected link between PTB and inflammation, it seems logical that eradication of urogenital tract bacteria might reduce the risk of early delivery. Numerous studies have therefore addressed the relationship between PTB and such microbes as *Trichomonas vaginalis*, bacterial vaginosis, *Candida*, *Chlamydia trachomatis*, gonorrhea, and group B *Streptococcus*. More importantly, as shown in **Table 2**, researchers have sought to determine whether treatment of such infections can reduce this risk.

In addition to treatment aimed at specific infections, antibiotic therapy in general has been proposed as an intervention to prevent PTB or at least prolong gestation. This strategy seems valid in the setting of preterm premature rupture of membranes, but such therapy does not seem to be effective in women with intact amniotic membranes. For example, in the ORACLE II trial, women in spontaneous preterm labor were randomized to receive erythromycin alone, amoxicillin and clavulanate potassium alone, erythromycin and amoxicillin and clavulanate potassium, or placebo.[40] No differences were shown in PTB rates or composite neonatal outcomes.[40] A similar study by Romero and colleagues[41] also failed to show a benefit to empiric antibiotic therapy. However, critics of such studies argue that perhaps the wrong antibiotic was used or the antibiotic was started too late in the process of parturition to make a difference. Regardless, the current literature does not support the use of empiric antibiotic therapy for prevention of PTB or prolongation of gestation.

In addition, the presence of infection and/or inflammation distant from the urogenital tract is also associated with increased PTB rates. Moderate to severe periodontitis is associated with an approximately 2-fold increased risk of PTB.[42,43] Despite this association, treatment of periodontal disease does not reduce the risk of a woman delivering prematurely and should currently be recommended only as part of routine health maintenance.[44–46]

Pessary

Use of the cervical pessary has been touted as a noninvasive cerclage. The Arabin pessary, a flexible ringlike silicone device, has been most effective in published trials. The smaller inner diameter of this device should fit around the cervix snugly, thereby minimizing exposure of fetal membranes to the vaginal flora.[47] The inclination of the cervical canal is also changed, directing it posteriorly so that the weight of the pregnancy centers on the anterior lower segment.[47]

Since its first use, multiple studies have been published investigating the efficacy of this intervention, with varying pessary types, research designs, and patient populations reported. The PECEP (Pesario Cervical Para Evitar Prematuridad) trial, the largest trial to date, was a randomized controlled trial that enrolled women with cervical shortening (cervical length ≤25 mm). Of women assigned to the pessary arm, 6% delivered before 34 weeks' gestation; an 82% reduction compared with the 27% of women who delivered prematurely in the expectant management arm.[48] This trial has been criticized because of a higher-than-expected rate of PTB in the control arm, questionable ability to generalize, and lack of administration of progestin therapy.

Table 2
The link between urogenital infections and PTB

Infection	PTB Association	Treatment Effect	Recommendation
T vaginalis	Increased risk of PTB with infection	Treatment of asymptomatic infection may increase the risk of PTB[20]	Routine screening and treatment in asymptomatic women not recommended
Bacterial vaginosis	Strong predictor of PTB (up to a 7.6-fold increased risk)[21]	No benefit seen in several RCTs using clindamycin or metronidazole[22-25]	Routine screening and treatment in asymptomatic women not recommended
Vaginal candidiasis	No clear association[26]	One RCT showed a reduction in PTB rates (RR, 0.34; 95% CI, 0.15–0.79) in asymptomatic women screened and treated in the second trimester[27]	More research needed
C trachomatis	Inconsistent literature	Retrospective cohort study showing an RR of 0.54 (95% CI, 0.37–0.8) for delivery at 32–36 wk gestation in patients treated at <20 wk[28] RCT showed no reduction in PTB rates with treatment between 23 and 29 wk of gestation[29]	Treatment indicated to prevent neonatal morbidity
Neisseria gonorrhea	Two retrospective studies showing an association[30,31]	No studies evaluating treatment effect	Definitive research cannot be performed because of public health issues
Group B Streptococcus colonization	Meta-analysis of cohort studies showed no relationship Meta-analysis of cross-sectional and case-control studies showed an association[32]	No benefit in prevention of PTB[33]	Treatment should follow CDC guidelines to prevent neonatal morbidity and mortality[34]
Asymptomatic bacteriuria	Inconsistent literature[35]	Cochrane Review showed no reduction in PTB rates with treatment[36]	Treatment recommended for reduction of maternal morbidity and mortality
Cystitis	Three retrospective studies showing an increased risk of PTB (RR, 1.03–1.38)[37,38]	No studies showing a reduction in PTB rates after treatment	Treatment recommended for reduction of maternal morbidity and mortality
Pyelonephritis	Associated with an increased risk of PTB (OR, 1.3; 95% CI, 1.2–1.5)[39]	No studies to date showing a reduction in PTB rates with treatment	Treatment recommended for reduction of maternal morbidity and mortality

Abbreviations: CDC, US Centers for Disease Control and Prevention; OR, odds ratio; RCT, randomized controlled trial.

The ProTWIN trial then evaluated the prophylactic use of Arabin pessaries in multiple-gestation pregnancies, showing no differences in PTB rates or a composite of poor perinatal outcomes in women randomized to receive a pessary compared with controls.[49] These findings prompted the investigators to conclude that, "in unselected women with a multiple pregnancy, prophylactic use of a cervical pessary does not reduce poor perinatal outcome."[49]

Despite these critiques, pessaries have several advantages compared with surgical cerclage. As a nonsurgical alternative, pessary use can be expected to result in decreased hospital costs and anesthesia exposure. Complications such as bleeding, infection, and rupture of membranes are also likely to be less common with pessary than cerclage. In addition, few complications and/or side effects have been reported with the use of cervical pessaries, with patients primarily complaining of increased vaginal discharge and discomfort with placement and removal of the device.[48]

Pessary use is currently a promising but unproven therapy for prevention of preterm labor. Multiple trials are currently in process to better define the populations that may benefit from this device.

SUCCESSFUL THERAPY
Lifestyle Modifications

Women should be counseled about simple and cost-effective interventions that may reduce their risk of early delivery. For example, smoking is a known risk factor for PTB. Although there are no randomized controlled trials that show a reduction in PTB rates with smoking cessation, all pregnant women who admit to tobacco use should be encouraged to quit and provided with resources to assist with cessation. In addition, because PTB is most common in women with an interpregnancy interval of less than 6 months, women should be counseled about safe pregnancy spacing.

However, the expected treatment effect is not seen for all interventions. For example, although poor prenatal care is linked to PTB, enhanced prenatal care with more frequent visits and improved education does not necessarily improve outcomes. For example, the March of Dimes Multicenter Prematurity Prevention Trial showed no difference in PTB rates in women assigned to a program of enhanced care involving frequent visits and increased education; a finding that was confirmed by a later Cochrane Review.[50,51] Likewise, interventions designed to enhance social support do not seem to effectively prolong gestational length.[52,53] Regardless, prenatal care and social support are recommended because of other benefits on maternal and fetal health.

Progestational Agents

Current evidence supports the use of progestin prophylaxis in certain populations for prevention of PTB. One group that seems to benefit from this therapy is women with a history of a prior spontaneous PTB. In 2003, Meis and colleagues[54] showed that 17-alpha-hydroxyprogesterone caproate (17OHPC) significantly reduced the risk of recurrent preterm delivery before 37 weeks' gestation with a relative risk (RR) of 0.66 (confidence interval [CI], 0.54–0.81). A trial by da Fonseca and colleagues[55] then showed a reduction in recurrent PTB rates using progesterone administered via a vaginal suppository: 13.8% of women in the progesterone group delivered before 37 weeks of gestation compared with 28.5% in the placebo group ($P = .03$), with incidences of delivery before 34 weeks of gestation of 2.8% versus 18.6% respectively ($P = .002$).[55] However, a trial by O'Brien and colleagues[56] failed to show a reduction in recurrent PTB rates using a progesterone gel, but a Cochran Review including 36 randomized controlled trials subsequently showed statistically significant reduction in risks of such important outcomes as PTB at less than 34 weeks (RR, 0.31; 95% CI, 0.14–0.69), PTB at less than 37 weeks (RR, 0.55; 95% CI, 0.42–0.74), and perinatal mortality (RR, 0.50; 95% CI, 0.33–0.75).[57]

Progestin prophylaxis is not effective in women with multiple gestations,[58–62] but another group that may benefit from therapy is women with cervical shortening. Fonseca and colleagues[63] in 2007 showed a reduction in preterm delivery before 34 weeks of gestation (RR, 0.56; 95% CI, 0.36–0.86) using progesterone suppositories in asymptomatic women with cervical shortening. A subsequent study by Hassan and colleagues[64] showed a similar reduction in PTB before 33 weeks of gestation (RR, 0.55; 95% CI, 0.33–0.92) using progesterone gel in this population. Grobman and colleagues[65] failed to show a reduction in preterm delivery rates in women with cervical shortening who were exposed to 17OHPC, but a meta-analysis by Romero and colleagues[66] showed that vaginal progesterone supplementation reduced the risk of PTB (RR, 0.69 with 95% CI, 0.55–0.88 for delivery <35 weeks; RR, 0.50 with 95% CI 0.30–0.81 for delivery <28 weeks) and associated morbidity in asymptomatic, otherwise low-risk women with cervical shortening.

Progestin prophylaxis therefore seems to be an important tool in the armamentarium to prevent PTB. As shown in **Fig. 1**, this therapy should be considered in women with prior preterm deliveries and those with cervical shortening less than 20 mm, but current research does not support its use in other clinical situations.[67]

Cerclage

The indications for cerclage placement have changed over the decades, with current practices more concerned with placement of indicated cerclages in women with cervical shortening despite progestin prophylaxis rather than placement of cerclages in the early second trimester based solely on a history of PTB.

Although none of the individual randomized controlled trials show an improvement in PTB rates with cerclage placement, a meta-analysis by Berghella and colleagues[68,69] found that cerclage placement was associated with an RR of 0.70 (95% CI, 0.55–0.89) for recurrent PTB before 35 weeks' gestation.[70–73] Cerclage placement was also associated with a decreased risk for recurrent PTB before 37 weeks' gestation (RR, 0.7 with 95% CI, 0.58–0.83), 32 weeks' gestation (RR, 0.66 with 95% CI, 0.48–0.91), 28 weeks' gestation (RR, 0.66 with 95% CI, 0.43–0.96), and 24 weeks' gestation (95% CI, 0.48 with 95% CI, 0.26–0.9), as well as a reduction in composite mortality and morbidity (RR, 0.64 with 95% CI, 0.45–0.91).[69]

Women enrolled in the trials discussed earlier were not concurrently treated with supplemental progesterone. No randomized controlled trial has been performed to date evaluating the efficacy of cerclage placement in women also treated with progestins. Rafael and colleagues[74] retrospectively examined this issue, showing no difference in the rate of recurrent PTB before 35 weeks' gestation with concurrent therapy (odds ratio, 1.72 with 95% CI, 0.5–5.89), suggesting that there may not be a cumulative effect with these two treatment modalities. Again, further research is needed to better define the utility of combined therapy.

Interventions to Limit Nonindicated Deliveries Before 39 Weeks of Gestation

One of the most successful quality improvement campaigns in obstetrics recently has involved a push toward elimination of elective deliveries before 39 weeks of gestation. This change reflects the growing understanding of the morbidity and mortality associated with late preterm and early term births, including increased risks of such complications as hypothermia, respiratory distress, hypoglycemia, infection, apnea of the newborn, hyperbilirubinemia, and feeding difficulties.[75] There also seems to be

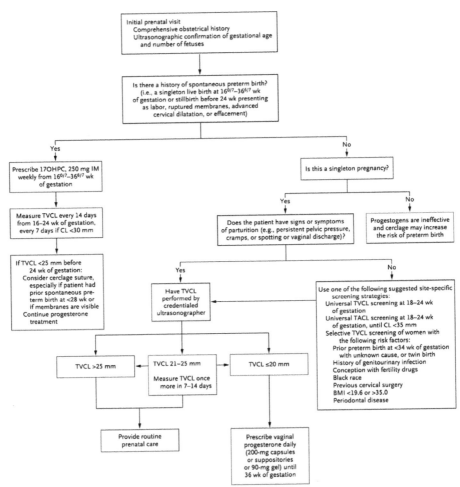

Fig. 1. Clinical use of progestin prophylaxis. BMI, body mass index; CL, cervical length; TACL, transabdominal cervical length; TVCL, transvaginal cervical length. (*From* Iams JD. Prevention of preterm parturition. N Engl J Med 2014;370:1861; with permission.)

long-term morbidity, particularly neurodevelopmental issues, associated with these births before 39 weeks.[75]

Such initiatives primarily focus on the timing of either elective deliveries or those in the setting of obstetric complications (ie, preeclampsia, intrauterine growth restriction, oligohydramnios, diabetes mellitus).[76] Deliveries related to spontaneous preterm labor or preterm premature rupture of membranes are less likely to be affected by these quality improvement programs, but they still represent an important milestone in the quest to reduce PTB rates overall.

SUMMARY

Preterm labor is a complex disease characterized by the interplay of multiple different pathways. As such, prevention of preterm labor and delivery is complicated as well, and it is highly likely that no single intervention will be effective for every woman. In addition to this complexity, one of the major obstacles to prevention is the early identification of women at risk, who do not usually present with symptoms until weeks or even months after the underlying process first started. Successful therapy therefore needs to be initiated far in advance of symptoms, examination findings, or even ultrasonography findings. To be effective worldwide, such therapy also needs to be inexpensive and easily obtainable. Researchers and clinicians must collaborate to achieve all of these essential qualifications if a cure for PTB is to be found.

REFERENCES

1. Hamilton BE, Martin JA, Ventura SJ. In: Births: preliminary data for 2011. National vital statistics reports, vol. 61. Hyattsville (MD): National Center for Health Statistics; 2012. no. 5.
2. Urquhart C, Currell R, Harlow F, et al. Home uterine monitoring for detecting preterm labour. Cochrane Database Syst Rev 2012;(5):CD006172.
3. Committee on Practice Bulletins–Obstetrics, The American College of Obstetricians and Gynecologists. Practice bulletin no. 130: prediction and prevention of preterm birth. Obstet Gynecol 2012;120:964.
4. Neilson JP, West HM, Dowswell T. Betamimetics for inhibiting preterm labour. Cochrane Database Syst Rev 2014;(2):CD004352.
5. Nanda K. Terbutaline pump maintenance therapy after threatened preterm labor for preventing preterm birth. Cochrane Database Syst Rev 2002;(4): CD003933.
6. Gaudet LM, Singh K, Weeks L, et al. Effectiveness of terbutaline pump for the prevention of preterm birth. A systematic review and meta-analysis. PLoS One 2012;7:e31679.
7. Available at: http://www.fda.gov/drugs/drugsafety/ucm243539.htm. Accessed January 21, 2014.
8. Conde-Agudelo A, Romero R, Kusanovic JP. Nifedipine in the management of preterm labor: a systematic review and metaanalysis. Am J Obstet Gynecol 2011;204:134.e1–20.
9. Roos C, Spaanderman M, Schuit E, et al. Effect of maintenance tocolysis with nifedipine in threatened preterm labor on perinatal outcomes. JAMA 2013; 309:41–7.
10. Niebyl JR, Blake DA, White RD, et al. The inhibition of preterm labor with indomethacin. Am J Obstet Gynecol 1980;136:1014.
11. King J, Flenady V, Cole S, et al. Cyclo-oxygenase (COX) inhibitors for treating preterm labour. Cochrane Database Syst Rev 2005;(2):CD001992.
12. Mercer BM, Merlino AA, Society for Maternal Fetal Medicine. Magnesium sulfate for preterm labor and preterm birth. Obstet Gynecol 2009;114:650.
13. Rouse DJ, Hirtz DG, Thom E, et al. A randomized, controlled trial of magnesium sulfate for the prevention of cerebral palsy. N Engl J Med 2008;359:895.
14. Papatsonis D, Flenady V, Cole S, et al. Oxytocin receptor antagonists for inhibiting preterm labour. Cochrane Database Syst Rev 2005;(3):CD004452.
15. Conde-Agudelo A, Romer R. Transdermal nitroglycerin for the treatment of preterm labor: a systematic review and meta-analysis. Am J Obstet Gynecol 2013; 209:551.e1–18.
16. Iams JD, Berghella V. Care for women with prior preterm birth. Am J Obstet Gynecol 2010;203:89–100.

17. Elliott JP, Miller HS, Coleman S, et al. A randomized multicenter study to determine the efficacy of activity restriction for preterm labor management in patients testing negative for fetal fibronectin. J Perinatol 2005;25:626–30.

18. Sosa C, Althabe F, Belizan J, et al. Bed rest in singleton pregnancies for preventing preterm birth. Cochrane Database Syst Rev 2004;(1):CD003581.

19. American College of Obstetricians and Gynecologists. Management of preterm labor. Practice Bulletin No. 127. Obstet Gynecol 2012;119:1308–17.

20. Klebanoff MA, Carey JC, Hauth JC, et al. Failure of metronidazole to prevent preterm delivery among pregnant women with asymptomatic Trichomonas vaginalis infection. N Engl J Med 2001;345:487–93.

21. Leitich H, Bodner-Adler B, Brunbauer M, et al. Bacterial vaginosis as a risk factor for preterm delivery: a meta-analysis. Am J Obstet Gynecol 2003;189:139–47.

22. Carey JC, Klebanoff MA, Hauth JC, et al. Metronidazole to prevent preterm delivery in pregnant women with asymptomatic bacterial vaginosis. National Institute of Child Health and Human Development Network of Maternal-Fetal Medicine Units. N Engl J Med 2000;342:534–40.

23. McDonald HM, Brocklehurst P, Gordon A. Antibiotics for treating bacterial vaginosis in pregnancy (Review). Cochrane Database Syst Rev 2007;(1): CD000262.

24. Brocklehurst P, Gordon A, Heatley E, et al. Antibiotics for treating bacterial vaginosis in pregnancy. Cochrane Database Syst Rev 2013;(1):CD000262.

25. Okun N, Gronau KA, Hannah ME. Antibiotics for bacterial vaginosis or Trichomonas vaginalis in pregnancy: a systematic review. Obstet Gynecol 2005;105:857–68.

26. Cotch MF, Hillier SL, Gibbs RS, et al. Epidemiology and outcomes associated with moderate to heavy Candida colonization during pregnancy. Vaginal infections and prematurity study group. Am J Obstet Gynecol 1998;178:374–80.

27. Kiss H, Petricevic L, Hussiein P. Prospective randomized controlled trial of an infection screening programme to reduce the rate of preterm delivery. Br Med J 2004;329:371.

28. Folger AT. Maternal Chlamydia trachomatis infections and preterm birth: The impact of early detection and eradication during pregnancy. Matern Child Health J 2014;18:1795–802.

29. Martin DH, Eschenbach DA, Cotch MF, et al. Double-blind placebo-controlled treatment trial of Chlamydia trachomatis endocervical infections in pregnant women. Infect Dis Obstet Gynecol 1997;5:10–7.

30. Johnson HL, Ghanem KG, Zenilman JM, et al. Sexually transmitted infections and adverse pregnancy outcomes among women attending inner city public sexually transmitted diseases clinics. Sex Transm Dis 2011;38:167–71.

31. Mann JR, McDermott S, Gill T. Sexually transmitted infection is associated with increased risk of preterm birth in South Carolina women insured by Medicaid. J Matern Fetal Neonatal Med 2010;23:563–8.

32. Valkenburg-van den Berg AW, Sprij AJ, Dekker FW, et al. Association between colonization with Group B Streptococcus and preterm delivery: a systematic review. Acta Obstet Gynecol Scand 2009;88:958–76.

33. Klebanoff MA, Regan JA, Rao AV, et al. Outcome of the Vaginal infections and Prematurity Study: results of a clinical trial of erythromycin among pregnant women colonized with group B streptococci. Am J Obstet Gynecol 1995;172:1540–5.

34. Centers for Disease Control and Prevention. Prevention of perinatal group B streptococcal disease. MMWR Recomm Rep 2010;59(RR-10):1–36.

35. Sheiner E, Mazor-Drey E, Levy A. Asymptomatic bacteriuria during pregnancy. J Matern Fetal Neonatal Med 2009;22:423–7.

36. Smaill F, Vazquez JC. Antibiotics for asymptomatic bacteriuria in pregnancy. Co-chrane Database Syst Rev 2007;(2):CD000490.
37. Banhidy F, ACS N, Puho EH, et al. Pregnancy complications and birth outcomes of pregnant women with urinary tract infections and related drug treatments. Scand J Infect Dis 2007;39:390–7.
38. Chen YK, Chen SF, Li HC, et al. No increased risk of adverse pregnancy out-comes in women with urinary tract infections: a nationwide population-based study. Acta Obstet Gynecol Scand 2010;89:882–9.
39. Wing DA, Fassett MJ, Getahun D. Acute pyelonephritis in pregnancy: an 18 year retrospective analysis. Am J Obstet Gynecol 2013.
40. Kenyon SL, Taylor DJ, Tarnow-Mordi W. Broad-spectrum antibiotics for spon-taneous preterm labour: the ORACLE II randomized trial. Lancet 2001;357:989–94.
41. Romero R, Sibai B, Caritis S, et al. Antibiotic treatment of preterm labor with intact membranes: a multicenter, randomized, double-blinded placebo-controlled trial. Am J Obstet Gynecol 1993;169:764–74.
42. Offenbacher S, Katz V, Fertik G, et al. Periodontal infection as a possible risk factor for preterm low birth weight. J Periodontol 1996;67:1103–13.
43. Jeffcoat MD, Geurs NC, Reddy MS, et al. Periodontal infection and preterm birth: results of a prospective study. J Am Dent Assoc 2001;132:875–80.
44. Polyzos NP, Polyzos IP, Zavos A, et al. Obstetric outcomes after treatment of periodontal disease during pregnancy: systematic review and meta-analysis. BMJ 2010;341:c7017.
45. Chambrone L, Pannuti CM, Guglielmetti MR, et al. Evidence grade associating periodontitis with preterm birth and/or low birth weight: II: a systematic review of randomized trials evaluating the effects of periodontal treatment. J Clin Perio-dontol 2011;38:902–14.
46. Kim AJ, Lo AJ, Pullin DA, et al. Scaling and root planing treatment for periodon-titis to reduce preterm birth and low birth weight: a systematic review and meta-analysis of randomized controlled trials. J Periodontol 2012;83:1508–19.
47. Arabin B, Halbesma JR, Vork F, et al. Is treatment with vaginal pessaries an op-tion in patients with a sonographically detected short cervix? J Perinat Med 2003;31:122.
48. Goya M, Pratcorona L, Merced C, et al. Cervical pessary in pregnant women with a short cervix (PECEP): an open-label randomised controlled trial. Lancet 2012;379(9828):1800–6.
49. Liem S, Schuit E, Hegeman M, et al. Cervical pessary for prevention of preterm birth in women with a multiple pregnancy (ProTWIN): a multicentre, open-label randomized controlled trial. Lancet 2013;382:1341–9.
50. Collaborative Group on Preterm Birth Prevention. Multicenter randomized, controlled trial of a preterm birth prevention program. Am J Obstet Gynecol 1993;169:352.
51. Whitworth M, Quenby S, Cockerill RO, et al. Specialised antenatal clinics for women with a pregnancy at high risk of preterm birth (excluding multiple preg-nancy) to improve maternal and infant outcomes. Cochrane Database Syst Rev 2011;(9):CD006760.
52. Orr ST. Social support and pregnancy outcome: a review of the literature. Clin Obstet Gynecol 2004;47:842.
53. Villar J, Farnot U, Barros F, et al. A randomized trial of psychosocial support dur-ing high-risk pregnancies. The Latin American Network for Perinatal and Repro-ductive Research. N Engl J Med 1992;327:1266.

54. Meis PJ, Klebanoff M, Thom E, et al. Prevention of recurrent preterm delivery by 17 alpha-hydroxyprogesterone caproate. N Engl J Med 2003;348:2379–85.
55. da Fonseca EB, Bittar RE, Carvalho MH, et al. Prophylactic administration of progesterone by vaginal suppository to reduce the incidence of spontaneous preterm birth in women at increased risk: a randomized placebo-controlled double-blind study. Am J Obstet Gynecol 2003;188:419.
56. O'Brien JM, Adair CD, Lewis DF, et al. Progesterone vaginal gel for the reduction of recurrent preterm birth: primary results from a randomized, double-blind, placebo-controlled trial. Ultrasound Obstet Gynecol 2007;30:687.
57. Dodd JM, Jones L, Flenady V, et al. Prenatal administration of progesterone for preventing preterm birth in women considered to be at risk of preterm birth. Cochrane Database Syst Rev 2013;(7):CD004947.
58. Combs CA, Garite T, Maurel K, et al. 17-Hydroxyprogesterone caproate for twin pregnancy: a double-blind, randomized clinical trial. Am J Obstet Gynecol 2011;204:221.e1–8.
59. Rouse DJ, Caritis SN, Peaceman AM, et al. A trial of 17 alpha-hydroxyprogesterone caproate to prevent prematurity in twins. N Engl J Med 2007;357:454–61.
60. Rode L, Klein K, Nicolaides KH, et al. Prevention of preterm delivery in twin gestations (PREDICT): a multicenter, randomized, placebo-controlled trial on the effect of vaginal micronized progesterone. Ultrasound Obstet Gynecol 2011;38:272–80.
61. Norman JE, Mackenzie F, Owen P, et al. Progesterone for the prevention of preterm birth in twin pregnancy (STOPPIT): a randomized, double-blind, placebo-controlled study and meta-analysis. Lancet 2009;373:2034–40.
62. Caritis SN, Rouse DJ, Peaceman AM, et al. Prevention of preterm birth in triplets using 17 alpha-hydroxyprogesterone caproate: a randomized controlled trial. Obstet Gynecol 2009;113:285.
63. Fonseca EB, Celik E, Parra M, et al. Progesterone and the risk of preterm birth among women with a short cervix. N Engl J Med 2007;357:462–9.
64. Hassan SS, Romero R, Vidyadhari D, et al, PREGNANT Trial. Vaginal progesterone reduces the rate of preterm birth in women with a sonographic short cervix: a multicenter, randomized, double-blind, placebo-controlled trial. Ultrasound Obstet Gynecol 2011;38:18.
65. Grobman WA, Thom EA, Spong CY, et al. 17 Alpha-hydroxyprogesterone caproate to prevent prematurity in nulliparas with cervical length less than 30 mm. Am J Obstet Gynecol 2012;207:390.e1.
66. Romero R, Nicolaides K, Conde-Agudelo A, et al. Vaginal progesterone in women with an asymptomatic sonographic short cervix in the midtrimester decreases preterm delivery and neonatal morbidity: a systematic review and metaanalysis of individual patient data. Am J Obstet Gynecol 2012;206:124.e1.
67. Iams JD. Prevention of preterm parturition. N Engl J Med 2014;370:1861.
68. Berghella V, Odibo AO, Tolosa JE. Cerclage for prevention of preterm birth in women with a short cervix found on transvaginal ultrasound examination: randomized controlled trial. Am J Obstet Gynecol 2004;191:1311–7.
69. Berghella V, Rafael T, Szychowski JM, et al. Cerclage for short cervix on ultrasonography in women with singleton gestations and previous preterm birth. Obstet Gynecol 2001;117:663–71.
70. Rust OA, Atlas RO, Reed J, et al. Revisiting the short cervix detected by transvaginal ultrasound in the second trimester: why cerclage therapy may not help. Am J Obstet Gynecol 2001;185:1098–105.

71. Althuisius SM, Dekker GA, Hummel P, et al. Final results of the Cervical Incompetence Prevention Randomized Cerclage Trial (CIPRACT): therapeutic cerclage with bed rest versus bed rest alone. Am J Obstet Gynecol 2001;185: 1106–12.
72. Owen J, Harnkins G, Iams JD, et al. Multicenter randomized trial of cerclage for preterm birth prevention in high-risk women with shortened midtrimester cervical length. Am J Obstet Gynecol 2009;201:375.e1–8.
73. To MS, Alfirevix Z, Heath VC, et al. Cervical cerclage for prevention of preterm delivery in women with short cervix: randomised controlled trial. Lancet 2004; 363:1849–53.
74. Rafael TJ, Mackeen AD, Berghella V. The effect of 17-alpha-hydroxyprogesterone caproate on preterm birth in women with an ultrasound-indicated cerclage. Am J Perinatol 2011;28:389–93.
75. Gyamfi-Bannerman C. The scope of the problem: the epidemiology of late preterm and early-term births. Semin Perinatol 2011;35:246–8.
76. Spong BY, Mercer BM, D'alton M, et al. Timing of indicated late-preterm and early-term birth. Obstet Gynecol 2011;188:323–33.

Challenges and Controversies in Fetal Diagnosis and Treatment
Hypoplastic Left Heart Syndrome

Michele A. Frommelt, MD

KEYWORDS

- Hypoplastic left heart syndrome • Fetal echocardiography
- Fetal aortic valvuloplasty • Norwood operation • Maternal hyperoxygenation

KEY POINTS

- Less than 2 decades ago, hypoplastic left heart syndrome (HLHS) was considered a lethal condition, with most babies dying within days of diagnosis.
- Pediatric cardiologists must be keenly aware of the flaws of staged palliation for the treatment of HLHS.
- Pediatric cardiologists should monitor the emerging data regarding fetal diagnosis and treatment.

INTRODUCTION

During the past 20 years, perhaps no form of congenital heart disease has generated more challenges and controversies than hypoplastic left heart syndrome (HLHS). The surgical approach, initially conceived by William Norwood in the late 1970s, was life-saving, but surgical mortality was high.[1] Rather than abandon the procedure, many centers adopted novel approaches in the management of these patients, resulting in dramatically improved survival (**Fig. 1**).[2–10] Although there is virtually no attrition following the second stage surgical procedure (bidirectional Glenn), the longer-term issues related to Fontan physiology are becoming much more apparent. Morbidities in children with HLHS status post Fontan palliation include exercise intolerance, ventricular dysfunction, progressive tricuspid and neoaortic valve insufficiency, arrhythmias, thromboembolic events, protein-losing enteropathy, plastic bronchitis and hepatic dysfunction, even hepatic carcinoma.[11–23] Of even greater concern is the identification of neurocognitive difficulties in many of these patients, the etiology of

Division of Cardiology, Children's Hospital of Wisconsin, 9000 West Wisconsin Avenue, Milwaukee, WI 53201, USA
E-mail address: mfrommelt@chw.org

Clin Perinatol 41 (2014) 787–798
http://dx.doi.org/10.1016/j.clp.2014.08.004   perinatology.theclinics.com
0095-5108/14/$ – see front matter © 2014 Elsevier Inc. All rights reserved.

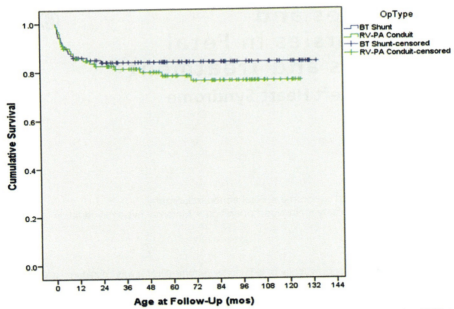

Fig. 1. Actuarial survival, Norwood operation. Children's Hospital of Wisconsin, 2003 to 2013. BT, Blalock-Taussig; RV-PA, right ventricle to pulmonary artery.

which is likely multifactorial.[24–26] Although medical therapy and ventricular assist devices can temper the situation, eventual cardiac replacement therapy for many of these patients seems inevitable. Unfortunately, the risk associated with cardiac transplantation in the Fontan population is high, as patients are frequently listed with significant chronic heart failure symptoms and end organ dysfunction, and there is no consensus on optimal timing of listing.[27–29] Pediatric cardiologists should be keenly aware of the flaws of staged palliation for treatment of HLHS, and need to monitor the emerging data regarding fetal diagnosis and treatment.

ETIOLOGY OF HYPOPLASTIC LEFT HEART SYNDROME

Before the advent of fetal echocardiography, the embryologic cause of HLHS was not entirely clear. However, in 1989 Allan and colleagues[30] observed the in utero evolution of HLHS in a fetus initially diagnosed with critical aortic stenosis. It is now postulated that many cases of HLHS are dynamic and progressive throughout gestation, resulting from altered left ventricular outflow as already described or, less commonly, altered left ventricular inflow (ie, mitral valve stenosis/foramen ovale restriction).[31–33]

In normal fetal circulation, the fetal left ventricle is predominantly filled with oxygenated blood that returns from the placenta and traverses the foramen ovale. If blood flow across the foramen ovale is diminished or reversed, the combined cardiac output is redistributed to the right ventricle and pulmonary artery, resulting in enlargement of the right heart structures and creating less impetus for normal growth of left heart structures. Perhaps the most well-recognized mechanism for decreased flow or reversal of flow through the foramen ovale in utero is the presence of severe aortic valve disease.[34] With significant aortic valve stenosis, alterations in left ventricular compliance occur, either secondary to the development of left ventricular hypertrophy or to the development of left ventricular dilation and dysfunction. Endocardial fibroelastosis, a poorly understood phenomenon whereby the endocardial lining of the left ventricle becomes fibrotic, may also be present. As the disease state progresses, with subsequent elevation in left atrial pressure, flow across the foramen ovale becomes bidirectional and eventually left to right, the result of which may be the cessation of left ventricular growth.

In a classic study by Hornberger and colleagues,[35] the prenatal and postnatal echocardiograms of 21 fetuses with left heart obstructive lesions were reviewed to identify possible prenatal indicators of postnatal disease severity. Prenatal indices that correlated with HLHS at birth included a smaller mitral valve and ascending aorta in the midtrimester, and a decreased rate of growth for all left heart structures. Other prenatal features of postnatal severity included reversal of flow across the foramen ovale and retrograde ductal supply of the distal aortic arch. In a more recent study, Makikallio and colleagues[36] reviewed the natural history of aortic stenosis in 43 fetuses initially referred before 30 weeks' gestation. At the time of the initial examination, the left ventricular to right ventricular length ratio was greater than 0.8:1, and aortic stenosis was the dominant lesion. The presence of moderate left ventricular dysfunction, retrograde transverse aortic arch flow, left-to-right atrial-level shunting, and a monophasic mitral inflow on the initial prenatal echocardiogram were found to be risk factors for the later development of HLHS (**Box 1**).

As more and more cases of "evolving" HLHS were reported, the fetal cardiology community began to consider the potential for intervention. Would it be feasible to perform fetal aortic balloon valvuloplasty at an acceptable risk to the fetus and minimal or no risk to the mother? Would this alter the natural history of HLHS by altering fetal blood flow patterns, potentially allowing for a biventricular circulation at the time of birth?

HYPOPLASTIC LEFT HEART SYNDROME: PRENATAL DIAGNOSIS AND PSYCHOSOCIAL IMPACT

During the past 20 years, advances in ultrasound technology have permitted the early prenatal diagnosis of complex congenital heart disease.[37] HLHS is one of the most common structural lesions diagnosed prenatally, as a screening obstetric ultrasonogram will preferentially identify lesions that dramatically alter the 4-chamber view (**Fig. 2**).[38] In the recent Single Ventricle Reconstruction Trial, which randomized

---

Box 1
Risk factors in hypoplastic left heart syndrome (HLHS)

Fetal risk factors for development of HLHS

1. Retrograde transverse aortic arch flow

2. Left to right foramen ovale flow

3. Monophasic mitral inflow pattern

4. Moderate to severe left ventricular dysfunction

Fetal risk factors predicting unsuccessful fetal aortic valvuloplasty

1. Aortic atresia

2. Left ventricular long-axis z score less than -2

3. Lower left ventricular pressure as estimated by the mitral insufficiency jet

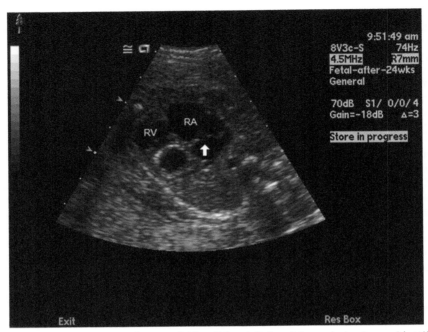

Fig. 2. Screening obstetric ultrasound identifying left heart hypoplasia. Arrow identifies bowing of atrial septum from left to right. RA, right atrium; RV, right ventricle.

patients with HLHS to a modified Blalock-Taussig shunt versus right ventricular to pulmonary artery conduit during stage I palliation (Norwood) procedure, 75% of the patients were diagnosed prenatally.[39] Prenatal diagnosis has resulted in complex decision making before the birth of the baby, ranging from termination of pregnancy to alteration in care and delivery plans, and, in a select few, referral for fetal cardiac intervention.

There is no doubt that the presence of any significant abnormality identified prenatally can result in a variety of emotions including grief, anxiety, and stress.[40,41] In a recent study by Larsson and colleagues,[42] 16 parents (mothers and fathers) were interviewed after their fetus had been diagnosed with an abnormality. Although the initial identification of the anomaly resulted in broken expectations ("You are very sad and shocked in the beginning…because the dream of a perfect child is broken) and anxiety ("I was laying there and becoming more anxious about everything"), parents quickly became involved in change and adaptation. The parents wanted accurate information about the anomaly, without a prolonged delay, and in a suitable environment. In the author's experience, the best way to approach this is the development of a multidisciplinary fetal heart program that includes fetal cardiologists, maternal fetal medicine experts, cardiac surgeons, and, importantly, a dedicated fetal cardiac nurse coordinator (**Box 2**). Having a team immediately available to consult with these families seems to help them cope with what will be a difficult period of time in their life. The dedicated nurse coordinator guides the family through the prenatal experience, fielding any questions or concerns that arise, and coordinating care, which often includes a change in delivery plan. Families are also referred to other parents who have gone through a similar experience, who are therefore able to give them

---

Box 2
Key elements of multidisciplinary fetal cardiac program

Nurse coordinator

24/7 intake; gathering of data; greet and welcome at visit; observation of counseling with all providers; coordination of care and follow-up appointments; tours of cardiac intensive care unit; dedicated follow-up as needed for continued support of family.

Fetal cardiologist

24/7 availability for performance and interpretation of complete fetal echocardiogram; same-day counseling and education in a quiet, suitable environment with the availability of descriptive images and data; knowledge of institutional surgical volume and outcomes; serial echocardiographic follow-up as indicated by heart diagnosis.

Maternal fetal medicine expert

24/7 availability for performance/interpretation of high-risk scan identifying any associated extracardiac anomalies; discussion of genetic screening; assessment of fetal growth and fetal well-being; plans for delivery with discussion of delivery options.

Cardiothoracic surgery

Available for consultation with family during pregnancy to answer any specific surgical questions that the family may have; part of planning for IMPACT (Immediate Postnatal Access to Cardiac Therapy) if necessary.

Additional support

Genetics, neonatology, social work, lactation, child life, interstage home monitoring program, research coordinators, and, if indicated, other pediatric specialties including pediatric surgery.

---

first-hand knowledge of raising a child with HLHS. All of these services provide the reality that their baby does have a chance of a good outcome.

HYPOPLASTIC LEFT HEART SYNDROME: RISK FACTORS FOR ADVERSE OUTCOME

Extracardiac anomalies, including genetic disorders, occur in 15% to 30% of patients with HLHS.[43,44] A few of the identifiable heritable syndromes and genetic disorders associated with HLHS include Kabuki syndrome, Noonan syndrome, trisomy 13, trisomy 18, Turner syndrome, and Jacobsen syndrome. Prenatal detection may affect parental decision making, as it is well known that any additional anomaly will decrease survival after Norwood palliation.[45] To better identify these associated problems, the author recommends a complete fetal ultrasonography examination by maternal fetal medicine colleagues, in addition to a genetics evaluation, again supporting the multidisciplinary team approach (see **Box 2**).

Parents may also have questions regarding surgical volumes and outcomes, as they do have the ability to access this information through many avenues, especially the Internet. Several recent publications suggest that smaller center and surgeon volumes are associated with adverse outcomes in children undergoing a variety of surgical procedures, including the Norwood operation.[46,47] Based on these findings, the investigators postulate that overall outcomes in the United States may be improved through regional collaboration and the development of quality improvement initiatives within and across centers. This notion also raises the controversial question, "Should we have centers of excellence?", an approach taken in some European countries.

Although the operative survival for infants born with HLHS has improved significantly over time, the subgroup of patients with a highly restrictive or intact atrial septum continues to experience a higher mortality.[48,49] These infants can be profoundly cyanotic at the time of delivery and are often unresponsive to medical intervention. Even with prompt resuscitation and adequate decompression of the atrial septum, there is ongoing morbidity and mortality, likely related to secondary anatomic changes in the lung. Some investigators have reported "arterialization" of the pulmonary veins and lymphatic dilation in this setting; others have postulated that there is associated pulmonary artery hypoplasia.[50]

The ability to diagnose a restrictive atrial septal defect before birth allows for more accurate prenatal counseling and planning of immediate postnatal intervention. Theoretically, prenatal catheter intervention in this subgroup of patients may alter the secondary anatomic changes in the lung, possibly improving long-term outcome. For all of these reasons, routine evaluation of the atrial septum should be performed in all fetuses with HLHS. Direct assessment of foramen ovale size has not correlated well with the degree of left atrial hypertension at the time of birth, likely a reflection of the inability to clearly visualize the defect, which often lies more superiorly and posteriorly in the left atrium.[51] Doppler interrogation of the pulmonary veins is technically much simpler, and the pattern of pulmonary venous flow in HLHS has correlated well with left atrial hemodynamics (**Fig. 3**).[52,53] The normal fetal pulmonary vein flow pattern consists of forward flow in systole and diastole, with cessation of flow or a small reversal

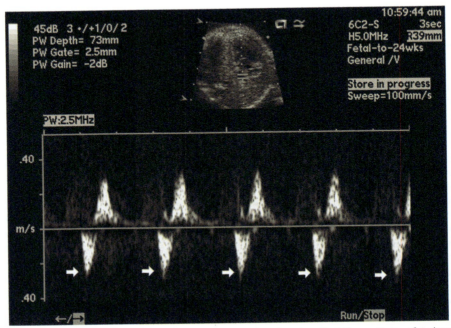

Fig. 3. Doppler interrogation of the pulmonary veins showing that the pattern of pulmonary venous flow in HLHS has correlated well with left atrial hemodynamics. Arrow demonstrates prominent reversal wave in pulmonary veins with atrial contraction.

wave with atrial systole. In a study by Taketazu and colleagues,[51] a pattern of a large reversal wave back into the pulmonary veins was associated with the need for immediate respiratory support and emergent atrial decompression. More specifically, calculation of the forward flow versus reverse flow Doppler derived velocity time integral has also been predictive of the need for immediate neonatal intervention, and should be routinely performed in all fetuses with HLHS.[54]

HYPOPLASTIC LEFT HEART SYNDROME: MANAGEMENT STRATEGIES
Delivery

When babies with HLHS are diagnosed de novo postnatally, they can present in extremis related to ductal closure and low cardiac output. If the atrial septum is restrictive, they can present with severe hypoxemia as well. When there is a prenatal diagnosis of HLHS, the author recommends delivery at the birthing center, so there can be immediate stabilization and initiation of prostaglandin to maintain ductal patency. This approach also allows the family to be in close contact with the physicians taking care of the baby, and allows for maternal bonding. One might expect that the improved preoperative condition of the baby with prenatally diagnosed HLHS would result in improved surgical outcome; however, recent studies suggest otherwise.[54] A retrospective study at the University of California in San Francisco evaluated 81 patients with HLHS who presented to their hospital between 1999 and 2010; more than half of the patients were diagnosed prenatally. Although the postnatally diagnosed patients had increased preoperative acidosis, multiorgan failure, right ventricular dysfunction, and tricuspid insufficiency on presentation, there was no difference in Norwood survival between groups. Long-term follow-up will be important, however, as there is a possibility that neurocognitive outcomes may be worse in those who present with cardiovascular collapse.

Maternal Hyperoxygenation

In the normal fetus, only a small proportion of the fetal cardiac output is directed to the lungs, with most flow directed across the ductus arteriosus to descending aorta. Studies have demonstrated that maternal hyperoxygenation later in pregnancy can increase pulmonary blood flow, and this has been used to assess pulmonary reactivity in fetuses with suspected pulmonary hypoplasia related to diaphragmatic hernia and severe renal disease.[55] In a recent study by Szwast and colleagues,[56] maternal hyperoxygenation was used to assess pulmonary reactivity in fetuses with HLHS and either an open atrial septum or a restrictive/intact atrial septum. The mother was administered 100% oxygen via a nonrebreather face mask for 10 minutes, and fetal Doppler assessment of pulmonary artery flow was measured at baseline, with maternal oxygen, and after recovery. The pulsatility index, a surrogate measure of vascular impedance, was used for assessment of pulmonary blood flow. Maternal hyperoxygenation led to a significant increase in pulmonary blood flow in fetuses with an open atrial septum; however, this was not the case in fetuses with atrial septal restriction that required immediate intervention on the atrial septum at birth. It seems that the fetal response to maternal hyperoxygenation is predictive of the need for urgent intervention at the time of birth, and the use of this diagnostic technique can be very helpful when planning the delivery. In the setting of a fetus with HLHS and restrictive or intact atrial septum and lack of pulmonary reactivity, the author recommends cesarean section in either the delivery room or operating room suite so that there can be Immediate Postnatal Access to Cardiac Therapy (IMPACT procedure), either surgical or interventional. The IMPACT procedure was designed to manage high-risk patients and assemble the multidisciplinary resources required to care for these critically ill neonates in the immediate postpartum period.[49]

Therapeutic use of maternal hyperoxygenation has also been proposed, as there has also been evidence that chronic intermittent maternal hyperoxygenation in late gestation may cause growth of hypoplastic cardiac structures. Thomas Kohl performed repetitive daily maternal hyperoxygenation in 15 pregnant women between 33 and 38 weeks' gestation.[57] The fetal cardiac disease was variable, but 13 of the 15 fetuses had hypoplasia of at least one left heart structure. Kohl demonstrated increases in cardiovascular dimensions (improvements in z scores for gestational age) in most fetuses with small ventricles and no inflow/outflow obstruction. The presence of inflow/outflow tract obstruction or a large ventricular septal defect seemed to ameliorate the effect of hyperoxygenation. Maternal hyperoxygenation is a new and exciting potential therapy in select fetal patients, especially considering its simplicity and universal availability. However, the long-term effects of hyperoxygenation on the fetus remain unknown.

Fetal Catheter Intervention

In 2000, Kohl and colleagues[58] reported the world experience of fetal aortic balloon valvuloplasty. The small early clinical experience (n = 12) was poor, with only 1 "long-term" survivor. However, more encouraging data were recently reported by McElhinney and colleagues[59] from the Children's Hospital of Boston and the Brigham and Women's Hospital. These data included 70 fetuses who underwent attempted aortic valvuloplasty for critical aortic stenosis with evolving HLHS between March 2000 and October 2008. There was a significant improvement in technical success (74%), and most procedures were performed with only percutaneous access (73%). Eight fetuses died in relation to the procedure (11% mortality). Although fetuses with a technically successful valvuloplasty had improved growth of the aortic valve and mitral valve, intervention did not effectively promote left ventricular growth. Therefore, fetuses with a larger left ventricular dimensions initially were more likely to sustain a biventricular circulation at the time of birth (n = 15). Based on these results, the investigators were able to create a multivariable scoring system to improve patient selection. Predictors of an unsuccessful fetal aortic valvuloplasty include the presence of aortic atresia, a left ventricular long axis z score of less than −2, and lower left ventricular pressure as estimated by the mitral insufficiency jet (see **Box 1**).

It is important to bear in mind that most fetuses with critical aortic stenosis will survive gestation. Therefore, fetal cardiac intervention in this setting does not serve as a life-saving procedure, but rather a procedure that may improve postnatal surgical options and outcomes. More specifically, the goal is that successful intervention will lead to a biventricular circulation at the time of birth. There is also an assumption that a biventricular circulation is better than a univentricular circulation. That being said, the possible benefits must be weighed against the risks of the procedure, which include fetal demise or extreme prematurity. One must also consider maternal risk, although no maternal deaths associated with fetal intervention have been reported in the United States. Because the risk/benefit ratio of fetal cardiac intervention in the setting of critical aortic stenosis is still largely unknown, it is not surprising that these procedures are not universally accepted. Some centers have advocated fetal cardiac intervention only when it is considered to be a life-saving procedure, such as in the setting of critical aortic stenosis with hydrops fetalis.

In utero therapy for HLHS with a severely restrictive or intact atrial septum has also been described. Successful decompression of the left atrium in utero may avoid severe hypoxemia at birth, and theoretically may also reduce prenatal lung damage and improve otherwise dismal outcomes. In a recent publication by Marshall and colleagues,[60] technically successful atrial septoplasty was performed in 19 of 21 fetuses between October 2001 and November 2007, with 2 episodes of fetal demise.[59] The investigators determined that creation of a larger defect was associated with better postnatal oxygenation; however, whether this confers a benefit to later survival is presently unknown.

SUMMARY

Less than 2 decades ago HLHS was considered a lethal condition, with most babies dying within days of diagnosis. Today it is estimated that almost 70% of patients with HLHS will survive into adulthood.[61] Despite this advance, there is significant long-term morbidity and mortality in this patient group, and clinicians are continually working to achieve better outcomes. At the same time there has been exciting progress in fetal diagnosis and intervention. Most babies with HLHS can be expected to be identified prenatally, with features likely to lead to a poor outcome able to be recognized, leading to improved counseling. It is now known that in utero dilatation of the aortic valve or atrial septum is technically feasible; however, these procedures require complex choreography, and there needs to be a dedicated team involved. One must bear in mind that 2 lives are at risk, and the safety of the mother is paramount. A salient point is that a biventricular circulation with multiple left-sided lesions has associated chronic morbidity and mortality, and there are essentially no long-term data on patients with a biventricular circulation after fetal intervention.

REFERENCES

1. Norwood WI, Kirkland JK, Sanders SP. Hypoplastic left heart syndrome: experience with palliative surgery. Am J Cardiol 1980;45:87–91.
2. Azakie A, Merklinger SL, McCrindle BW, et al. Evolving strategies and improving outcomes of the modified Norwood procedure: a 10-year single-institution experience. Ann Thorac Surg 2001;72:1349–53.
3. Sano S, Ishino K, Kawada M, et al. Right ventricle-pulmonary artery shunt in first-stage palliation of hypoplastic left heart syndrome. Semin Thorac Cardiovasc Surg Pediatr Card Surg Annu 2004;7:22–31.
4. Pizarro C, Malec E, Maher KO, et al. Right ventricle to pulmonary artery conduit improves outcome after stage I Norwood for hypoplastic left heart syndrome. Circulation 2003;108:II155–60.
5. Tweddell JS, Hoffman GM, Fedderly RT, et al. Phenoxybenzamine improves systemic oxygen delivery after the Norwood procedure. Ann Thorac Surg 1999;67:161–7.
6. Hoffman GM, Ghanayem NS, Kampine JM, et al. Venous saturation and the anaerobic threshold in neonates after the Norwood procedure for hypoplastic left heart syndrome. Ann Thorac Surg 2000;70:1515–20.
7. Tweddell JS, Hoffman GM, Mussatto KA, et al. Improved survival of patients undergoing palliation of hypoplastic left heart syndrome: lessons learned from 115 consecutive patients. Circulation 2002;106:182–9.
8. Tweddell JS, Ghanayem NS, Mussatto KA, et al. Mixed venous oxygen saturation monitoring after stage 1 palliation for hypoplastic left heart syndrome. Ann Thorac Surg 2007;84:1301–11.
9. Hoffman GM, Mussatto KA, Brosig CL, et al. Systemic venous oxygen saturation after the Norwood procedure and childhood neurodevelopmental outcome. J Thorac Cardiovasc Surg 2005;130:1094–100.

10. Tortoriello TA, Stayer SA, Mott AR, et al. A noninvasive estimation of mixed venous oxygen saturation using near-infrared spectroscopy by cerebral oximetry in pediatric cardiac surgery patients. Paediatr Anaesth 2005;15: 495–503.

11. Ranucci M, Isgró G, De La Torre T, et al. Near-infrared spectroscopy correlates with continuous superior vena cava oxygen saturation in pediatric cardiac surgery patients. Paediatr Anaesth 2008;18:1163–9.

12. Ghanayem NS, Hoffman GM, Mussatto KA, et al. Home surveillance program prevents interstage mortality after the Norwood procedure. J Thorac Cardiovasc Surg 2003;126:1367–75.

13. Kugler JD, Beekman Iii RH, Rosenthal GL, et al. Development of a pediatric cardiology quality improvement collaborative: from inception to implementation. From the Joint Council on Congenital Heart Disease Quality Improvement Task Force. Congenit Heart Dis 2009;4:318–28.

14. Anderson PA, Sleeper LA, Mahony L, et al. Contemporary outcomes after the Fontan procedure: a Pediatric Heart Network multicenter study. J Am Coll Cardiol 2008;52:85–98.

15. Shachar G, Fuhrman B, Wang Y, et al. Rest and exercise hemodynamics after the Fontan procedure. Circulation 1982;65:1043–8.

16. Cohen MS, Marino BS, McElhinney DB, et al. Neo-aortic root dilation and valve regurgitation up to 21 years after staged reconstruction for hypoplastic left heart syndrome. J Am Coll Cardiol 2003;42:533–40.

17. Ghaferi AA, Hutchins GM. Progression of liver pathology in patients undergoing the Fontan procedure: chronic passive congestion, cardiac cirrhosis, hepatic adenoma, and hepatocellular carcinoma. J Thorac Cardiovasc Surg 2005; 129:1348–52.

18. Kiesewetter CH, Sheron N, Vettukattill JJ, et al. Hepatic changes in the failing Fontan circulation. Heart 2007;93:579–84.

19. Crupi G, Locatelli G, Tiraboschi R, et al. Protein-losing enteropathy after Fontan operation for tricuspid atresia (imperforate tricuspid valve). Thorac Cardiovasc Surg 1980;28:359–63.

20. Feldt RH, Driscoll DJ, Offord KP, et al. Protein-losing enteropathy after the Fontan operation. J Thorac Cardiovasc Surg 1996;112:672–80.

21. Goo HW, Jhang WK, Kim YH, et al. CT findings of plastic bronchitis in children after a Fontan operation. Pediatr Radiol 2008;38:989–93.

22. Ghai A, Harris L, Harrison DA, et al. Outcomes of late atrial tachyarrhythmias in adults after the Fontan operation. J Am Coll Cardiol 2001;37:585–92.

23. Stephenson EA, Lu M, Berul CI, et al. Arrhythmias in a contemporary Fontan cohort: prevalence and clinical associations in a multicenter cross-sectional study. J Am Coll Cardiol 2010;56:890–6.

24. Mahle WT, Clancy RR, Moss EM, et al. Neurodevelopmental outcome and lifestyle assessment in school-aged and adolescent children with hypoplastic left heart syndrome. Pediatrics 2000;105:1082–9.

25. Goldberg CS, Schwartz EM, Brunberg JA, et al. Neurodevelopmental outcome of patients after the Fontan operation: a comparison between children with hypoplastic left heart syndrome and other functional single ventricle lesions. J Pediatr 2000;137:646–52.

26. Limperopoulos C. Disorders of the fetal circulation and the fetal brain. Clin Perinatol 2009;36:561–77.

27. Gamba A, Merlo M, Fiocchi R, et al. Heart transplantation in patients with previous Fontan operations. J Thorac Cardiovasc Surg 2004;127:555–62.

28. Bernstein D, Naftel D, Chin C, et al. Outcome of listing for cardiac transplantation for failed Fontan: a multi-institutional study. Circulation 2006;114:273–80.
29. Michielon G, Parisi F, Di Carlo D, et al. Orthotopic heart transplantation for failing single ventricle physiology. Eur J Cardiothorac Surg 2003;24:502–10.
30. Allan LD, Sharland GK, Tynan MJ. The natural history of hypoplastic left heart syndrome. Int J Cardiol 1989;25:341–3.
31. Feit LR, Copel JA, Kleinman CS. Foramen ovale size in the normal and abnormal human fetal heart: an indicator of transatrial flow physiology. Ultrasound Obstet Gynecol 1991;1:313–9.
32. Chin AJ, Weinberg PM, Barber G. Subcostal two-dimensional echocardiographic identification of anomalous attachment of septum primum in patients with left atrioventricular valve underdevelopment. J Am Coll Cardiol 1990;15:678–81.
33. Lurie PR. Changing concepts of endocardial fibroelastosis. Cardiol Young 2010; 20:115–23.
34. Danford DA, Cronican P. Hypoplastic left heart syndrome: progression of left ventricular dilation and dysfunction to left ventricular hypoplasia in utero. Am Heart J 1992;123:1712–3.
35. Hornberger LK, Sanders SP, Rein AJ, et al. Left heart obstructive lesions and left ventricular growth in the midtrimester fetus: a longitudinal study. Circulation 1995;92:1531–8.
36. Makikallio K, Levine JC, Marx GR, et al. Fetal aortic valve stenosis and the evolution of hypoplastic left heart syndrome: patient selection for fetal intervention [abstract]. Circulation 2004;110:III690.
37. Allan LD, Crawford DC, Chita SK, et al. Prenatal screening for congenital heart disease. BMJ 1986;292:1717–9.
38. Copel JA, Pilu G, Green J, et al. Fetal echocardiographic screening for congenital heart disease: the importance of the four chamber view. Am J Obstet Gynecol 1987;157(3):648–55.
39. Atz AM, Travison TG, Williams IA, et al. Prenatal diagnosis and risk factors for preoperative death in neonates with single right ventricle and systemic outflow obstruction: screening data from the Pediatric Heart Network Single Ventricle Reconstruction Trial. J Thorac Cardiovasc Surg 2010;140(6):1245–50.
40. Brosig CL, Whitstne BN, Frommelt MA, et al. Psychological distress in parents of children with severe congenital heart disease: the impact of prenatal versus postnatal diagnosis. J Perinatol 2007;27:687–92.
41. Sklansky M, Tang A, Levy D, et al. Maternal psychological impact of fetal echocardiography. J Am Soc Echocardiogr 2002;15:159–66.
42. Larrson AK, Svalenius EC, Lundqvist A, et al. Parents' experiences of an abnormal ultrasound examination – vacillating between emotional confusion and sense of reality. Reprod Health 2010;7:1–10.
43. Ye M, Coldren C, Liang X, et al. Deletion of ETS-1, a gene in the Jacobsen syndrome critical region, causes ventricular septal defects and abnormal ventricular morphology in mice. Hum Mol Genet 2010;19:648–56.
44. Natowicz M, Chatten J, Clancy R, et al. Genetic disorders and major extracardiac anomalies associated with the hypoplastic left heart syndrome. Pediatrics 1988;82:698–706.
45. Stasik CN, Goldberg CS, Bove EL, et al. Current outcomes and risk factors for the Norwood procedure. J Thorac Cardiovasc Surg 2006;131:412–7.
46. Hornik CP, He X, Jacobs JP, et al. Relative impact of surgeon and center volume on early mortality after the Norwood procedure. Ann Thorac Surg 2012;93(6): 1992–7.

47. Checchia PA, McCollegan J, Daher N, et al. The effect of surgical case volume on outcome after the Norwood procedure. J Thorac Cardiovasc Surg 2005; 129(4):754–9.
48. Vlahos AP, Lock JE, McElhinney DB, et al. Hypoplastic left heart syndrome with intact or highly restrictive atrial septum: outcome after neonatal transcatheter atrial septostomy. Circulation 2004;109:2326–30.
49. Glatz JA, Gaynor JW, Rome JJ, et al. Hypoplastic left heart syndrome with atrial level restriction in the era of prenatal diagnosis. Ann Thorac Surg 2007;84(5): 1633–8.
50. Rychik J, Rome JJ, Collins MH, et al. The hypoplastic left heart syndrome with intact atrial septum: atrial morphology, pulmonary vascular histopathology and outcome. J Am Coll Cardiol 1999;34:554–60.
51. Taketazu M, Barrea C, Smallhorn JF, et al. Intrauterine pulmonary venous flow and restrictive foramen ovale in fetal hypoplastic left heart syndrome. J Am Coll Cardiol 2004;43:1902–7.
52. Better DJ, Apfel HD, Zidere V, et al. Pattern of pulmonary venous blood flow in the hypoplastic left heart syndrome in the fetus. Heart 1999;81:646–9.
53. Michelfelder E, Gomez C, Border W, et al. Predictive value of fetal pulmonary venous flow patterns in identifying the need for atrial septoplasty in the newborn with hypoplastic left ventricle. Circulation 2005;112(19):2974–9.
54. Kipps AK, Feuille C, Azakie A, et al. Prenatal diagnosis of hypoplastic left heart syndrome in current era. Am J Cardiol 2011;108(3):421–7.
55. Broth RE, Wood DC, Rasanen J, et al. Prenatal prediction of lethal pulmonary hypoplasia: the hyperoxygenation test for pulmonary artery reactivity. Am J Obstet Gynecol 2002;187:940–5.
56. Szwast A, Tian Z, McCann M, et al. Vasoreactive response to maternal hyperoxygenation in the fetus with hypoplastic left heart syndrome. Circ Cardiovasc Imaging 2010;3(2):172–8.
57. Kohl T. Chronic intermittent materno-fetal hyperoxygenation in late gestation may improve on hypoplastic cardiovascular structures associated with cardiac malformations in human fetuses. Pediatr Cardiol 2010;31:250–63.
58. Kohl T, Sharland G, Allan LD, et al. World experience of percutaneous ultrasound-guided balloon valvuloplasty in human fetuses with severe aortic valve obstruction. Am J Cardiol 2000;85:1230–3.
59. McElhinney DB, Marshall AC, Wilkins-Haug LE, et al. Predictors of technical success and postnatal biventricular outcome after in utero aortic valvuloplasty for aortic stenosis with evolving hypoplastic left heart syndrome. Circulation 2009;120:1482–90.
60. Marshall A, Levine J, Morash D, et al. Results of in utero atrial septoplasty in fetuses with hypoplastic left heart syndrome. Prenat Diagn 2008;28:1023–8.
61. Feinstein JA, Benson DW, Dubin AM, et al. Hypoplastic left heart syndrome: current considerations and expectations. J Am Coll Cardiol 2012;59(Suppl 1): S1–42.

Borderline Viability

Controversies in Caring for the Extremely Premature Infant

Steven R. Leuthner, MD, MA

KEYWORDS

- Extreme prematurity • Periviable • Viability • Ethics • Decision-making

KEY POINTS

- There is general consensus regarding threshold levels that describe the gray zone on the limits of viability, and gestational age alone should not be used solely in making a decision.
- There is no evidence to support a mandate on a trial of assessment and treatment in the gray zone, although it is permissible to take this approach with family agreement.
- Supporting parental decision-making in the gray zone before delivery and afterward in the NICU is ethically permissible and is the ideal.

INTRODUCTION

Controversy surrounding the decision to resuscitate at the limits or borderline of viability has been at the center of neonatal ethical debate for decades. This debate has led to numerous reports, from individual institutions, councils, and advisory committees, that all have remarkable consistency in the development of gestational age-based guidelines.[1–18] The consensus based on outcome data has led to recommendations and common practice of two threshold levels of care: a lower threshold of no resuscitation (<22 weeks), and an upper threshold of obligatory resuscitation (25 weeks). The 22- to 24-week range then becomes the gray zone. Although there are differing caveats among the guidelines regarding physician assessments or strength of recommendations from the ethical perspective, the gray zone has become the gestational age spectrum in which resuscitation is based on parental choice. The outer thresholds represent limits on parental authority to make a decision. The underlying goal in any of these guidelines is to limit overtreat and undertreat of the neonate, to support parents, yet rely on a best interest standard for the neonate. Decisions are centered on the dilemma that withholding resuscitation leads to certain death, yet resuscitation leads to an uncertain future with the possibilities ranging from death to

No conflicts of interest to disclose.
Medical College of Wisconsin, 999 North 92nd Street, Suite C410, Wauwatosa, WI 53226, USA
E-mail address: sleuthne@mcw.edu

Clin Perinatol 41 (2014) 799–814
http://dx.doi.org/10.1016/j.clp.2014.08.005
0095-5108/14/$ – see front matter © 2014 Elsevier Inc. All rights reserved.

considerable medical, emotional, societal, and financial risk to normal life. After decades of debate and reasonably consistent consensus statements regarding resuscitation, what if any are the remaining controversies?

Some might see controversy at the larger social or policy level, such as concerns of legal or regulatory conflicts with the guidelines, or suggestions that the guidelines as a whole are discriminatory. For most, however, controversy arises at an individual case-by-case perspective with disagreement on what is actually best for a particular neonate. This is often portrayed as a conflict between parental autonomy and the child's best interest.

This article reviews legal or regulatory concerns that may contradict ethical discussion and guidelines, discriminatory and scientific basis concerns with consensus guidelines, and personal controversy about how to determine best interest, and suggests that guidelines are a reasonable place to start in helping determine parental authority and autonomy. It also addresses controversies raised in counseling and costs.

LEGAL CONFLICT WITH GUIDELINES?

It is rare that when physicians and family agree on a plan there are any legal ramifications. Although it is beyond the scope of this article to review in detail the pertinent legal cases that might have an impact on this issue, there are at least four cases that deserve mention. One case is that of a father who withdrew support on his 26-week gestation infant after he was resuscitated against parental wishes. The father was acquitted of wrong-doing.[19] A second case involved a physician who started resuscitation per parental wishes, but stopped when the infant was not responding. The physician was accused of failure to provide full resuscitation and violating informed consent. He was acquitted.[20] Then there were two cases in which physicians unilaterally resuscitated the baby, one against parental wishes because of institutional pressure, and the other with later claims of violating informed consent.[21,22] In both cases parties were acquitted. The pattern in each of these cases is that of unilateral decision-making. Yet despite contradictory outcomes (two survived with some neurodevelopment impairment (NDI), and two died), all defendants were acquitted. Perhaps the message is the courts do not want to lay blame in these difficult situations, at least after they occur.

Despite the results of these individual legal cases, there is potential danger in the stacking of some federal regulations, namely the Born-Alive law, Emergency Medical Treatment & Labor Act (EMTALA), and CAPTA (Child Abuse Prevention and Treatment Act), that could lead to mandated emergency medical treatment.[23] The law has supported the idea that the periviable birth is an emergency.[21,22,24] The labor and delivery unit could be held to the same EMTALA requirements as an emergency room.[24] EMTALA makes no claim that resuscitation is necessary, only that there should be a screening examination. It does not define what that assessment entails, nor does it argue for mandated treatment.[24] A Texas case raised the question of whether a periviable birth should be considered an emergency exception to informed consent.[21] Some authors and even some of the guidelines seem to agree with this line of reasoning by leaving open the possibility of changing perinatal decisions after birth.[2,3,9,25] The stacking of some case law and federal regulations can lead to the claim that all infants should be given a trial of assessment and treatment.[23,25]

ARGUMENT 1 AGAINST GUIDELINES: A TRIAL OF ASSESSMENT AND TREATMENT FOR ALL

The emergency claim that would require a trial of assessment and treatment of all periviable newborns is based on four premises[25]: (1) assessment of gestational age after birth is more accurate; (2) assessment of vigorousness adds prognostic information; (3) testing treatment responses in first hours to days provides more facts or certainty to help determine long-term prognosis and therefore decreases speculation; and (4) treatment withdrawal is ethically equivalent to withholding, from the parents' perspective. Are these four premises all true for all cases at the limits of viability? If not, a mandate is not justified.

RESPONSE TO MANDATORY TRIAL OF ASSESSMENT AND TREATMENT
Premise 1: Assessment of Gestational Age After Birth Is Most Accurate

The argument for mandating a neonatal assessment of gestational age at delivery is essentially based on a belief in the uncertainty of gestational age measurements. Proponents argue that, although there can be some discussion and advanced care planning with prospective parents on their wishes, decisions should be contingent on the neonatologist's assessment at birth in the delivery room.[2–4,9] The argument is that estimates of gestational age can vary, sometimes up to 1 to 2 weeks gestation, which leads to uncertainty, and therefore may not be reliable for prognostication. This has important implications, especially if the range of accuracy can place a newborn at either end of the guideline thresholds.

There are, however, more and less accurate assessment tools (**Fig. 1**). There is evidence supporting that obstetric modalities of dating are superior to a well-trained neonatal clinician's assessment of gestational age by examination.[26–30] In fact, research on accuracy of the Ballard examination revealed that clinicians overestimated gestational age by 2 weeks, with a range of ±4 weeks.[29] This is evidence

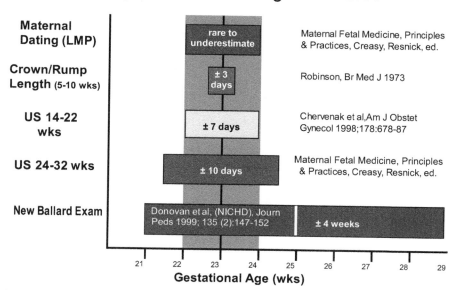

Fig. 1. Accuracy of gestational age assessment tools. Accuracy measurements of different gestational age assessment tools within the gray zone of borderline viability, assuming 23 weeks gestational age, graph demonstrates potential range of error in measurements. US, ultrasound; LMP, last menstrual period.

that the neonatal examination is the least accurate assessment, and should never override obstetric dating. Also, although obstetric dating has its level of uncertainty, it must be acknowledged that the epidemiologic outcome data used in developing existing consensus guidelines are based on similar uncertainties, and thus they remain applicable.[18] Finally, the most recent guidelines now acknowledge one should not look at gestational age alone, but take into account other factors that help predict outcome (weight, gender, singleton, steroids).[31] The fact remains that gestational age, albeit not solely, is still a factor in outcome predictions, and the most accurate measurement available should be used in discussions and decision-making. The only time this should be the neonatal examination is when there is no prenatal information available, thus making it a real emergency.

Premise 2: Assessment of Vigorousness Adds Prognostic Information and Therefore Decreases Uncertainty

Although it seems natural to assume that the more vigorous-looking preterm may be more mature acting and therefore do better, the data again do not support this premise. Using Apgar scores as a marker of vigorousness, neither the 1- nor 5-minute Apgar score can help predict survival or survival with or without morbidities.[32–34]

Premise 3: Testing Treatment Responses in First Hours to Days Provides More Facts or Certainty to Help Determine Long-Term Prognosis and Therefore Decreases Speculation

What responses in this time frame provide factual versus speculative predictions? Although there are some infants who are too immature to even survive this short period of time, the ability to support and keep alive babies for longer and longer time has certainly improved to the point that the average time to death has increased from 4 days to now weeks.[31,35–37] Certainly a grade 3 to 4 intraventricular hemorrhage increases risk, but the significance and certainty of any neurologic prediction remain speculative. At the same time one-third of infants with a normal head ultrasound at 1 week develop significant neurologic handicaps.[38] Physiologic response in these first days provides no prediction of other illnesses, such as necrotizing enterocolitis, bronchopulmonary dysplasia, patent ductus arteriosus, iatrogenic infection, and retinopathy of prematurity, which are also associated with significant NDI, and late death. Physiologic stability based on serial assessments for an individual infant are imperfect to begin with and grow less accurate each day.[39] Incorporating intuitions of "die before neonatal intensive care unit (NICU) discharge" and head ultrasound does improve prognostication. A child who has even a single day of corroborated prediction of "die before NICU discharge" and any degree of head ultrasound abnormality (grade 2 or worse) has only a 4% of being alive without NDI at 2 years.[40] This would require NICU teams to begin the practice of predicting death before discharge more routinely in their rounds. Although some facts may emerge, uncertainty remains, and so prognosis remains speculative.

Premise 4: Treatment Withdrawal Is Ethically Equivalent to Withholding (From the Parents' Perspective)

The equivalence of withdrawing and withholding life-sustaining medical treatment is well supported in ethics and the law.[41–47] To provide a trial of therapy with the option of withdrawal should the prognostication become worse is a reasonable and permissible process to undertake. Despite the ethical and legal support, however, data suggest that even physicians find it more difficult to withdraw than to withhold.[48,49] This should be reason enough to accept that at least some parents may psychologically feel different about choosing to withhold versus withdraw. Whether this feeling is based on a sense of moral responsibility about a more deliberate act (killing vs letting die), remaining uncertainty or disbelief in prognostication, or the commitment of time and effort they have already been through with the baby is not clear. What is clear is that all parents who can come to the decision to withdraw find it extremely difficult, and that not all parents may be able to come to this decision.

PRETERM BIRTH CAN BE BUT IS MOST OFTEN NOT AN EMERGENCY SITUATION

The science and ethics support that there are factual problems with each premise of emergency trial of assessment and treatment mandate. What is distinctively different in the perinatal care environment is that in most cases there are reasonable and accurate data on the fetus (gestational age, sex, weight, maternal steroids) that can help with prognosis, and time to counsel families about these issues before initiation. Perinatal data from surveys that include births at the margin of viability suggest that up to two-thirds of such pregnancies have complications that would bring the mother to the attention of the obstetrician days or weeks before delivery.[50] Only a small minority of births at the margins of viability occur so precipitously that there are insufficient data or time. Prenatal prognostication and decision-making, although not perfect, are not based on ignorance. Because there have been no legal cases against physicians and parents who collaborate in these decisions, the legal concerns should be minimal.

The consensus guidelines suggest that if the situation is emergent because facts are not known or there is no time to talk, one should resuscitate first, evaluate, and talk later. The medical team needs to start treatment if they are ever going to be able to have the conversation about family values and wishes. Finally, even though there is no medical evidence to support a mandate on a trial of assessment and treatment in the gray area, it does not mean a family cannot be supported in this decision (discussed later).

ARGUMENT 2 AGAINST GUIDELINES: THEY ARE DISCRIMINATORY AND LACK ETHICAL AND SCIENTIFIC BASIS

Several authors have challenged the ethical and scientific basis for setting up these thresholds, claiming they set up too simple of rules for a complicated ethical decision.[51–55] They argue that preterm infants seem to have a different moral status than everyone else. There are few to no other policy statements in the literature regarding resuscitation from an age perspective for any other life-threatening situation (eg, head trauma, near-drowning, meningitis, stroke, or burns).[52] Survey literature has shown that despite similar outcome data, preterm infants are less likely to be resuscitated than older children and adults, and the authors argue that the best-interest standard is not applied to these infants.[56] This raises concern of discrimination or gestational ageism.[18]

Ageism Within and at the Border of the Gray Zone

Meadow suggests that there is some level of ageism even within the gray zone. There are four possible outcomes for the borderline viable preterm infant: (1) palliative comfort care leading to death; (2) resuscitation and NICU intervention, but the infant dies anyway; (3) resuscitation and NICU intervention with survival but significant NDI; and (4) resuscitation and NICU intervention with eventual discharge and no significant NDI.[57,58]

Most clinicians would like to avoid numbers 2 and 3. For some parents, however, having an infant in group 2 is not necessarily the worst thing. For these parents, "giving your baby a chance," even if he or she dies, is sad but may not be worse than the alternative of not trying at all. For these parents, the worst outcome is group 3. He rightly states that for this scenario, there is a different calculation that should come into play during antenatal counseling: the proportion of NICU survivors (not all births) who survive without NDI. Although the traditional outcomes of survival and intact survival combined are steeply dependent on gestational age, the percentage of NICU survivors who are free of NDI is flat over the 22- to 25-week gestational range at approximately 50%.[57,58] If this is true, then why do some neonatologists and guidelines declare treatment as obligatory at 25 weeks, yet permissible or not at 23 weeks? Why should the parent of a 23-week gestation infant have the choice of resuscitation or not, yet the parent of the 25-week infant may not? There seems to be discrimination against the 23-week infant.

Response to Ageism

Responses to ageism could go in one of two directions. First, assume all these 23- to 25-week infants should be treated equally and with consistency. This would require changes in current medical practice. There are two ways there could be more consistency. Either there should be a mandated trial of assessment and treatment for all preterm infants in the gray zone, or parents should have a choice on whether they want a trial of assessment and treatment or palliative care. If there is a mandate, this essentially eliminates any upper threshold of any consensus guideline. If one allows a trial based on parental choice, the upper threshold might have to be raised for consistency.[5]

When comparing the neonate with the older patient, it is argued one is undervaluing the preterm infant. However, one could turn it around and suggest that parental permissibility is the correct ethical way, and perhaps could be a model for the older population. The second direction to take is to explore whether there are differences between the preterm infant within the gray zone and with older patients that justify a different approach.

Wilkinson[18] suggests there are three potential reasons for a justified difference. First, there is the possibility of greater harm or burden of treatment. In the short term, these infants require 3 to 4 months in the hospital, with many requiring 10 to 16 painful or stressful procedures a day.[59] He makes an argument that for a newborn a "keep alive" mistake is potentially worse than a "let die" mistake.[60] His claim is that death for a newborn is not as bad a death as for an older child because they have not established relationships, nor developed preferences, plans, or hopes. It deprives them of their future life, but they will not be aware to regret it. What is bad is the absence of experience rather than the experience of a negative. A "keep alive" mistake is potentially worse because if it is a life not worth living it is a net burden and caused greater harm.[60]

A second difference is that typically there is time and opportunity for counseling and discussions in advance that may not be there for the comparative scenarios of the older patient suggested in the literature.[52] Perhaps the neonatal community is ahead of its time, and other groups could consider whether they would want to create consensus guidelines, but again most of these might be on withdrawal based on prognosis, unless nonemergent situations.

Third, perhaps there is a difference in how one makes a best interest judgment for the preterm versus the older patient. Although for some parents the calculus and value of outcome that Meadow presents might be true, there are others who might believe that NICU care and death is a bad outcome they would like to prevent their child from experiencing. Wilkinson[60] claims parents have a weightier role based on their own interests.

ARGUMENT 3: DOCTOR KNOWS BEST

Often the real moral controversies come up on a case-by-case basis at the borderline viable newborn. Batton[51] acknowledged the difficulty for the American Academy of Pediatrics (AAP) Committee on Fetus and Newborn in formulating guidelines because of individual personal convictions. The goal in this article cannot be to change anyone's mind. However, thinking about constructs of pediatric surrogate decision-making, and recognition of conflicting interests and uncertainties, might help physicians become more comfortable in being tolerant and flexible within the guidelines.

BEST INTEREST

All consensus statements, and all those who have concerns about those consensus statements, would likely agree that the goal of neonatal medicine is to minimize undertreatment and overtreatment of the extremely premature infant. All advocate that the decision-making process ought to be based on the concept of the infant's best interest. The best interest standard, theoretically a beneficence-based decision for the patient whose wishes are unknowable, is the core ethical principle in neonatal surrogate decision-making. Because the newborn is immature and vulnerable, an adult is to make decisions on behalf of it. It is considered the right and responsibility of the parents to be the ones to make these best interest decisions.[46,61] However, there are limitations placed on parental authority based on the idea that children need to be protected from unwise parental decisions, such as in cases of abuse or neglect. Controversy arises when parents and health care staff might view a child's best interests differently, often based on their own model or interpretation of what is best.[62] The argument often becomes circular. Although the concept of parental autonomy and parental permission suggests the parents, based on their values, are the ones to weigh the benefits and burdens of medical therapy for their child in determining what is best, there are times parental autonomy can be overridden.

Although best interest is central to the ethical language in neonatology, there are those who argue it is incoherent, unrealistic, unknowable, or overly individualistic.[63,64] On the one hand the principle is meant to be objective. One is to ignore or negate all other interests except that of the infant's self-regarding interest. In doing this, however, one has a tendency to pit the parental and family interests against the infant's interest as if they are not interrelated. If, on the other hand, one is to allow parental and family interests and values to define best interest, then it seems subjective. Finally, there are provider interests that must be acknowledged in neonatal care, such as personal ego, program development, or financial payment.

Others argue best interest is a pragmatic standard of reasonableness.[65] If one thinks of best interest as a simple narrow concept on how to make decisions for any incompetent patient it becomes too restrictive. Instead, if one understands best interest as a construct of action-guiding principles, it can be helpful. What the words or construct of best interest should do is make medical professionals think.[66] Medical experts have the expertise on disease processes and data. They need to acknowledge that parental values provide the meaning to that prognosis.[62] "The best interest principle is to serve as a regulative ideal, not as a strict and literal requirement, because parents' obligations toward their other children as well as their own legitimate self-interests can conflict with doing what maximizes the child's well-being, and sometimes takes precedence over it."[67]

CONSTRAINED PARENTAL AUTONOMY

Another construct for pediatric decision-making is that of constrained parental autonomy.[64] In this construct, the infant's interests are not taken in isolation, but within the framework of an intimate family. If the self-regarding interests of a child conflict with the family goals or interests, the parents may compromise the interests of the child, as long as it is not sacrificing the child's basic needs. The constraining of parental autonomy is based on respect for persons. Respect is (1) owed to all individuals based on the individual's personhood; (2) is owed proportionate to actualized capacities and potential: and (3) varies depending on the relationship. This construct permits wide parental autonomy and respects the freedom of parents to balance competing claims of family members, provided that each has basic needs met. This rings true in everyday parenting as limits are set, and sacrifices are asked, of children and parents every day.

UNCERTAINTY AND HARM

When making a decision for an extremely preterm infant there are actually many levels of uncertainty.[60] On one level there is medical prognostic uncertainty. What complicates predictions includes variations in an individual's genetic or physical susceptibilities, their psychological ability to cope with the physical, neuroplasticity, and the environment. These help determine experiential uncertainty; how happy or unhappy will the survivor be, how difficult will they find their outcome, how much pain will they experience? This is why for some significant NDI is tolerable and for others mild cerebral palsy or attention-deficit issues may seem insurmountable.[52] Finally, there is moral uncertainty; what ought we to do, what ethical framework or rules should we apply, or how do we weigh values to consider what is right or wrong to do, and what risks do we take?

One of the problems with any advancing technology is that the vector of technical success may not necessarily be in sync with the vector of outcomes valued. Except for the rare, true biologic vitalist, most would agree with the premise that death can be preferable to a life with severe, intolerable deficits.[68] In other words, there is a life not worth living because the current and future burdens for the individual outweigh the future benefits.[69] As neonatal care pushes the limits of viability, infants who would have died now survive, many with significant NDI, and those that would have survived with significant NDI are now surviving with moderate to little NDI. Yet the value ordering is that in some cases death may be preferable. The uncertainties in this model include (1) what is the definition of intolerable deficits (experiential uncertainty), (2) at the time of intervention it is not known whether the baby has been benefited or harmed (prognostic uncertainty), and (3) it is not clear how to judge what ratio between the best and worst outcome (9:1 vs 2:8) is acceptable. In the end, who decides what risk to take for an individual infant (moral uncertainty)?[60,68]

If one accepts that the preterm infant's interests are intertwined with the potentially competing family interests, there are added uncertainties. Although there are stories of how the surviving infant has enriched the family experience, there are costs to families of a surviving infant with significant NDI. For prospective parents these might include a higher divorce rate; higher rates of psychological or physical health issues; and increasing care needs leading to parents being unable to work or work fewer hours, which leads to lower income. At the same time, the costs of an impaired newborn are estimated at more than three times that of a nonimpaired child.[60,70] Siblings lives can be enriched by greater psychological maturation, empathy, and appreciation, or they can develop depression, loneliness, anxiety, and have lower self-esteem and social functioning.[60]

Thinking more about the models of surrogate decision-making and the different levels and forms of uncertainty can help the individual physician in dealing with their opinions and concerns about these vulnerable infants and families. When facing uncertainty in clinical situations, the clinician must form a partnership with their patient and the parent; explore values to negotiate the meaning of a prognosis, incorporating the objective and subjective components of best interest; and weigh competing interests.[62,64,69] Sometimes a truly best or right decision might be unknowable. Instead, when dealing with hard choices the notion of "satisficing," that is to satisfy to some extent and suffice, given the constraints on the decision-making process might be the best that can be done ethically.[71] By adopting an approach that accepts the finite limits of what can be known at any given moment, uncertainty is less formidable.

DEBATE ABOUT COUNSELING

NICUs have moved toward the concept of family-centered care. Much of this was in response to parent advocates voicing concerns about families being at the mercy of accelerated technology. Although it is easy at some level to think about family-centered care as supporting parental involvement through education and understanding of their infant and child, it's basis was about being involved in decision-making.[72,73] It seems the acceptance of the concept of family-centered care, combined with the acceptance that clinicians should counsel about outcomes in these scenarios, is secondary to the underlying assumption that parents actually do need to participate in decision-making, which means parents should have a choice. Again, where is the controversy?

I defer to the article on informing and educating parents about the risks and outcomes of prematurity elsewhere in this issue by Kim and Basir. It is worth mentioning, however, that there is some discussion, if not debate, about what counseling should entail. The AAP provides guidance in suggesting the prospective parents receive detailed information on range of survival rates and of the types and rates of short- and long-term disabilities that can be expected, and the treatments necessary to achieve this.[10] There are those who are concerned about the AAP's recommended approach. They argue that people do not understand statistics and percentages or groups, there is a well-known "framing effect," that informed consent discussions in stressful situations are not well remembered, and that emotions play a significant role in decision-making.[74,75]

Decision analysis shows that two things are required to make decisions about patient care: probability (P) and utility (value).[76] Properly defined values help dictate the necessary accuracy of probability estimates needed for making diagnoses, prognoses, and treatment decisions. (How certain does our diagnosis have to be before we decide to act?) The decision to resuscitate is said to be sensitive to the probability of handicap, so the use of accurate probability estimates is imperative. Assigning different values to the same set of outcome probabilities can result in different decisions. The decision to resuscitate is sensitive to the values-assigned outcomes. Evidence-based medicine experts point out that values are important because individuals present with subjective outcome descriptions (or their own set of values) to outcomes. Helping parents explore and in some way assign values is essential to practicing evidence-based medicine. This is consistent with the negotiated model of best interest.[62]

There is evidence about what parental values versus physician or health care team values might be. There are detailed and rigorous assessments of health status, health utilities, and health-related quality of life for premature infants.[77–80] These studies reveal that many parents adapt and judge their child's quality of life to be good. At the same time, however, there are concerns raised regarding quality of life studies in general.[60,81] These might include a reporting bias, where only the healthier patients who can report actually do, whereas the more ill survivors either have died or are so low in functioning they cannot participate. Parents may rate the child's quality of life more positively as a defense mechanism to avoid cognitive dissonance.[82]

Knowing many of those involved in the debate, it is not clear to me that there is much controversy. Most, if not all, agree and recommend framing the data in the positive and negative way. Most, if not all, acknowledge that comprehension of some short- and long-term outcomes is only part of the story. Most, if not all, acknowledge that an important part of counseling is not only giving the data as best can be done, but also includes listening to hopes and goals the parents have for their child, exploring values to add meaning to a probability outcome. This means more than accepting the simple goal of "doing everything," hoping their child can survive without suffering and get through it all without deficits. It is also the beginning of an exploration of possible thresholds of what a parent might consider success, or a life worth living. For many, the 50% chance at survival and then a 50% chance of being "OK" is worth a trial of therapy, but counseling must move beyond this. There is a need to develop a trusting relationship of mutual respect, one where clinicians can openly hear from parents their values, their hopes, and their thresholds. Only then can clinicians also respectfully help guide them in decision-making for resuscitation, but also on level of care once in the NICU, including the possibility of withdrawal of support.

DEBATE ABOUT COST

The issue of cost often arises during discussions regarding the resuscitation of the borderline viable infant. Writings on the ethics of extreme prematurity frame this as a complex issue of balancing interests of infants, parents, professionals, and society. The United Kingdom's Nuffield Council on Bioethics states "There is now much broader public awareness of the need for difficult choices to be made by the providers of national healthcare... Contentiously, this has caused questioning of whether funds spent on resuscitating or prolonging the life of babies where the prognosis is very poor are spent appropriately."[6]

What are some facts about NICU cost? Direct costs of NICUs are in the billions of dollars range. In 2004 it was estimated at $21 billion.[20] NICUs are often profit centers for hospitals and departments of pediatrics in academic centers.[20] This has led to the high number of neonatologists per live birth in the United States compared with other countries.[20] Within the NICU costs increase with decreasing gestational age and birthweight, with approximately 7% of cases accounting for 90% of the total costs.[83]

Despite these costs, there are arguments that a policy to limit neonatal care to this population saves little costs, whereas lives will be lost.[84] When compared with medical ICUs, neonatal treatment and care is more cost-effective because those who die do so early, therefore 90% of the costs are spent on survivors.[85] Thus, why pick on the premie? Rationing should be done elsewhere.

In response to this, others share some concerns. First, as medical treatments are getting better, and some of the dying infants are living longer, efficiency may be getting less.[86] Second, Medicaid and other community resources are almost never limited to what is spent in the NICU.[6,86,87] Economic studies of this population have difficulty in measuring post-NICU costs, for example, of day-care services, respite care, schools, voluntary organizations, and families as a result of modifications of their everyday activities.[6] An EPICure study that looked at spending in hospital inpatient, outpatient, community health, drugs, education, additional family expenses, and indirect costs over 12 months at age 6, reported a range of two to six times the cost for extremely low-birth-weight children compared with a control group of term infants.[88]

Finally, the claim that rationing certain levels of care in the NICU would save fewer dollars than rationing in other areas of medicine is not a reason to spend resources disproportionately in the NICU. Camosy[86] argues that a person's dignity is not violated by refusing him or her a disproportionately large share of community resources, but giving someone just such a share does violate the right to equal treatment of those left with a disproportionately small share. Perhaps just as in the development of guidelines, the NICU can be a leader, encouraging a more just medical service.

SUMMARY

Although there continues to be ethical discussion about extremely premature infants, it is not clear there are many hotly debated controversies. There is a broad consensus on guidelines that are available as just that, guidelines. There are excellent conversations in the literature about counseling and how it can be improved, in how to provide data, and how to assess values. The real controversies regarding the borderline viable neonate are when an individual physician may disagree with the consensus or the parent. However, understanding the concepts of a negotiated model of best interest or constrained parental autonomy, along with an acceptance of the medical, experiential, and moral uncertainties on a case-by-case basis perhaps can help each participant be more comfortable.

Guidelines can be helpful as a framework and a starting place, but also have their limitations.[89] "It is tough to have a single guiding principle when (i) you are not sure what is actually in the patient's best interest and (ii) any decision you make has negative consequences for somebody else's interests. The hard cases are those where ethical principles come into conflict – when 'best interests' bangs up against 'do no harm'; when 'respect for autonomy' is challenged by 'medical professionalism'. Then, concern for the 'best interests of the child' may need to be tempered by other legitimate ethical claims. The child's interests come first, but when it is unclear what is in the child's interest, then we must consider the interests of parents, siblings, doctors, nurses and even of society."[90]

REFERENCES

1. Allen MC, Donohue PK, Dusman AE. The limit of viability: neonatal outcome of infants born at 22 to 25 weeks' gestation. N Engl J Med 1993;329:1597–601.
2. Hack M, Fanaroff AA. Outcomes of extremely immature infants - a perinatal dilemma. N Engl J Med 1993;329:1649–50.
3. Yellin PB, Fleischman AR. DNR in the DR? J Perinatol 1995;15:232–6.
4. Pinkerton JV, Finnerty JJ, Lombardo PA, et al. Parental rights at the birth of a near-viable infant: conflicting perspectives. Am J Obstet Gynecol 1997;177:283–90.
5. Kaempf JW, Tomlinson M, Arduza C, et al. Medical staff guidelines for periviability pregnancy counseling and medical treatment of extremely premature infants. Pediatrics 2006;117(1):22–9.
6. Nuffield Council on Bioethics. Critical care and decisions in fetal and neonatal medicine: ethical issues. London: Nuffield Council on Bioethics; 2006. Available at: www.nuffieldbioethics.org/go/ourwork/neonatal/introduction.
7. Wilkinson AR, Ahluwalia J, Cole A, et al. Management of babies born extremely preterm at less than 26 weeks of gestation: a framework for clinical practice at the time of birth. Arch Dis Child Fetal Neonatal Ed 2009;94(1):f2–5.

8. Jeffries AL, Kirpalani HM, Canadian Paediatric Society Fetus and Newborn Committee. Counselling and management for anticipated extremely preterm birth. Paediatr Child Health 2012;17(8):443. Available at: www.cps.ca/en.
9. Kattwinkel J, Perlman JM, Aziz K, et al, American Heart Association. Neonatal resuscitation: 2010 American Heart Association guidelines for cardiopulmonary resuscitation and emergency cardiovascular care. Pediatrics 2010;126(5): e1400–13.
10. MacDonald H, American Academy of Pediatrics, Committee on Fetus and Newborn. Perinatal care at the threshold of viability. Pediatrics 2002;110(5): 1024–7.
11. Verloove-Vanhorick SP. Management of the neonate at the limits of viability: the Dutch viewpoint. BJOG 2006;113(Suppl 3):13–6.
12. Raju TN, Mercer BM, Burchfield DJ, et al. Periviable birth: executive summary of a Joint Workshop by the Eunice Kennedy Shriver National Institute of Child Health and Human Development, Society for maternal-Fetal Medicine, American Academy of Pediatrics, and American College of Obstetricians and Gynecologists. J Perinatol 2014;34(5):333–42.
13. Lui K, Bajuk B, Foster K, et al. Perinatal care at the borderlines of viability: a consensus statement based on a NSW and ACT consensus workshop. Med J Aust 2006;185(9):495–500.
14. Swiss Society of Neonatologists. Guidelines. Recommendation for the care of infants born at the limit of viability (GA 22–26 weeks). Available at: http://www.neonet.ch/Infants_born_at_the_limit_of_viability_-_english_final.pdf. Accessed September 23, 2014.
15. Moriette G, Rameix S, Azria E, et al, Groupe de réflexion sur les aspects éthiques de la périnatologie. Very premature births: dilemmas and management, second part: ethical aspects and recommendations. Arch Pediatr 2010;17(5): 527–39 [in French].
16. International Liaison Committee on Resuscitation. The International Liaison Committee on Resuscitation (ILCOR) consensus on science with treatment recommendations for pediatric and neonatal patients: neonatal resuscitation. Pediatrics 2006;117:e978–88.
17. Pignotti MS, Donzelli G. Perinatal care at the threshold of viability: an international comparison of practical guidelines for the treatment of extremely preterm births. Pediatrics 2008;121(1):e193–8.
18. Wilkinson DJ. Gestational ageism. Arch Pediatr Adolesc Med 2012;166(6): 567–72.
19. Children and infants-case discussion: the messenger case. Available at: www.msu.edu/course/hm/546/messenger.htm. Accessed September 23, 2014.
20. Lantos JD, Meadow WL. Neonatal bioethics; the moral challenges of medical innovation. Baltimore (MD): The John Hopkins University Press; 2006.
21. Miller v HCA, Inc. 118 S.W. 3d 758 (Tex. 2003).
22. Montalvo v Borkovec. 647 N.W. 2d 413 (Wis.App. 2002).
23. Sayeed SA. Baby doe redux? The Department of Health and Human Services and the Born-Alive Infants Protection Act of 2002: a cautionary note on normative neonatal practice. Pediatrics 2005;116:e576–85.
24. Preston v Meriter Hospital. 678 N.W. 2d 347 (Wis.App. 2004).
25. Robertson JA. Extreme prematurity and parental rights after baby doe. Hastings Cent Rep 2004;34(4):32–9.
26. Creasy RK, Resnick R, Iams J, editors. Maternal fetal medicine: principles & practices. 5th edition. Philadelphia: Saunders; 2004. p. 321–2.

27. Robinson HP. Sonar measurement of fetal crown-rump length as means of assessing maturity in first trimester of pregnancy. Br Med J 1973;4(5883): 28–31.
28. Chervenak FA, Skupski DW, Romero R, et al. How accurate is fetal biometry in the assessment of fetal age? Am J Obstet Gynecol 1998;178(4):678–87.
29. Donovan EF, Tyson JE, Ehrenkranz RE, et al. Inaccuracy of Ballard scores before 28 weeks' gestation. J Pediatr 1999;135:147–52.
30. Mercurio MR. Physicians' refusal to resuscitate at borderline gestational age. J Perinatol 2005;25:685–9.
31. Tyson JE, Parikh NA, Langer J, et al, National Institute of Child Health and Human Development Neonatal Research Network. Intensive care for extreme prematurity: moving beyond gestational age. N Engl J Med 2008;358(16): 1672–81.
32. Singh J, Fanaroff J, Andrews B, et al. Resuscitation in the "gray zone" of viability: determining physician preferences and predicting infant outcomes. Pediatrics 2007;120(3):519–26.
33. Lee HC, Subeh M, Gould JB. Low Apgar score and mortality in extremely preterm neonates born in the United States. Acta Paediatr 2010;99(12):1785–9.
34. Lagatta J, Yan K, Hoffman R. The association between 5-min Apgar score and mortality disappears after 24 h at the borderline of viability. Acta Paediatr 2012; 101(6):e243–7.
35. Meadow W, Reimshisel T, Lantos J. Birth weight-specific mortality for extremely low birth weight infants vanishes by four days of life: epidemiology and ethics in the neonatal intensive care unit. Pediatrics 1996;97(5):636–43.
36. Meadow W, Lee G, Lin L, et al. Changes in mortality for extremely low birth weight infants in the 1990s: implications for treatment decisions and resource use. Pediatrics 2004;113:1223–9.
37. Donohue PK, Boss RD, Shepard J, et al. Interventions at the border of viability; perspective over a decade. Arch Pediatr Adolesc Med 2009;163(10):902–6.
38. Broitman E, Ambalavanan N, Higgins RD, et al. Clinical data predict neurodevelopmental outcome better than head ultrasound in extremely low birth weight infants. J Pediatr 2007;151(5):500–5.
39. Meadow W, Frain L, Ren Y, et al. Serial assessment of mortality in the neonatal intensive care unit by algorithm and intuition: certainty, uncertainty, and informed consent. Pediatrics 2002;109(5):878–86.
40. Meadow W, Lagatta J, Andrews B, et al. Just in time: ethical implications of serial pre- dictions of death and morbidity for ventilated premature infants. Pediatrics 2008;121(4):732–40.
41. President's Commission for the Study of Ethical Problems in Medicine and Biomedical and Behavioral Research. Deciding to forego life-sustaining treatment: a report on the ethical, medical, and legal issues in treatment decisions. Washington, DC: US Government Printing Office; 1983.
42. Position of the American Academy of Neurology on certain aspects of the care and management of the persistent vegetative state patient. Adopted by the Executive Board, American Academy of Neurology, April 21, 1988, Cincinnati, Ohio. Neurology 1989;39:125–6.
43. Truog RD, Brackett SE, Burns JP, et al. Recommendations for end-of-life care in the intensive care unit: the ethics committee of the society of critical care medicine. Crit Care Med 2001;29(12):2332–48.
44. American Academy of Pediatrics Committee on Bioethics. Guidelines on forgoing life-sustaining medical treatment. Pediatrics 1994;93:532–6.

45. Council on Ethical and Judicial Affairs, American Medical Association. Code of medical ethics: current opinions and annotations, 2006-2007 edition. Chicago: American Medical Association; 2006.
46. American Academy of Pediatrics Committee on Fetus and Newborn, Bell EF. Noninitiation or withdrawal of intensive care for high-risk newborns. Pediatrics 2007;119:401–3.
47. Berlinger N, Jennings B, Wolf SM. The Hastings Center guidelines for decisions on life-sustaining treatment and care near the end of life: revised and expanded second edition. New York: Oxford University Press; 2013.
48. Dickenson DL. Are medical ethicists out of touch? Practitioner attitudes in the US and UK towards decisions at the end of life. J Med Ethics 2000;26(4): 254–60.
49. Feltman DM, Du H, Leuthner SR. Survey of neonatologists' attitudes toward limiting life-sustaining treatments in the neonatal intensive care unit. J Perinatol 2012;32(11):886–92.
50. Costeloe K, Hennessy E, Gibson AT, et al, EPICure Study Group. The EPICure study: outcomes to discharge from hospital for infants born at the threshold of viability. Pediatrics 2000;106:659–71.
51. Batton D. Resuscitation of extremely low gestational age infants: an advisory committee's dilemmas. Acta Paediatr 2010;99(6):810–1.
52. Janvier A, Barrington KJ, Aziz K, et al. Ethics ain't easy: do we need simple rules for complicated ethical decisions? Acta Paediatr 2008;97(4):402–6.
53. Janvier A, Barrington KJ, Aziz K, et al. CPS position statement for prenatal counselling before a premature birth: simple rules for complicated decisions. Paediatr Child Health 2014;19(1):22–4.
54. Meadow W, Lantos J. Moral reflections on neonatal intensive care. Pediatrics 2009;123(2):595–7.
55. Turillazzi E, Fineschi V. How old are you? newborn gestational age discriminates neonatal resuscitation practices in the Italian debate. BMC Med Ethics 2009;10:19.
56. Janvier A, Leblanc I, Barrington KJ. The best-interest standard is not applied for neonatal resuscitation decisions. Pediatrics 2008;121(5):963–9.
57. Meadow W. Ethics at the margins of viability. Neoreviews 2013;14:e588.
58. Andrews B, Lagatta J, Chu A, et al. The nonimpact of gestational age on neurodevelopmental outcome for ventilated survivors born at 23–28 weeks of gestation. Acta Paediatr 2012;101:574–8.
59. Carbajal R, Rousset A, Danan C, et al. Epidemiology and treatment of painful procedures in neonates in intensive care units. JAMA 2008;300(1):60–70.
60. Wilkinson DJ. Death or disability? The 'carmentis machine' and decision-making for critically ill children. Oxford (UK): Oxford University Press; 2013. p. P125–45.
61. Informed consent, parental permission, and assent in pediatric practice. Committee on Bioethics, American Academy of Pediatrics. Pediatrics 1995;95:314–7.
62. Leuthner SR. Decisions regarding resuscitation of the extremely premature infant and models of best interest. J Perinatol 2001;21:193–8.
63. Brody H, Bartholome WG. In the best interest of. Hastings Cent Rep 1988;18: 37–40.
64. Ross LF. Children, families, and health care decision making. Oxford (UK): Clarendon Press; 1998.
65. Kopelman LM. The best-interests standard as threshold, ideal, and standard of reasonableness. J Med Philos 1997;22:271–89.
66. Coggon J. Best interests, public interest, and the power of the medical profession. Health Care Anal 2008;16:219–32.

67. Buchanan AE, Brock DW. Deciding for others: the ethics of surrogate decision making. Cambridge (United Kingdom): Cambridge University Press; 1989.
68. Kipnis K. Harm and uncertainty in newborn intensive care. Theor Med Bioeth 2007;28(5):393–412.
69. Wilkinson DJ. A life worth giving? The threshold for permissible withdrawal of life support from disabled newborn infants. Am J Bioeth 2011;11(2):20–32.
70. Curran AL, Sharples PM, White C, et al. Time costs of caring for children with severe disabilities compared with caring for children without disabilities. Dev Med Child Neurol 2001;43(8):529–33.
71. Carter BS, Leuthner SR. Decision-making in the NICU: strategies, statistics, and "satisficing". Bioethics Forum 2002;18(3–4):7–15.
72. Harrison H. Parents and handicapped infants. N Engl J Med 1983;309(11):664–5.
73. Harrison H. The principles for family-centered care and the pediatrician's role. Pediatrics 2003;112(3):691–6.
74. Janvier A, Lorenz JM, Lantos JD. Antenatal counseling for parents pacing an extremely preterm birth: limitations of the medical evidence. Acta Paediatr 2012;101:800–4.
75. Hayward MF, Murphy RO, Lorenz JM. Message framing and perinatal decisions. Pediatrics 2008;122(1):109–18.
76. Schumacher RE. Myth: neonatology is evidence-based. Semin Fetal Neonatal Med 2011;16:288–92.
77. Streiner DL, Saigal S, Burrows E, et al. Attitudes of parents and health care professionals toward active treatment of extremely premature infants. Pediatrics 2001;108:152–7.
78. Saigal S, Feeny D, Rosenbaum P, et al. Self-perceived health status and health-related quality of life of extremely low birth-weight infants at adolescence. JAMA 1996;276:453–9.
79. Saigal S, Rosenbaum PL, Feeny D, et al. Parental perspectives of the health status and health-related quality of life of teen-aged children who were extremely low birth weight and term controls. Pediatrics 2000;105:569–74.
80. Feeny D, Furlong W, Saigal S, et al. Comparing directly measured standard gamble scores to HUI2 and HUI3 utility scores: group- and individual-level comparisons. Soc Sci Med 2004;58:799–809.
81. Harrison H. Making lemonade: a parent's view of 'quality of life' studies. J Clin Ethics 2001;12:239–50 when life gives you lemons.
82. Patrick DL, Danis M, Southerland LI, et al. Quality of life following intensive care. J Gen Intern Med 1988;3(3):218–23.
83. Schmitt SK. Costs of newborn care in California: a population-based study. Pediatrics 2006;117:154–60.
84. Stolz J, McCormick M. Restricting access to neonatal intensive care: effect on mortality and economic savings. Pediatrics 1998;101:344.
85. Lantos JD, Mokalla M, Meado W. Resource allocation in neonatal and medical ICUs. Epidemiology and rationing at the extremes of life. Am J Respir Crit Care Med 1997;156:185–9.
86. Camosy C. Too expensive to treat? Finitude, tragedy, and the neonatal ICU. Grand Rapids (MI): Wm. B. Eerdmans Press; 2010. p. P189–91.
87. Hack M. Chronic conditions, functional limitations, and special health care needs of school-aged children born with extremely low birth weight in the 1990's. JAMA 2005;294:318–25.
88. Camosy CC. Just distribution of health-care resources and the neonatal ICU. Pediatr Rev 2011;32(5):205–7.

89. Leuthner SR, Lorenz JM. Can rule-based ethics help in the NICU? Available at: http://virtualmentor.ama-assn.org/2008/10/pdf/ccas2-0810.pdf. Accessed June 2, 2014.

90. Lantos J, Meadow W. Re: 'Decisions about life-sustaining measures in children: in whose best interests?'. Acta Paediatr 2012;101(4):337.

Fetal Programming, Epigenetics, and Adult Onset Disease

Robert H. Lane, MD, MS

KEYWORDS

- DNA methylation • Developmental origins of disease • Epigenetics • Food desert
- Histone covalent modifications • Insulin growth factor 1 • Insulin resistance
- Obesity

KEY POINTS

- Early life events program the occurrence of significant adult diseases, including obesity and insulin resistance.
- Although our understanding started with issues that seem remote now, relevant current issues such as food deserts and prematurity continue to make programming a priority if adult disease is to be prevented, as opposed to treating it.
- Environmental epigenetics describes how our chromatin adapts to surroundings and is a likely mechanism central to programming.
- Environmental epigenetics involves changes to chromatin structure that changes the DNA accessibility as well as nontranslated RNAs.
- A key characteristic of environmental epigenetics is that it can be manipulated, so that it is a potential target for both personalized medicine and population health.

INTRODUCTION

Significant early life events program individuals toward adult health and disease. Epidemiologic evidence exists for this concept within communities across the globe as well as developed and developing countries.[1–4] Biological programming is defined as the process in which cells develop, function, and adapt to the environment in response to an entrained set of executable commands, often emanating from the cell's chromatin. Cells normally contain these programs. Significant early life events reformulate these programs, likely as adaptations to ensure early survival at the price of later disease.

Disclosures: We have no relationships with commercial companies that have a direct financial interest in the subject matter or materials discussed in the article.
Department of Pediatrics, Children's Hospital of Wisconsin, Medical College of Wisconsin, Suite 720, PO Box 1997, Milwaukee, WI 53201-1997, USA
E-mail address: rlane@mcw.edu

Clin Perinatol 41 (2014) 815–831
http://dx.doi.org/10.1016/j.clp.2014.08.006
0095-5108/14/$ – see front matter © 2014 Elsevier Inc. All rights reserved.

EARLY LIFE PROGRAMMING PROVIDES A CONCEPTUAL INFRASTRUCTURE FOR HOW PEDIATRIC NEEDS TO CHANGE

The diseases associated with programming include those that cost the most in terms of human suffering and resources. The concept that early life events predict adult health and disease guides everything we do as a pediatric community. Moreover, this concept touches all 4 legs of the stool on which academic pediatrics stands.

- In term of education, young clinicians need to actively consider later life consequences of clinical interventions, and not just the immediate consequences. This statement is particularly true considering the paucity of prospective data informing us on how common interventions in the neonatal intensive care (NICU) affect long-term outcomes.
- In terms of research, investigators need to anticipate later life health and disease outcomes in the planning of their studies. Present funding fails to support this anticipation, but the presence of conceptual investigational infrastructure that accounts for later life health and disease outcomes keeps options open for key questions.
- In terms of community health, health care organizations need to think proactively on not only how to treat a community's disease but also how to maintain and sustain a community's health.[5] This proactive thinking requires the removal or at least the moderation of environmental elements that prevent and threaten community health before disease becomes tenured.
- In terms of clinical care, clinicians need to act on the truism that preventing disease improves individual and community health more than treating disease (**Box 1**). A challenge to this truism resides in the reality that we do not know

---

Box 1
A community pediatrician's dilemma

Johnny is a reasonably happy 6 year old. His height is 44 inches (10th percentile), and his weight is 50 pounds (75th percentile). His past medical history is remarkable for being a 28-week former premature infant. His course in the NICU was relatively benign, with the most significant events including a few days of bubble CPAP, TPN, and antibiotics. He was discharged home to his single mother, who is working an hourly job. She cannot afford a car, and as such, she is limited to public transportation. He and his mother live in an economically depressed neighborhood, and they are the third generation of his family to live in this neighborhood. His mother is sincerely motivated to support positive changes for her family. She is involved in Johnny's care, and she can verbalize the many risks associated with prematurity.

Running 15 minutes behind schedule, you enter the room to discover Johnny eating a bag of chips and drinking a large sugared soda. You are discouraged, but you try to understand why your efforts to encourage more healthy behaviors seem to be failing.

You learn that Johnny and his mother live in a neighborhood characterized by high rates of violent crime and school dropout. There are no supermarkets within walking distance; only stores that sell a few very expensive items of produce or calorie-dense low nutrition food are near their residence. She walks with him to school in the morning, but her job does not allow her to often be home after school. Fearing for his safety, she entices Johnny with video games to come home right away after school and to stay inside. This keeps him to some extent from the violence inherent to this neighborhood. For Johnny's mother to be home, let alone make his appointments, she must take off work. Because she is an hourly worker, she loses pay and opportunities for advancement if she takes off. Johnny is presently eating chips because he was hungry because he missed lunch to catch the bus to clinic, and his mother obtained snacks from the vending machine in the lobby of the clinic. Moreover, the snacks serve as a reward for Johnny to be willing to come to clinic without a fuss (because Johnny really likes school).

how to do that yet secondary to the lack of clinically relevant prospective long-term studies, the broad continuum of the human experience, and the mathematical challenge of predicting multifactorial diseases. The mathematical challenge exists secondary to the matrixed set of confounding factors that impact the human experience, such as genetics, current environment, and family exposures across generations. Despite this challenge, a foundation exists that provides insight into the relevance and scope of the problems associated with fetal programming.

EARLY LIFE PROGRAMMING OCCURS SECONDARY TO SIGNIFICANT ENVIRONMENTAL EXPOSURES

Large epidemiologic studies and cohorts that involve multiple generations provide the foundation for understanding fetal programming. These initial studies focus on how maternal malnutrition, as an environmental exposure from a fetal stand point, program adult health and disease.[6–11] These studies take advantage of spontaneous and sometimes tragic population-wide "experiments" induced by extreme environmental exposures (**Table 1**). Subsequently, these "malnutrition"-based studies provide utility by demonstrating common themes that build a conceptual foundation on which to understand fetal programming. These themes also become evident when looking at other environmental exposures, such as maternal stress, maternal smoking, pollution, and toxic exposures.

- Maternal malnutrition, usually defined by insufficient intake of macronutrients or micronutrients, affects adult health of the offspring regardless of the country of origin or ethnicity. Although the impact may differ based on the country, likely because of confounding environmental and genetics factors, an impact still occurs. Two concepts are basic to interpreting these studies as well as future studies in the field. The first concept is that most of these studies use birth weight as a surrogate measure of maternal malnutrition, as opposed to direct measure of maternal intact (the "Dutch Famine" studies are a population-wide exception). The second concept is that the definition of maternal malnutrition includes excess and not just deprivation.
- Maternal malnutrition's timing during the gestation determines the impact on offspring adult health (**Fig. 1**). For example, in the Dutch Famine, offspring experiencing maternal malnutrition early in gestation suffer from an increased incidence of coronary artery disease, hypertension, and obesity as adults.[12]

Table 1
Tragic population—wide exposures

Name	Country	Time Period	Exposure
Dutch Famine	Netherlands	1944	Daily rations of 400–800 kcal
Leningrad Siege	Russia	1941–1944	Daily rations of 300 kcals (most severe in winter of 1941–1942)
Occupation of Guernsey	UK Channel Islands	1940–1945	Daily rations of 1200 kcal
Great Chinese Famine (Three Bitter Years)	China	1959–1961	Unknown: extreme variability particularly between Rural and urban communities
North Korean Famine (Arduous March)	North Korea	1994–1998	Unknown

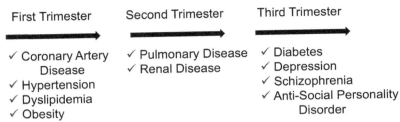

Fig. 1. Compilation of adult disease predisposition with trimester of affected pregnancy from the Dutch Famine. Although variation in the timing of maternal malnutrition and offspring predisposition's exists, the important concept is that the timing of the insult is an important variable in offspring outcome.

Offspring experiencing maternal malnutrition during mid gestation suffer from an increased incidence of obstructive airway disease.[13] Finally, offspring experiencing maternal malnutrition during late gestation suffer from insulin resistance.[14] The absolute relationship between timing of the malnutrition during the gestation and outcome differs between studies, communities, and countries, but the theme remains true.

- Maternal malnutrition affects the adult health of more than one organ system. Indeed, all of the morbidities noted in the previous statement require interactions of multiple organ systems. For example, in terms of coronary artery disease, this morbidity results from an interaction of the coronary arteries themselves, the immune system, and the liver (through its regulation of serum lipid homeostasis).
- Maternal malnutrition affects adult morbidities, such as coronary artery disease, insulin resistance, and obesity, which are among the most costly on a population basis. Indeed, obesity owns the nickname of "public health enemy number one" in the United States by extracting greater than $147 billion a year in health care expenditures.[15]

Health care expenditures toward diseases such as obesity affect the economies of all countries, diverting resources away from social improvement that may lead to prevention. As we grow into a "world" economy, an increase in adult morbidities due to fetal programming in one country distributes the impact across borders. A potential example of this exists in aftershock of the "Chinese Famine."[16-20] The Chinese Famine lasted 3 years from 1958 to 1961. Conservatively, 30 million deaths occurred during this time.[20] The Chinese Famine differs from the Dutch Famine by spanning a longer period of time, affecting a population already struggling under the weight of chronic malnutrition, and varying across regions in terms of severity.

Subsequently, the impact of the Chinese Famine reaches extremes that the Dutch Famine fails to reach. On a population-wide basis, decreased adult height and neurodevelopmental outcomes characterize first-generation adults who survived in utero during the Chinese Famine.[17,21] Greater than normal birth weights characterized second-generation grandchildren.[22] The impact of the Chinese Famine stretches across generations to increase the incidence of large-for-gestational age infants (LGA). LGA predisposes toward adult insulin resistance and obesity in affected individuals. Moreover, women suffering from insulin resistance and obesity are more likely to give birth to an LGA infant. Considering the millions of individuals impacted by the famine, the cost in terms of health and health care expenditures for this second generation and the subsequent third generation will be felt across the world economy, diverting essential resources from other priorities.

Diversion of resources also needs to occur in the United States if we are to learn from the Chinese Famine. This diversion needs to occur in 2 arenas. The first arena exists with the concept of food deserts. The second arena exists in our growing population of former premature infants.

Food deserts play a role perpetrating the racial disparities in health that occur in the United States, such as with obesity (http://www.cdc.gov/obesity/data/adult.html) (**Table 2**).[23] The United States Department of Agriculture defines a food desert as "a census tract with a substantial share of residents who live in low-income areas that have low levels of access to a grocery store or healthy affordable food retail outlet." In New York City, the most severe food deserts exist within East and Central Harlem as well as North and Central Brooklyn. These communities contain a high proportion of low-income African Americans.[24] In contrast, food oases within New York City exist in the Upper East Side, which contains middle and upper income families.

Children stranded within a food desert suffer from an increased risk of obesity. Children that live in communities enduring higher priced fruits and vegetables develop higher body mass indexes (BMIs) than children that live in communities with lower priced produce.[25] A 10% increase in the price of produce associates with a 0.7% increase in childhood BMI.[25,26] For the community pediatrician, the realities of the food desert go beyond the abstract nature of statistics because it predicts both present and future health. Childhood obesity predicts adult coronary artery disease, hypertension, and adult onset obesity.[27–29] Maternal and paternal obesity predisposes toward obesity in their offspring, although the statistical link is stronger for maternal obesity.[30] Maternal obesity increases the risk for preeclampsia and gestational diabetes.[31] Moreover, maternal obesity increases the risk for spontaneous preterm birth, although the association is complex and involves ethnicity, parity, and environmental factors such as smoking.[32–34]

Preterm births still account for approximately 12.5% of deliveries in the United States.[35] Medical care services of premature infants cost the United States approximately $26.2 billion in 2005. Indirect costs involving early intervention services and lost household productivity additionally cost the United States another $7 billion. It is suspected that costs are not less in 2014. Moreover, evidence continues to slowly accumulate, suggesting that prematurity programs toward adult diseases. In referencing programming, pathophysiologies that involve direct cell damage are excluded, such as what happens with hypoxia-ischemia encephalopathy. Our insight into the relevant programming remains foggy secondary to the relative youth of neonatology as a field, the temporal and regional heterogeneity of neonatal practice, and the confounders of environment and genetics. Nevertheless, a couple of themes pierce the fog, albeit bluntly.

Table 2
Racial disparity and obesity

Ethnic Group	Incidence of Obesity (Age-Adjusted Rates) (%)
Non-Hispanic Blacks	47.8
Hispanics	42.5
Non-Hispanic Whites	32.6
Non-Hispanic Asians	10.8

From the CDC. Available at: http://www.cdc.gov/obesity/data/adult.html. Accessed June 01, 2014.

- Prematurity predisposes toward childhood adiposity. Preterm children demonstrate increased waist circumferences despite decreased BMI relative to nonpreterm children.[36,37] These findings indicate a shift in adipose mass distribution toward visceral fat, which is significant considering the association between excess visceral fat and insulin resistance.
- Prematurity predisposes toward childhood and adult hypertension.[33,38,39] The pathophysiology of the association likely lies in multiple mechanisms on the tissue level, including decreased nephron number, decreased vascular density, endothelial dysfunction, and increased arterial stiffness.[40–42] The latter appears to affect smaller preresistance and resistance vessels relative to the large elastic arteries.[42] An important observation in the relationship between prematurity and hypertension is that arterial stiffness proceeds the appearance of clinically relevant hypertension.
- Prematurity possibly predisposes toward insulin resistance, although the findings are conflicting, likely confounded by the many factors ranging from genetics to variation in care practices, among others.[43,44] The relationship between prematurity and insulin resistance appears to be regulated at least in part by postnatal growth.[45]
- Prematurity possibly predisposes to multiple other morbidities when rapid infancy weight gain exceeds relative gain in length. Evidence exists to support this paradigm for obesity, dyslipidemia, blood pressure, carotid intima-media thickness, and insulin resistance.[46–48] If it is presumed that premature infants endure malnutrition early in their hospital course (although not for lack of trying, just that the isolette will never be better than mom), the observation that rapid infancy weight gain increases the risk for disease teleologically suggests the following.

Programming reformatted by the premature environment fails to accommodate for the surplus nutrition that is traditionally inflicted on NICU graduates. However, the conundrum exists that supplemented nutrition appears to improve neurodevelopmental outcomes, particularly when associated with good linear growth.[49–53] Therefore, no clear answer exists in how much the premature infant should be fed in terms of quantity or quality that balances with certainty the risks for adult diseases versus the goal of optimizing neurodevelopmental outcomes. Eventually, this becomes a rich soil for the seed of personalized medicine.

The challenge in interpreting the field is that more reviews exist than hypothesis-driven double-blinded prospective data (the author recognizes the paradox of that statement). The challenge in treating infants is that little evidence-driven data exist to guide the clinician. As alluded to above, much of the data reflect confounding factors resulting in contradictory or ambiguous implications. Moreover, to design studies that aim to clarify the data, 2 truisms need to be acknowledged.

- The first truism is that multiple mechanisms play a role in early life programming and subsequent adult disease. Evidence of varying degrees of confidence implicates mechanisms such as microbiome dyshomeostasis,[54] mitochondrial dysfunction, apoptosis, genetic vulnerability, and epigenetics. Likely, all of these mechanisms play some role in early life programming toward adult disease. Subsequently, study design struggles to easily define a specific hypothesis based on mechanism, either directly or indirectly.
- The second truism is that we need to pragmatically focus our hypotheses so that our studies generate reliable answers. This truism requires 2 steps: a commitment to a specific mechanism and a knowledge basis that informs us of the right questions. Epigenetics deserves this commitment.

EPIGENETICS PRIMER

Epigenetics regulates eukaryotic gene expression. Changes in epigenetic character-istics potentially change gene expression without affecting DNA sequence.

Epigenetics as a field divides conceptually into developmental epigenetics and envi-ronmental epigenetics. Developmental epigenetics studies the maintenance and execution of rigid patterns of gene expression involved in development, maturation, and tissue specificity. Environmental epigenetics studies how cells respond to the environment by changing chromatin structure or expressing small RNAs. This response changes gene expression by affecting the threshold toward how easy it is for a gene to be expressed (**Fig. 2**). A generally applicable difference between environ-mental epigenetics and developmental epigenetics is that changes in developmental epigenetics turn genes off and on. No one needs a neuron to turn into a hepatocyte. Changes attributed to environmental epigenetics modify gene expression in a more subtle and incremental manner. Responses to the environment that turn off an impor-tant gene are unlikely to benefit the cell or organism. The response is too drastic. In contrast, finely tuning expression in response to the environment does confer a sur-vival advantage. In a broader sense, environmental epigenetics describes how the environment determines phenotype by modulating gene expression.

EPIGENETIC TOOLS

Cells use several epigenetic tools to regulate gene expression. These epigenetic tools can be divided into modifications of chromatin structure versus production of different species of small RNAs (**Table 3**). The scientific community's understanding of epige-netics exists at an infancy stage, despite significant progress over the last 2 years. The scientific community's understanding of how the different epigenetic tools influence and interact with each other is even more immature. Despite this immaturity, the ef-forts of many contribute to a foundation of understanding on which we continue to build; this is particularly true for the tools involving modifications of chromatin struc-ture, DNA cytosine phosphate guanine (CpG) methylation, and histone covalent

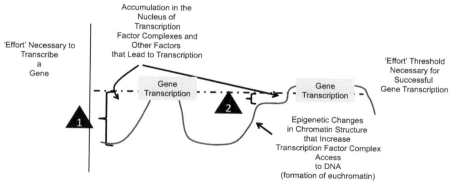

Fig. 2. Conceptualization of "effort" necessary to transcribe a gene and the role environ-mental epigenetics plays. Transcription requires synchronized effort of multiple processes, including (1) intercellular signaling, (2) synthesis and accumulation of transcription factor complexes, and (3) synthesis and accumulation of chromatin-modifying enzymes that impart epigenetic changes. Conceptually, this can be seen in the difference between number 1 and number 2. The delta of number 2 is less than number 1 because of environmental epige-netics. Environmental epigenetics can also increase the delta.

Table 3
Examples of epigenetic modifications

Chromatin-modifying Epigenetic	Non-coding RNAs
DNA CpG methylation	Micro-RNAs (17–25 nucleotides)
DNA CpG hydroxymethylation	Piwi-interacting RNA (26–31 nucleotides)
Histone covalent 3′ N-terminal tail modification: methylation[a]	Promoter RNAs (90–200 nucleotides)
Histone covalent 3′ N-terminal tail modification: acetylation	Promoter RNAs (90–200 nucleotides)
Histone covalent 3′ N-terminal tail modification: phosphorylation	LncRNAs (>200 nucleotides)
Histone Covalent 3′ N-terminal tail modification: ubiquitination	Telomeric repeat containing RNAs (100–9000 nucleotides)
Histone covalent 3′ N-terminal tail modification: citrullination	

[a] Histone methylation can be mono-, di-, or tri-.

modification. These tools generally affect how accessible DNA is to transcription factor complexes or how efficiently transcription proceeds, including both initiation and elongation.

- DNA CpG methylation involves placing a methyl group on the cytosine of CpG dinucleotides. CpG dinucleotides occur disproportionately in CpG islands. Two-thirds of human promoters reside with CpG islands. Most promoters residing in these islands stay relatively unmethylated if the gene is expressed at any level within the tissue of question. DNA CpG methylation does characterize silenced genes, but initiation of silencing does not require methylation and most likely represents maintenance of transcriptional repression.
- Histone covalent modification involves modifying one N-terminal tail of a histone protein. Histone proteins form the nucleosome core around which DNA wraps. Nucleosomes and DNA form the backbone of eukaryotic chromatin. The pattern and combination of histone covalent modifications assimilate into the histone code. The histone code appears to participate directly in 3 basic functions.
  - Some combinations of histone codes modulate the charge of histone lysine residues and thereby regulate charge-dependent associations between nucleosomes and DNA. This association affects the affinity of chromatin-modifying and transcription-related protein to the chromatin's DNA. A histone covalent modification that often associates with this function is histone acetylation of the N-terminal tail of histone 3.
  - Some combinations of histone code modulate the physical accessibility of chromatin-modifying and transcription-related proteins to the chromatin's DNA. A histone covalent modification that often associates with this function is histone methylation of the N-terminal of histone 3.
  - Some combinations of histone code modulate the charge histone lysine residues and physical accessibility of chromatin-modifying and transcription-related proteins to the chromatin's DNA. A histone covalent modification that often associates with this function is histone phosphorylation.

Interpreting and subsequently understanding the histone code remains a mystery overall, particularly when considering the challenges of integrating the possibility of a histone modification affecting transcription from a distance of hundreds of thousands of base-pairs. Further contributing to the mystery is that the histone code within a single cell contains more than 4×10^{30} possible permutations. Based on varying combinations of histone covalent modifications, 51 distinct chromatin states exist. Further adding to the complexity, these states affect transcription and expression based on the individual complexs interacting with the chromatin and its DNA. Although daunting, this level of complexity and capacity offers opportunity as an information storage system that continually records in detail the impact of the environment on our chromatin.

Subsequently, reviewing how an early life event affects the epigenetics of a relevant gene generates value by providing a paradigm to build on when interpreting future investigations. A relevant gene to review is insulinlike growth factor 1 (IGF-1). IGF-1 is a polypeptide whose homology resembles pro-insulin. Hepatic production of IGF-1 determines serum levels, although local production of IGF-1 plays an important paracrine role for many tissues such as the lung. Several lines of evidence point to IGF-1 as a likely effector of early programming toward adult disease, particularly when considering the common theme morbidities of insulin resistance and coronary artery disease from above.

- In terms of insulin resistance, hepatic IGF-1 plays a significant role in modulating postnatal glucose homeostasis. In mice, elimination of hepatic IGF-1 production increases serum levels of insulin without affecting glucose.[55] In humans, severe IGF-1 deficiency leads to clinically relevant insulin resistance, and the latter can be reversed with recombinant IGF-1.[56] Finally, within the context of a more normal situation, euglycemic clamp studies in adolescents demonstrate that serum IGF-1 levels significantly correlated with insulin sensitivity.[57]
- In terms of coronary artery disease, a recent nested case control study found that low IGF-1 levels predict increased risk for developing ischemic heart disease. Moreover, polymorphisms of the IGF-1 gene impact on coronary artery disease susceptibility.[58] Evidence exists that suggests one mechanism through which IGF-1 reduces the risk of coronary artery disease occurs through opposing the effects of C-reactive protein on endothelial cell activation.[59]

Epigenetic mechanisms play a role in regulating IGF-1 gene expression. A red flag for the role of epigenetic mechanisms in the regulating of IGF-1 gene expression is that the IGF-1 gene generates multiple transcribed products based on differential exon usage. Variation like this represents a key characteristic that differentiates mammalian gene expression from simpler organisms.

The hepatic IGF-1 gene generates multiple transcribed products that lead to a single protein product. IGF-1 promoter 1 (IGF-1 P1) initiates transcription from multiple start sites (**Fig. 3**). Hepatic IGF-1P1 usage predominates early in life. IGF-1 promoter 2 (IGF-1P2) also initiates transcription from multiple start sites as well as contains growth hormone response elements. IGF-1P2 becomes active in postnatal life and responds to both diet and growth hormone stimulation. The hepatic IGF-1 transcript may or may not contain exon 5. Transcripts that do not include exon 5 are designated IGF-1A. Transcripts that do include exon 5 are designated IGF-1B transcripts. The relevance of this alternative exon usage involves the production of 2 E-peptides, EA and EB, respectively. Although still open to debate, studies exist proposing that these peptides play roles in cell proliferation, migration, and survival.[60]

To further build our paradigm of how an early life event affects IGF-1 epigenetic mechanisms, the extensive use of animal models needs to be acknowledged. Indeed, most our present insight on early life events and epigenetic mechanisms arises from animal models because of increased accessibility to tissue, briefer gestations, and

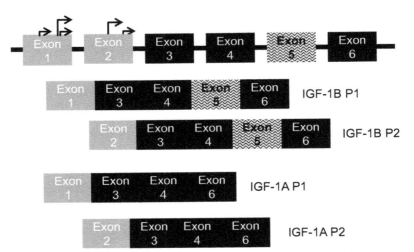

Fig. 3. Organization of the rat IGF-1 gene. This gene produces up to 4 different transcripts. Transcription may initiate in promoter 1 and subsequently include exon 1. Transcription may initiate in promoter 2 and subsequently include exon 2. Inclusion of exon 5 in the transcript produces the IGF-1B transcript.

shorter life spans. A common animal model of early life events predisposing to adult insulin resistance involves the induction of uteroplacental insufficiency in the rat. Uteroplacental insufficiency in rats and humans leads to a fetal in utero environment characterized by malnutrition. Moreover, uteroplacental insufficiency in humans and rats associates with adult insulin resistance and obesity.

In humans, uteroplacental insufficiency decreases fetal and early postnatal serum IGF-1 levels. Later in life, there appears to be a dysregulation of IGF-1 homeostasis possibly varying with the extent of postnatal catch-up growth.

In rats, uteroplacental insufficiency decreases serum IGF-1 levels and hepatic IGF-1 transcripts, although the effect is transcript-specific, further pointing toward epigenetic mechanisms. For example, uteroplacental insufficiency decreases IGF-1P1 and EA transcripts at day 0 of life. In contrast, uteroplacental insufficiency decreases IGF-1P2 and IGF-1B transcripts at both day of life 0 and day of life 21 (**Fig. 4**). The latter represents the time when rat pups wean from their mothers.

The impact of uteroplacental insufficiency on hepatic IGF-1 expression corresponds with changes in the epigenetic characteristics of the whole rat hepatic IGF-1 gene. For example, uteroplacental insufficiency enriches DNA CpG methylation at IGF-1P2 at day of life 21. Uteroplacental insufficiency also decreased lysine 36 trimethylation on histone 3 across the whole gene, with the greatest impact toward the 3′ region of the gene (**Fig. 5**). In vitro studies postulate that lysine 36 trimethylation on histone 3 facilitates RNA polymerase elongation of transcripts.[61] Unfortunately, technology does not exist that presently allows for the generation of a transgenic animal that specifically decreases hepatic IGF-1 3′ lysine 36 trimethylation. However, another rat model that uses maternal hyperglycemia as an early life event to induce adult cardiovascular disease similarly finds decreased lysine 36 trimethylation of the hepatic IGF-1 gene.[62,63]

The paradigm that these and other studies (both in vivo and in vitro) generate includes the following principles, which are helpful when interpreting epigenetic studies:

- Environmental challenges often initiate different responses between the genders.

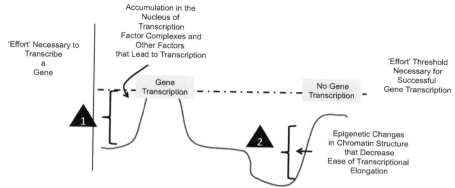

Fig. 4. Hypothetical impact of uteroplacental insufficiency on the "effort" necessary to transcribe the hepatic IGF-1 gene. Similar to **Fig. 2**, delta 1 represents the normal effort to transcribe hepatic IGF-1, the gene presented as a paradigm within this review. Delta 2 represents the similar effort, but after uteroplacental insufficiency-induced chromatin changes increase the effort necessary for successful transcription of a functional transcript.

- Environmental challenges rarely affect only strong promoters or other key regulators of gene expression. The impact of environmental challenges occurs along the length of the gene. Looking at only a single site within an epigenetic study limits the informative nature of the study.
- Environmental challenges and their impact on chromatin cannot be interpreted via a single site of change. Changes in DNA methylation or the histone covalent modifications affect transcription based on the (1) location within a gene's organization; (2) context of other surrounding epigenetic modifications; and (3) the nuclear milieu of chromatin-modifying enzymes and transcription factor complexes.
- Environmental challenges impact epigenetics characteristics early in life and later in life relative to a control or nonexposed group. However, the differences between the groups may be different early in life versus the differences later in life, and likely due to the reality that epigenetic characteristics change as mammals mature. An early change therefore leads to a different progression of epigenetic maturation.
- Environmental challenges impact epigenetic characteristics early in life, but the impact in terms of gene expression or phenotype does not become evident until much later. A relevant example of this involves epigenetic changes involving sex

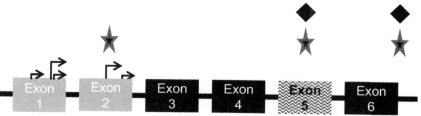

Fig. 5. Effect of uteroplacental insufficiency on IGF-1 gene histone covalent modifications. Location of the star designates where intrauterine growth retardation decreased hepatic IGF-1 lysine 36 trimethylation on histone 3 enrichment. Location of the diamond designates where maternal hyperglycemia decreased offspring postnatal hepatic IGF-1 lysine 36 trimethylation on histone 3 enrichment.

steroid response elements, likely due to transcription machinery that interacts with epigenetic mechanisms changes as the animal matures. An easy example of this resides within sex steroid biology. A corollary of this tenant is that the impact of a specific set of epigenetic changes on gene expression and phenotype may be different in later life relative to the impact early in life.

Other epigenetic mechanisms exist through the expression of different species of noncoding RNAs.[64–67] Our present understanding of the relevance of these noncoding RNAs in vivo is descriptive, although in vitro studies suggest that these noncoding RNAs provide another layer of epigenetic regulation. Considering where the epigenetic community is in terms of translating the significance of these molecules toward human disease, only 2 of these noncoding RNAs are briefly described in later discussion. These noncoding RNAs arise from the 98% of our genome that does not encode proteins.[68] The biological significance of these noncoding RNAs becomes apparent when acknowledging that the ratio of non-protein-encoding DNA to protein-encoding DNA correlates with biological complexity. Most of these noncoding RNA appear to mediate posttranscriptional regulation of gene expression. For example, micro-RNAs contain approximately 22 nucleotides, and they affect expression of up to 60% of our genome. They silence expression by binding to complementary base-pairs of mRNA, thereby preventing translation.

Another small RNA epigenetic mechanism includes long noncoding RNAs (lncRNAs), which is a diverse class of transcripts that lack an open reading frame. LncRNAs are typically greater than 200 nucleotides, and cells express tens of thousands of these transcripts. LncRNAs regulate several of the serial steps involved in transcriptional regulation, including modifying transcription factor activity and regulating the association with chromatin. LncRNAs may also function as an interface between transcriptome and proteosome.

ENVIRONMENTAL EPIGENETICS AS FIT FOR AND PERSONALIZED MEDICINE AND FITNESS

The future of epigenetics lies in its potential as a tool to apply toward personalized medicine. Personalized medicine proposes the customization of health care, with decisions, practices, and products being tailored to individual patients. The future of epigenetics lies in this field because environmental epigenetics represents the recording of the interactions between our genome and our environment. Environmental epigenetics contains the capacity and specificity to do the following:

- Allows for tissue-specific and gender-specific responses to early life environmental events.
- Allows for the variability and complexity of the human experience (the capacity of the histone code is particularly exciting for this reason).
- Incorporates and acknowledges the pivotal role non-protein-encoding DNA plays in determining gene expression and subsequent phenotype.

Environmental epigenetics also allows for the concept of Lamarckian inheritance. Lamarckian inheritance exists as the idea that mammals pass on adaptations acquired during a lifetime of environmental exposures to their offspring with the teleologic goal of increasing the survival odds. Describing research as Lamarckian used to be considered diminutive, but evidence of cross-generational impact of early life events such as with the Chinese Famine suggests important applicability to the concept. Intuitively, several keen observers of the human condition, including the author's children, note that individuals cannot change their genetics, but they can change their epigenetics.

EPIGENETICS AS A BIOMARKER AND AN INTERVENTION TARGET

The concept that epigenetic characteristics can be purposefully and strategically modified belies a key characteristic of environmental epigenetics as a future basis for personalized medicine. Our present studies focus on the use of epigenetics as a biomarker, as either a pattern via high through-put studies or detailed characteristics of an individual gene. For example, life variables, such as maternal macronutrient and micronutrient consumption, multiple gestations, mode of conception, mode of delivery, and maternal smoking, associate with various differences in DNA CpG methylation. With rare exception, the present understanding of epigenetics and technology, in terms of both the biology and mathematical computation, suffer from naïve but well-intended reductionism in terms of many of these studies, providing actionable data. However, this will change.

The field will progress through the fruitful efforts of many. Future studies will allow us to take the next steps to specifically intervene and thereby soften the adult impact of an early life event. Because all interventions carry some aspect of risk, identifying the right intervention for the right person stands as the end prize to make personalized medicine real on a population-wide basis. Caution must be used in terms of intervening until our knowledge base increases. Interventions that aim at changing epigenetic characteristics of a specific gene or subset of genes in a specific tissue for a specific disease may result in either immediate or long-term unintended consequences. Presently, few studies account for this contingency.

Despite this caution, environmental epigenetics represents hope for biomarkers and intervention in diseases acquired by programming. This hope resides in the primary difference between genetics and epigenetics, which has been paraphrased by several pundits in the following observation, "you can't change your parents, but you can change your epigenetics."

How early life events program adult disease is undergoing a transition from the broad field of maternal malnutrition to the currently relevant issues of food deserts and prematurity. Although many adult diseases and morbidities associate with various early life events and programming, the morbidities of insulin resistance, cardiovascular disease, and obesity appear to be common end points of many early life events despite potential confounders. Environmental epigenetics as a mechanism becomes particularly relevant because it contains the capacity to account for the complexity intrinsic to mammalian biology and environmental factors, while allowing for adaptation and change.

ACKNOWLEDGMENTS

The author acknowledges the Developmental Origin Team at the Medical College of Wisconsin and Children's Hospital of Wisconsin, particularly Amber Majnik, PhD, for her editing, and Veronica Gunn, MD, MPH, for her input on the plight of the community pediatrician.

REFERENCES

1. Barker DJ, Hales CN, Fall CH, et al. Type 2 (non-insulin-dependent) diabetes mellitus, hypertension and hyperlipidaemia (syndrome X): relation to reduced fetal growth. Diabetologia 1993;36(1):62–7.
2. Gupta R, Misra A, Vikram NK, et al. Younger age of escalation of cardiovascular risk factors in Asian Indian subjects. BMC Cardiovasc Disord 2009;9:28.
3. Fan Z, Zhang ZX, Li Y, et al. Relationship between birth size and coronary heart disease in China. Ann Med 2010;42(8):596–602.

4. Lackland DT, Bendall HE, Osmond C, et al. Low birth weights contribute to high rates of early-onset chronic renal failure in the Southeastern United States. Arch Intern Med 2000;160(10):1472–6.
5. Cubbin C, Sundquist K, Ahlen H, et al. Neighborhood deprivation and cardio-vascular disease risk factors: protective and harmful effects. Scand J Public Health 2006;34(3):228–37.
6. Painter RC, Roseboom TJ, Bleker OP. Prenatal exposure to the Dutch famine and disease in later life: an overview. Reprod Toxicol 2005;20(3):345–52.
7. Roseboom TJ, van der Meulen JH, Osmond C, et al. Adult survival after prenatal exposure to the Dutch famine 1944–45. Paediatr Perinat Epidemiol 2001;15(3):220–5.
8. Painter RC, Osmond C, Gluckman P, et al. Transgenerational effects of prenatal exposure to the Dutch famine on neonatal adiposity and health in later life. BJOG 2008;115(10):1243–9.
9. Barker DJ, Osmond C. Infant mortality, childhood nutrition, and ischaemic heart disease in England and Wales. Lancet 1986;1(8489):1077–81.
10. Stampfer MJ, Colditz GA, Willett WC, et al. A prospective study of moderate alcohol drinking and risk of diabetes in women. Am J Epidemiol 1988;128(3):549–58.
11. Rich-Edwards JW, Colditz GA, Stampfer MJ, et al. Birthweight and the risk for type 2 diabetes mellitus in adult women. Ann Intern Med 1999;130(4 Pt 1):278–84.
12. de Rooij SR, Painter RC, Phillips DI, et al. Hypothalamic- pituitary-adrenal axis activity in adults who were prenatally exposed to the Dutch famine. Eur J Endocrinol 2006;155(1):153–60.
13. Lopuhaa CE, Roseboom TJ, Osmond C, et al. Atopy, lung function, and obstructive airways disease after prenatal exposure to famine. Thorax 2000;55(7):555–61.
14. Ravelli AC, van der Meulen JH, Michels RP, et al. Glucose tolerance in adults after prenatal exposure to famine. Lancet 1998;351(9097):173–7.
15. Finkelstein EA, Trogdon JG, Cohen JW, et al. Annual medical spending attributable to obesity: payer-and service-specific estimates. Health Aff (Millwood) 2009;28(5):w822–31.
16. Yang Z, Zhao W, Zhang X, et al. Impact of famine during pregnancy and infancy on health in adulthood. Obes Rev 2008;9(Suppl 1):95–9.
17. Wang Y, Wang X, Kong Y, et al. The Great Chinese Famine leads to shorter and overweight females in Chongqing Chinese population after 50 years. Obesity (Silver Spring) 2010;18(3):588–92.
18. Li Y, Jaddoe VW, Qi L, et al. Exposure to the Chinese famine in early life and the risk of metabolic syndrome in adulthood. Diabetes Care 2011;34(4):1014–8.
19. Li Y, Jaddoe VW, Qi L, et al. Exposure to the Chinese famine in early life and the risk of hypertension in adulthood. J Hypertens 2011;29(6):1085–92.
20. Wang PX, Wang JJ, Lei YX, et al. Impact of fetal and infant exposure to the Chinese Great Famine on the risk of hypertension in adulthood. PLoS One 2012;7(11):e49720.
21. Huang C, Phillips MR, Zhang Y, et al. Malnutrition in early life and adult mental health: evidence from a natural experiment. Soc Sci Med 2013;97:259–66.
22. Huang C, Li Z, Narayan KM, et al. Bigger babies born to women survivors of the 1959-1961 Chinese famine: a puzzle due to survival selection. J Dev Orig Health Dis 2010;1(6):1–7.
23. Cannuscio CC, Weiss EE, Asch DA. The contribution of urban foodways to health disparities. J Urban Health 2010;87(3):381–93.

24. Gordon C, Purciel-Hill M, Ghai NR, et al. Measuring food deserts in New York City's low-income neighborhoods. Health Place 2011;17(2):696–700.
25. Morrissey TW, Jacknowitz A, Vinopal K. Local food prices and their associations with children's weight and food security. Pediatrics 2014;133(3):422–30.
26. Powell LM, Bao Y. Food prices, access to food outlets and child weight. Econ Hum Biol 2009;7(1):64–72.
27. Virdis A, Ghiadoni L, Masi S, et al. Obesity in the childhood: a link to adult hypertension. Curr Pharm Des 2009;15(10):1063–71.
28. Magnussen CG, Koskinen J, Chen W, et al. Pediatric metabolic syndrome predicts adulthood metabolic syndrome, subclinical atherosclerosis, and type 2 diabetes mellitus but is no better than body mass index alone: the Bogalusa Heart Study and the Cardiovascular Risk in Young Finns Study. Circulation 2010;122(16):1604–11.
29. Kelsey MM, Zaepfel A, Bjornstad P, et al. Age-related consequences of childhood obesity. Gerontology 2014;60(3):222–8.
30. Linabery AM, Nahhas RW, Johnson W, et al. Stronger influence of maternal than paternal obesity on infant and early childhood body mass index: the Fels Longitudinal Study. Pediatr Obes 2013;8(3):159–69.
31. Sukalich S, Mingione MJ, Glantz JC. Obstetric outcomes in overweight and obese adolescents. Am J Obstet Gynecol 2006;195(3):851–5.
32. Shaw GM, Wise PH, Mayo J, et al. Maternal prepregnancy body mass index and risk of spontaneous preterm birth. Paediatr Perinat Epidemiol 2014;28(4):302–11.
33. Bonamy AK, Kallen K, Norman M. High blood pressure in 2.5-year-old children born extremely preterm. Pediatrics 2012;129(5):e1199–204.
34. Torloni MR, Betran AP, Daher S, et al. Maternal BMI and preterm birth: a systematic review of the literature with meta-analysis. J Matern Fetal Neonatal Med 2009;22(11):957–70.
35. Behrman RE, Butler AS, editors. Preterm birth: causes, consequences, and prevention. Washington, DC: National Academies Press; 2007. Available at: http://www.ncbi.nlm.nih.gov/books/NBK11362.
36. Roswall J, Karlsson AK, Allvin K, et al. Preschool children born moderately preterm have increased waist circumference at two years of age despite low body mass index. Acta Paediatr 2012;101(11):1175–81.
37. Stokes TA, Holston A, Olsen C, et al. Preterm infants of lower gestational age at birth have greater waist circumference-length ratio and ponderal index at term age than preterm infants of higher gestational ages. J Pediatr 2012;161(4):735–41.e1.
38. Luyckx VA, Bertram JF, Brenner BM, et al. Effect of fetal and child health on kidney development and long-term risk of hypertension and kidney disease. Lancet 2013;382(9888):273–83.
39. Kerkhof GF, Breukhoven PE, Leunissen RW, et al. Does preterm birth influence cardiovascular risk in early adulthood? J Pediatr 2012;161(3):390–6.e1.
40. Kandasamy Y, Smith R, Wright IM, et al. Extra-uterine renal growth in preterm infants: oligonephropathy and prematurity. Pediatr Nephrol 2013;28(9):1791–6.
41. Sutherland MR, Gubhaju L, Moore L, et al. Accelerated maturation and abnormal morphology in the preterm neonatal kidney. J Am Soc Nephrol 2011;22(7):1365–74.
42. McEniery CM, Bolton CE, Fawke J, et al. Cardiovascular consequences of extreme prematurity: the EPICure study. J Hypertens 2011;29(7):1367–73.
43. Wang G, Divall S, Radovick S, et al. Preterm birth and random plasma insulin levels at birth and in early childhood. JAMA 2014;311(6):587–96.

44. Yanni D, Darendeliler F, Bas F, et al. The role of leptin, soluble leptin receptor, adiponectin and visfatin in insulin sensitivity in preterm born children in prepubertal ages. Cytokine 2013;64(1):448–53.

45. Finken MJ, Keijzer-Veen MG, Dekker FW, et al. Preterm birth and later insulin resistance: effects of birth weight and postnatal growth in a population based longitudinal study from birth into adult life. Diabetologia 2006;49(3): 478–85.

46. Casey PH, Bradley RH, Whiteside-Mansell L, et al. Evolution of obesity in a low birth weight cohort. J Perinatol 2012;32(2):91–6.

47. Kerkhof GF, Willemsen RH, Leunissen RW, et al. Health profile of young adults born preterm: negative effects of rapid weight gain in early life. J Clin Endocrinol Metab 2012;97(12):4498–506.

48. Leunissen RW, Kerkhof GF, Stijnen T, et al. Effect of birth size and catch-up growth on adult blood pressure and carotid intima-media thickness. Horm Res Paediatr 2012;77(6):394–401.

49. Ramel SE, Demerath EW, Gray HL, et al. The relationship of poor linear growth velocity with neonatal illness and two-year neurodevelopment in preterm infants. Neonatology 2012;102(1):19–24.

50. Nash A, Dunn M, Asztalos E, et al. Pattern of growth of very low birth weight preterm infants, assessed using the WHO Growth Standards, is associated with neurodevelopment. Appl Physiol Nutr Metab 2011;36(4):562–9.

51. Lucas A, Fewtrell MS, Morley R, et al. Randomized trial of nutrient-enriched formula versus standard formula for postdischarge preterm infants. Pediatrics 2001;108(3):703–11.

52. Neubauer AP, Voss W, Kattner E. Outcome of extremely low birth weight survivors at school age: the influence of perinatal parameters on neurodevelopment. Eur J Pediatr 2008;167(1):87–95.

53. Lucas A, Morley R, Cole TJ. Randomised trial of early diet in preterm babies and later intelligence quotient. BMJ 1998;317(7171):1481–7.

54. Hansen CH, Krych L, Buschard K, et al. A maternal gluten-free diet reduces inflammation and diabetes incidence in the offspring of NOD mice. Diabetes 2014;63(8):2821–32.

55. Isaksson OG, Jansson JO, Sjogren K, et al. Metabolic functions of liver-derived (endocrine) insulin-like growth factor I. Horm Res 2001;55(Suppl 2): 18–21.

56. Guler HP, Zapf J, Froesch ER. Short-term metabolic effects of recombinant human insulin-like growth factor I in healthy adults. N Engl J Med 1987; 317(3):137–40.

57. Moran A, Jacobs DR Jr, Steinberger J, et al. Association between the insulin resistance of puberty and the insulin-like growth factor-I/growth hormone axis. J Clin Endocrinol Metab 2002;87(10):4817–20.

58. Lin HL, Ueng KC, Wang HL, et al. The impact of IGF-I gene polymorphisms on coronary artery disease susceptibility. J Clin Lab Anal 2013;27(2):162–9.

59. Liu SJ, Zhong Y, You XY, et al. Insulin-like growth factor 1 opposes the effects of C-reactive protein on endothelial cell activation. Mol Cell Biochem 2014; 385(1–2):199–205.

60. Brisson BK, Barton ER. Insulin-like growth factor-I E-peptide activity is dependent on the IGF-I receptor. PLoS One 2012;7(9):e45588.

61. Fu Q, Yu X, Callaway CW, et al. Epigenetics: intrauterine growth retardation (IUGR) modifies the histone code along the rat hepatic IGF-1 gene. FASEB J 2009;23(8):2438–49.

62. Agoudemos M, Reinking BE, Koppenhafer SL, et al. Programming of adult cardiovascular disease following exposure to late-gestation hyperglycemia. Neonatology 2011;100(2):198–205.
63. Zinkhan EK, Fu Q, Wang Y, et al. Maternal hyperglycemia disrupts histone 3 lysine 36 trimethylation of the IGF-1 gene. J Nutr Metab 2012;2012:930364.
64. Smythies J, Edelstein L, Ramachandran V. Molecular mechanisms for the inheritance of acquired characteristics-exosomes, microRNA shuttling, fear and stress: Lamarck resurrected? Front Genet 2014;5:133.
65. Stuwe E, Toth KF, Aravin AA. Small but sturdy: small RNAs in cellular memory and epigenetics. Genes Dev 2014;28(5):423–31.
66. Peschansky VJ, Wahlestedt C. Non-coding RNAs as direct and indirect modulators of epigenetic regulation. Epigenetics 2014;9(1):3–12.
67. Bhan A, Mandal SS. Long noncoding RNAs: emerging stars in gene regulation, epigenetics and human disease. ChemMedChem 2014;9(9):1932–56 [Epub ahead of print].
68. Lander ES, Linton LM, Birren B, et al. Initial sequencing and analysis of the human genome. Nature 2001;409(6822):860–921.

Comparative Effectiveness and Practice Variation in Neonatal Care

Joanne Lagatta, MD, MS[a],*, Michael Uhing, MD[a],
Julie Panepinto, MD, MSPH[a,b]

KEYWORDS

- Comparative effectiveness • Neonatology • Clinical research methods

KEY POINTS

- Components of comparative effectiveness research (CER) include comparisons of alternative standards of care, evaluating outcomes important to individuals, and incorporating varied settings and participants.
- Neonatal clinical research contains examples of CER with strengths in clinical trials and metaanalyses comparing alternative standards of care.
- Future work in neonatal CER could focus on patient-centered outcomes in both prospective and retrospective studies.

INTRODUCTION

There is increasing discussion in medical literature and among grant funding agencies about the need for comparative effectiveness research (CER). CER is defined by the Institute of Medicine as "the generation and synthesis of evidence that compares the benefits and harms of alternative methods to prevent, diagnose, treat, and monitor a clinical condition or to improve the delivery of care."[1] At first glance, this definition is broad enough that it potentially encompasses all types of clinical research, because the prevention, diagnosis, and treatment of illness is the ultimate goal of any clinical research team. In fact, neonatal clinical research literature already contains many examples of research that fit into the broad framework of CER. This article describes the main types of CER research methods using recent examples from existing neonatology literature, and highlights challenges in conducting CER specific to neonatal research.

Disclosures: None.
[a] Department of Pediatrics, Medical College of Wisconsin, 999 North 92nd Street, Suite C410, Milwaukee, WI 53226, USA; [b] Center for Clinical Effectiveness Research, Department of Pediatrics, Medical College of Wisconsin, 8701 Watertown Plank Road, Milwaukee, WI 53226, USA
* Corresponding author.
E-mail address: jlagatta@mcw.edu

Clin Perinatol 41 (2014) 833–845
http://dx.doi.org/10.1016/j.clp.2014.08.007
0095-5108/14/$ – see front matter © 2014 Elsevier Inc. All rights reserved.
perinatology.theclinics.com

WHAT IS COMPARATIVE EFFECTIVENESS RESEARCH?

The focus of CER is to assist patients, clinicians, and policymakers in making informed decisions to improve health care. Although a variety of research methods can be used to accomplish these goals, 4 key elements of CER have been identified.

Direct Comparison of Potential Alternative Standards of Care

In contrast with an efficacy trial of a novel intervention versus a placebo, an effectiveness study compares the outcome of at least 2 existing interventions that a patient or clinician could reasonably choose in day-to-day clinical practice. Specifically, an effectiveness study aims to determine if an intervention does work, whereas a traditional efficacy study aims to determine if it can work.[2]

Evaluating a Broad Array of Health-related Outcomes that Are Important to Individuals

Although there is often overlap, CER targets individual decision making by the patient or clinician, whereas public health decision making focuses on a population. CER studies assess both benefits and harms of interventions, and the measurement of clinical outcomes (as opposed to surrogate markers) that are important to decision-makers such as survival, daily functioning, symptoms, and health-related quality of life.

Incorporating a Wide Variety of Settings and Participants

In contrast with carefully controlled clinical trials evaluating a select group of patients, CER is meant to focus on a typical patient in a typical practice setting. In addition to estimating an average treatment effect across an entire study population, a goal of CER is to study heterogeneous effects within clinically relevant subgroups to help predict which individuals most benefit from treatment.[3]

Prioritizing Topics of Interest to Stakeholders

Involvement from patients, clinicians, policymakers, and other relevant participants in health care delivery is seen as key to guiding investment in research that reflects the priorities of the public.

HOW DOES COMPARATIVE EFFECTIVENESS RESEARCH RELATE TO QUALITY IMPROVEMENT?

Neonatal research has documented numerous examples of variation in neonatal care practices, such as use of inotropic agents,[4] use of home oxygen and diuretics for infants with bronchopulmonary dysplasia,[5,6] and antenatal counseling for preterm infants.[7] Likewise, there are numerous examples of variation in important clinical outcomes, such as mortality for extremely preterm infants,[8] bronchopulmonary dysplasia,[9] and length of hospital stay.[10] Quality improvement efforts focus on reducing variation in care and implementing best process and practice within individual neonatal intensive care units (NICUs) via education, monitoring changes in care and outcome, and benchmarking of outcomes against national standards.[11] For example, there have been multiple quality improvement efforts to reduce rates of bloodstream infections in the NICU in which multicenter groups work collaboratively to standardize and implement best practices identified through review of care at the centers with the lowest reported rates of bloodstream infections.[12–14]

CER, on the other hand, can be thought of as research directed at identifying best practices among the wide variation present in medical care. This is especially true when there are multiple treatments or processes available to treat the same condition.

In contrast to the quality improvement examples cited, a CER study on preventing bloodstream infection would compare outcomes after use of differing handwashing agents, types of catheters, or approaches to line placement, while using similar risk adjustment measures that are used for benchmarking outcomes in quality reporting.[11,15,16] For an outcome that is clearly positive or negative, such as line infection rates, the goal of CER is to provide evidence that can be implemented to optimize outcomes, and not necessarily directed at standardizing practice.

For outcomes in which family or clinician preferences vary, or optimal treatments differ by patient subgroup, a goal of CER is to provide enough evidence to allow clinicians and families to tailor their approach to achieve the outcomes that are best for the patient. In neonatology, tailored approaches to care based on parent preferences are discussed most commonly in the context of resuscitation for extremely preterm infants,[17] but could be applied to other medical decision making as well. For example, a NICU that allows more home nasogastric feedings, places gastrostomy tubes earlier, or prescribes home oxygen or apnea monitors more readily might have a shorter length of stay, but this shorter length of stay is not necessarily preferable to a family with more limited home resources. This is the rationale behind measuring a broad array of outcomes for any given intervention, as well as focusing on outcomes that are directly interpretable to families.

STUDY DESIGNS FOR COMPARATIVE EFFECTIVENESS RESEARCH

Any traditional clinical study design can be used to answer research questions that can be categorized as CER. Neonatal literature contains examples that highlight CER principles across categories of study designs and data sources. This article highlights 3 major categories: Randomized controlled trials (RCT), systematic reviews of existing literature, and observational studies. These examples are not meant as an exhaustive review of the literature, but rather to highlight existing neonatal research as examples of CER.

Randomized, Controlled Trials

RCTs are traditionally designed to evaluate the efficacy of therapies in a specific population of subjects, analyzing an intervention by comparing randomized groups to receive either a treatment or a blinded placebo under standardized conditions. RCTs are also used to determine effectiveness by comparing treatments or procedures. Successful randomization and blinding minimizes confounding, and is the reason that RCTs are considered the gold standard of clinical research.

The media controversy after the SUPPORT trial makes it seem as though effectiveness trials in neonatology are new,[18] but numerous neonatal RCTs are examples of effectiveness trials. Although comparisons of oxygen saturation targets are the most publicized recent clinical trials in this category,[19–21] many other studies fit this description. Trials comparing modes of ventilation for preterm infants can be considered comparative effectiveness trials, because there could be no ethical or practical placebo group receiving no respiratory support. Examples include prophylactic intubation and surfactant versus nasal continuous positive airway pressure (NCPAP) at resuscitation, or noninvasive ventilation comparisons, such as synchronized nasal intermittent positive pressure ventilation versus NCPAP or high-flow nasal cannula versus NCPAP.[22–24] Even in evaluations of drug therapies, neonatal literature has relevant examples, such as comparisons of bevacizumab versus laser therapy for retinopathy of prematurity,[25] dopamine versus epinephrine for hypotension,[26] and high versus low amino acid levels in parenteral nutrition for extremely low birth weight infants.[27] Developing new therapies and testing them against a placebo is obviously crucial to major progress in care for critically ill infants; initial evaluations of surfactant and antenatal steroids led to enormous improvements in neonatal mortality and morbidity.[28,29] However, effectiveness trials such as optimizing the timing and preparation of surfactant and antenatal steroids,[30–32] and improving key components of neonatal intensive care management such as ventilation, blood pressure, and nutritional support, are needed to continue the significant improvements in mortality and morbidity seen since 2000.[33,34]

RCTs have limitations in the context of CER, which focuses on identifying the best treatment of available options individualized to relevant subgroups. "Standardized conditions" may have differing effects on the generalizability of trial results to a broader population. A larger sample size is often required to power a study comparing 2 treatment outcomes than to compare a single treatment to placebo, which makes enrollment more difficult. Inclusion criteria and the consent process may result in a different set of baseline characteristics between the trial cohort and the general population. This was noted most recently during enrollment for the SUPPORT trial, which noted differences between enrolled and nonenrolled patients by receipt of prenatal antibiotics, antenatal steroids, delivery room interventions, and outcomes including mortality, bronchopulmonary dysplasia (BPD) and severe intraventricular hemorrhage.[35,36] As a result, interpreting the study findings of higher mortality in the lower oxygen saturation target group has been difficult, because both groups had lower mortality than nonenrolled patients.[21,37,38] Measuring the effect of an intervention versus a placebo may require changes to "standard care" by altering the timing of the primary intervention and its associated care. Placebo effects may change the outcome in either a treatment or a control group. The process of selecting measurable outcome criteria with a limited sample size may or may not result in trial results that reflect the key factors used by a clinician in weighing treatment options.[39]

One criticism of RCTs in CER is that enrolled patients may be a narrow group without comorbidities. In neonatology, clinical trials often enroll patients in a stratified fashion based on gestational age (for diseases of prematurity) rather than excluding patients with comorbid conditions. Gestational age or birth weight groups are often the clinically relevant subgroup analysis. This was demonstrated in initial comparisons of prophylactic surfactant versus early NCPAP, which suggested that infants born at earlier gestational ages treated with early NCPAP may have higher incidence of pneumothorax,[40] which prompted more recent studies.[24]

Another potential limitation of RCTs for the purposes of CER is the site of care. Most patients in RCTs are treated in academic medical centers, and may have different baseline characteristics than patients treated in other settings. This may be less of an issue in neonatology than in other areas of medicine, such as primary care, because patients with high-risk conditions such as extreme prematurity or conditions requiring mechanical ventilation or surgical intervention are concentrated in level III/IV units. Because the enrollment criteria for many RCTs are based on gestational age, the study populations in academic and nonacademic centers are often comparable.[33,41] For patients with uncommon conditions requiring multiple subspecialty care, the only (and therefore typical practice environment) is an academic center. Although most RCTs are conducted at academic-affiliated centers, the Vermont Oxford Network has conducted trials that enroll patients within private centers, such as comparisons of ventilatory and heat loss prevention strategies during resuscitation of preterm infants.[30,42] For patients who do not require level III care, it would be of interest to compare outcomes for infants treated in lower acuity centers to be able to generalize results to the setting under which most of those infants are treated. As with other fields of medicine, most lower acuity centers do not have the infrastructure or the volume to support prospective clinical trials.

Systematic Review and Metaanalysis

Systematic reviews and metaanalyses are overlapping methods of evaluating existing evidence. Systematic reviews use prespecified search methods to evaluate and synthesize eligible studies on a specific clinical question. Metaanalysis refers to a quantitative re-analysis of pooled data from individual studies.[43] These techniques allow results from multiple independent studies to be combined into a quantitative estimate of effect, such as combining results of multiple RCTs or epidemiologic studies. Neonatology has a strong history of systematic review, beginning with the Oxford Database of Perinatal Trials in the 1980s and continuing as the Cochrane Neonatal Group.[44,45] Numerous systematic reviews and metaanalyses are updated through the Cochrane Neonatal Reviews, which serve different goals within the framework of CER.[46,47] Many analyze direct comparisons of alternative potentially standard therapies, such as dopamine versus dobutamine for hypotensive preterm infants.[48] In addition, the synthesis of multiple similar studies can increase power to detect a treatment effect when not all individual studies have found statistical significance. They are advantageous in studying rare or adverse events, and can also highlight effects in relevant subgroups, which may be too small in single RCTs. The Cochrane review of ibuprofen for the treatment of patent ductus arteriosus provides an example of several of these advantages. Treatment with ibuprofen versus indomethacin showed equivalent effectiveness in patent ductus arteriosus closure, but less risk of necrotizing enterocolitis in pooled estimates, although no single trial showed a significant difference.[49] Although not strictly CER because it reviewed comparisons of an intervention with placebo, a significant example of neonatal research metaanalysis showing subgroup benefits was in the use of antenatal corticosteroids for prevention of respiratory distress syndrome. Crowley identified RDS reduction in infants less than 31 weeks by metaanalysis, although outcomes from individual studies were not significant.[50] Systematic reviews and metaanalyses can also report observational studies, although this is less common owing to differences in study design that limit pooled estimates.[51]

Observational Study Design in Comparative Effectiveness Research

The recent funding availability for CER has resulted in increased attention to observational studies. This raises controversy because of bias limitations inherent in observational study design. One of the most common problems with nonrandomized studies is the uneven distribution of unmeasured confounders. Another major issue is confounding by indication, meaning that the patients believed most likely to benefit from a treatment are the ones most likely to receive it, which exaggerates the actual treatment effect in the analysis. Time frames of the study cohort can present difficulties, with new entrants and attrition. Finally, practice and policy changes that occur during data collection can affect analysis. The data source can affect applicability to other settings, such as the characteristics of that population, local practice patterns, and resource availability.[52] Although quantitative methods to minimize the effect of bias are beyond the scope of this paper, the Institute of Medicine has recommended explicit attention to methodologic considerations of observational study design.[1,53]

Despite these limitations, observational studies provide a mechanism for answering clinical questions for which RCTs are not feasible for a variety of reasons. Observational studies offer potential benefit for clinical questions in which the required sample size would be prohibitive.[54] This could include evaluations of adverse events, such as comparing the effect of differing lengths of initial antibiotic therapy on subsequent development of necrotizing enterocolitis.[55] Studies have found that confounding by indication is less problematic for evaluating unanticipated harms than for evaluating beneficial effects.[47] The large number of patients available for observational studies also facilitates studies of relatively rare diseases, such as the effect of antifungal therapy in extremely low birth weight infants with invasive candidiasis.[56] It can be useful in comparing the effects of similar therapies for which the sample size to detect treatment differences may be prohibitive, such as comparing types of antenatal corticosteroids on subsequent hearing and neurodevelopmental impairment.[57] Observational studies are also important when randomization is not feasible owing to ethical considerations, or practical issues related to the study question at hand, such as questions of treatment adherence or usage outside of trials, such as during evaluation of total body cooling for hypoxic ischemic encephalopathy,[58] or geographic or demographic effects on treatment results.[54] Finally, observational studies, particularly those using already existing data, are far less expensive and time consuming than RCTs. For clinical questions where an RCT would be cost or time prohibitive, observational data represent an alternative to expedite advancing the evidence basis for clinical decision making.[54]

Data Sources for Observational Study Design

Observational studies can be conducted as a prospective cohort, as was done in comparing antihypotensive therapies for extremely preterm infants.[59] In this example, an observational design was chosen over an RCT owing to lack of physician equipoise in treating hypotension, wide practice variability complicating identification of inclusion and exclusion criteria, and the potential for enrollment or selection bias when enrolling a vulnerable patient population shortly after birth.[35,59] More commonly, to obtain the sample size that confers an advantage to observational studies, they can be accomplished via secondary analysis of already collected data. Data sources include disease registries, electronic health records data, and administrative data.

Very low birth weight registries such as the National Institute of Child Health and Human Development Neonatal Research Network and Vermont Oxford Network, or disease registries such as the Extracorporeal Life Support Organization database and the Congenital Diaphragmatic Hernia Study Group, are gathered via primary data abstraction of prespecified data elements. Benefits to this approach include trained abstractors, ongoing quality assurance regarding data collection, and discrete coded variables that relate to the disease of interest. Limitations to this approach include lack of granularity of the data fields, differences in definitions between data sources, and differences in the way that detailed individual data (eg, serial laboratory values) are aggregated into discrete variables. For example, the Vermont Oxford Network collects information on an infant's respiratory support at 36 weeks postmenstrual age. This type of data does then not allow comparison of therapies that require the need to discriminate between the differences in respiratory requirements that may be relevant only before or after this particular data point.

Following the US government meaningful use incentives for use of electronic health records systems, chart review for clinical research is rapidly becoming a more viable large-scale option.[60] Secondary analyses of clinical data can be more easily facilitated in single centers as well as in emerging collaborative arrangements.[61] Detailed clinical data are available, although accurate abstraction depends on consistency in documenting the start and resolution of illnesses, and limiting diagnostic variability between centers for common illnesses such as apnea.[62,63] In addition to difficulties inherent in obtaining research data from a clinical chart, challenges to study design include identification of interventions and outcomes, a study population and follow-up interval, and a plan for active versus passive data capture.[64] One of the most established sources of secondary analysis using medical records data in neonatology comes from the Pediatrix Medical Group, whose Clinical Data Warehouse automatically facilitates export of de-identified, discrete data elements from patient charts.[65] Several comparative effectiveness studies have come from this group, including comparisons of adverse events after differing preparations of surfactant[32] and different empiric antibiotic regimens.[66]

In many fields of medicine, administrative data taken from billing claims are commonly used for CER. Compared with patient registry or electronic health record data, these data sources are more likely to be limited by lack of completeness of the listed diagnoses. Acute and particularly surgical conditions are more likely to be coded appropriately. Neonatology, as in many other fields, has some discrepancies between clinical diagnoses and coding terminology for common diseases, such as bronchopulmonary dysplasia and respiratory distress syndrome, which limits the clinical detail needed to design CER studies.[67] Public use data files, such the National Inpatient Sample and its associated Kids Inpatient Database available from the Agency for Healthcare Research and Quality, have similar limitations in diagnosis availability because they are derived from billing data. However, billing files are a potential source of post-NICU follow-up data on rehospitalizations or costs of outpatient care, which could provide useful outcome measures. Linked data sets that pair the longitudinal data collection of billing data with the appropriate amount of neonatal coding accuracy, such as the California Perinatal Quality Care Collaborative,[68] the Kaiser Permanente Neonatal Minimum Data Set,[69] or the Children's Hospitals Association Neonatal Database,[63] could be used to conduct this type of research.

CHALLENGES IN NEONATAL COMPARATIVE EFFECTIVENESS RESEARCH
Comparing Treatment with Placebo: Efficacy Versus Effectiveness

Perhaps more commonly than in other clinical fields of medicine, for many diseases of prematurity, a potential "standard of care" is observation without intervention. There are no noted differences in mortality or morbidity whether a hypotensive extremely low birth weight infant with reasonable end-organ perfusion receives a vasopressor or clinical observation alone.[59] Thus, in some circumstances, comparing an intervention with observation alone could be considered an effectiveness study. Historically, some treatments that were adopted as standard practice without controlled trials, such as bicarbonate for metabolic acidosis, turned out to be worse than placebo.[70] Although there are other instances in medicine where observation alone is a viable treatment option (early stage prostate cancer), very few other specialties see an individual patient grow 5- to 7-fold over the course of a single hospitalization, making observation without intervention potentially a more relevant therapeutic option in neonatology than in other fields.

Defining and Measuring Patient-Centered Outcomes

The Institute of Medicine has identified "patient-centered outcomes" as outcomes that are directly relevant to stakeholders, rather than proxy measures. Depending on the research question, a stakeholder could be a patient or parent, a practicing clinician, or a health system administrator developing practice standards. In outlining standards for patient-centered research, the Patient Centered Outcomes Research Institute encourages providing information supporting the selection of outcomes as clinically meaningful, such as input from patients and their families.

Deciding which stakeholder's perspective drives outcome selection makes a difference in study design. For example, leaders of a NICU wishing for their hospital to compare favorably in outcomes reporting across the Vermont Oxford Network or their multi-unit practice group may be interested in strategies to reduce their unit's rate of BPD. However, families may be less concerned about whether their infant requires oxygen at 36 weeks' postmenstrual age, versus whether their infant requires home oxygen at discharge or requires rehospitalization after leaving the NICU. When a reduction in a proximal morbidity such as BPD results in a better long-term health outcome, all stakeholders are mutually satisfied. However, a recent publication from the SUPPORT trial highlights the fact that proximal and distal outcomes are not necessarily equivalent: The study found no difference in the primary composite outcome of death or bronchopulmonary dysplasia, but significant differences in more functional outcomes, such as wheezing.[71] In this case, it seems straightforward for a clinician to choose the treatment option that results in better patient outcomes. But functional outcomes such as wheezing, or even health care utilization measures such as readmissions after NICU discharge, are more variably defined and reported than proximal morbidities such as BPD.[72] Obtaining consensus on best treatment strategies based on patient-centered outcomes requires more effort in selecting and defining outcomes that matter to a broader range of stakeholders.

In general, designing and powering studies that measure patient-centered outcomes in neonatal CER will continue to be a challenge. RCTs are often powered for a set of primary endpoints, such as death or BPD, and measure multiple secondary endpoints, such as respiratory symptoms. Interpreting results of multiple secondary outcomes is difficult when adjusting for multiple comparisons. Involving families explicitly in study design could provide additional insights into selection of outcomes from the multiple available options. In the United Kingdom, many health research funding bodies require patient involvement in study design. Consumer involvement has been reported in convincing funders of study relevance, developing clear and relevant study questions and outcomes, providing insights into patients' views of trial logistics, advising on recruitment, and developing patient information materials.[73,74] Neonatal research has noted differences in parent and clinician perspectives about neonatal treatments for extremely preterm infants and infants with trisomy 13 and 18[75,76]; differing perspectives are also likely present and insightful for decision making that involves less life-and-death situations.

If the large sample size available for observational studies could facilitate evaluation of multiple outcomes, it could be easier to evaluate enough patient-centered outcomes to appeal to multiple stakeholders. Currently, many observational data sources lack discrete data on patient-centered outcomes besides mortality and length of stay. Measuring symptoms such as pain and fatigue rather than laboratory values or definitions (BPD) presents unique issues in a very young pediatric population because they require either clinician assessment or parent report, and there are no validated multidomain quality of life measures for infants under 1 month of age. Two-year neurodevelopmental assessments are often used as proxy measures for long-term functioning, although the correlation between 2-year assessments and later functioning is imperfect.[77] There are many longitudinal studies of quality of life in survivors of preterm birth,[78] but none have been used yet for CER. However, this could be an area for future development in neonatal patient-centered outcomes research. Nurses already record discrete pain scores, and therapists perform standardized motor assessments, which are part of the health record and could be abstracted for observational research.[79] For infants older than 1 month of age there are validated tools for infants and young children, as well as for caregivers related to their child's illness.[80,81] In adult populations with wider use of patient-reported outcome measures, such as the National Institutes of Health-supported Patient-reported Outcomes Measurement Information System (PROMIS) measures, there are increasing efforts to embed patient-reported outcomes assessments into the electronic health record for clinical and research purposes.[82,83] There is a need for more work on defining key patient-centered measures for infants in the NICU and in postdischarge follow-up to help focus efforts in neonatal CER.

SUMMARY

CER is a relatively new focus area that encompasses principles of clinical research that to some extent have been present in neonatal research for some time. Identifying best practices within the wide variation of NICU care can enable clinicians and quality improvement efforts to either standardize care across groups, or tailor efforts to specific patients that benefit from particular approaches. This increased emphasis on evidence to direct decision making ties in well with neonatology's already strong efforts in quality improvement, systematic reviews, patient registries and multicenter efforts. Many data sources exist with the potential to increase CER efforts within neonatology. Future work is needed to define patient-centered outcomes to focus prospective clinical studies, and embed appropriate tools within observational data to facilitate analysis of patient-centered outcomes.

REFERENCES

1. Sox HC, Greenfield S. Comparative effectiveness research: a report from the Institute of Medicine. Ann Intern Med 2009;151:203–5.
2. Luce BR, Drummond M, Jonsson B, et al. EBM, HTA, and CER: clearing the confusion. Milbank Q 2010;88:256–76.
3. Varadhan R, Segal JB, Boyd CM, et al. A framework for the analysis of heterogeneity of treatment effect in patient-centered outcomes research. J Clin Epidemiol 2013;66:818–25.
4. Wong J, Shah PS, Yoon EW, et al. Inotrope use among extremely preterm infants in Canadian neonatal intensive care units: variation and outcomes. Am J Perinatol 2014. [Epub ahead of print].
5. Lagatta J, Clark R, Spitzer A. Clinical predictors and institutional variation in home oxygen use in preterm infants. J Pediatr 2012;160:232–8.
6. Slaughter JL, Stenger MR, Reagan PB. Variation in the use of diuretic therapy for infants with bronchopulmonary dysplasia. Pediatrics 2013;131:716–23.
7. Mehrotra A, Lagatta J, Simpson P, et al. Variations among US hospitals in counseling practices regarding prematurely born infants. J Perinatol 2013;33:509–13.
8. Alleman BW, Bell EF, Li L, et al. Individual and center-level factors affecting mortality among extremely low birth weight infants. Pediatrics 2013;132:e175–84.
9. Ambalavanan N, Walsh M, Bobashev G, et al. Intercenter differences in bronchopulmonary dysplasia or death among very low birth weight infants. Pediatrics 2011;127:e106–16.
10. Murthy K, Dykes FD, Padula MA, et al. The Children's Hospitals neonatal database: an overview of patient complexity, outcomes and variation in care. J Perinatol 2014;34(8):582–6.
11. Horbar JD. The Vermont Oxford Network: evidence-based quality improvement for neonatology. Pediatrics 1999;103:350–9.

12. Schulman J, Stricof R, Stevens TP, et al. Statewide NICU central-line-associated bloodstream infection rates decline after bundles and checklists. Pediatrics 2011;127:436–44.
13. Aly H, Herson V, Duncan A, et al. Is bloodstream infection preventable among premature infants? A tale of two cities. Pediatrics 2005;115:1513–8.
14. Kilbride HW, Wirtschafter DD, Powers RJ, et al. Implementation of evidence-based potentially better practices to decrease nosocomial infections. Pediatrics 2003;111:e519–33.
15. Rogowski JA, Horbar JD, Staiger DO, et al. Indirect vs direct hospital quality indicators for very low-birth-weight infants. JAMA 2004;291:202–9.
16. Richardson D, Tarnow-Mordi WO, Lee SK. Risk adjustment for quality improvement. Pediatrics 1999;103:255–65.
17. Mercurio MR. Parental authority, patient's best interest and refusal of resuscitation at borderline gestational age. J Perinatol 2006;26:452–7.
18. Lantos JD. Learning the right lessons from the SUPPORT study controversy. Arch Dis Child Fetal Neonatal Ed 2014;99:F4–5.
19. Group BIUKC, Group BIAC, Group BINZC, et al. Oxygen saturation and outcomes in preterm infants. N Engl J Med 2013;368:2094–104.
20. Schmidt B, Whyte RK, Asztalos EV, et al. Effects of targeting higher vs lower arterial oxygen saturations on death or disability in extremely preterm infants: a randomized clinical trial. JAMA 2013;309:2111–20.
21. SUPPORT Study Group of the Eunice Kennedy Shriver NICHD Neonatal Research Network, Carlo WA, Finer NN, Walsh MC, et al. Target ranges of oxygen saturation in extremely preterm infants. N Engl J Med 2010;362:1959–69.
22. Bhandari V, Finer NN, Ehrenkranz RA, et al. Synchronized nasal intermittent positive-pressure ventilation and neonatal outcomes. Pediatrics 2009;124:517–26.
23. Yoder BA, Stoddard RA, Li M, et al. Heated, humidified high-flow nasal cannula versus nasal CPAP for respiratory support in neonates. Pediatrics 2013;131:e1482–90.
24. Early CPAP versus surfactant in extremely preterm infants. N Engl J Med 2010;362:1970–9.
25. Mintz-Hittner HA, Kennedy KA, Chuang AZ. Efficacy of intravitreal bevacizumab for stage 3+ retinopathy of prematurity. N Engl J Med 2011;364:603–15.
26. Valverde E, Pellicer A, Madero R, et al. Dopamine versus epinephrine for cardiovascular support in low birth weight infants: analysis of systemic effects and neonatal clinical outcomes. Pediatrics 2006;117:e1213–22.
27. Burattini I, Bellagamba MP, Spagnoli C, et al. Targeting 2.5 versus 4 g/kg/day of amino acids for extremely low birth weight infants: a randomized clinical trial. J Pediatr 2013;163:1278–82.e1.
28. Seger N, Soll R. Animal derived surfactant extract for treatment of respiratory distress syndrome. Cochrane Database Syst Rev 2009;(2):CD007836.
29. Roberts D, Dalziel S. Antenatal corticosteroids for accelerating fetal lung maturation for women at risk of preterm birth. Cochrane Database Syst Rev 2006;(3):CD004454.
30. Dunn MS, Kaempf J, de Klerk A, et al. Randomized trial comparing 3 approaches to the initial respiratory management of preterm neonates. Pediatrics 2011;128:e1069–76.
31. Guinn DA, Atkinson MW, Sullivan L, et al. Single vs weekly courses of antenatal corticosteroids for women at risk of preterm delivery: a randomized controlled trial. JAMA 2001;286:1581–7.

32. Trembath A, Hornik CP, Clark R, et al. Comparative effectiveness of surfactant preparations in premature infants. J Pediatr 2013;163:955–60.e1.
33. Horbar JD, Carpenter JH, Badger GJ, et al. Mortality and neonatal morbidity among infants 501 to 1500 grams from 2000 to 2009. Pediatrics 2012;129: 1019–26.
34. Fanaroff AA, Stoll BJ, Wright LL, et al. Trends in neonatal morbidity and mortality for very low birthweight infants. Am J Obstet Gynecol 2007;196:147.e1-8.
35. Rich W, Finer NN, Gantz MG, et al. Enrollment of extremely low birth weight infants in a clinical research study may not be representative. Pediatrics 2012;129:480–4.
36. Rich WD, Auten KJ, Gantz MG, et al. Antenatal consent in the SUPPORT trial: challenges, costs, and representative enrollment. Pediatrics 2010;126:e215–21.
37. Bancalari E, Claure N. Oxygenation targets and outcomes in premature infants. JAMA 2013;309:2161–2.
38. Polin RA, Bateman D. Oxygen-saturation targets in preterm infants. N Engl J Med 2013;368:2141–2.
39. Schwartz D, Lellouch J. Explanatory and pragmatic attitudes in therapeutical trials. J Clin Epidemiol 2009;62:499–505.
40. Morley CJ, Davis PG, Doyle LW, et al. Nasal CPAP or intubation at birth for very preterm infants. N Engl J Med 2008;358:700–8.
41. Stoll BJ, Hansen NI, Bell EF, et al. Neonatal outcomes of extremely preterm infants from the NICHD neonatal research network. Pediatrics 2010;126:443–56.
42. Vohra S, Reilly M, Rac VE, et al. Study protocol for multicentre randomized controlled trial of HeLP (Heat loss prevention) in the delivery room. Contemp Clin Trials 2013;36:54–60.
43. Akobeng AK. Understanding systematic reviews and meta-analysis. Arch Dis Child 2005;90:845–8.
44. Chalmers I, Hetherington J, Newdick M, et al. The Oxford database of perinatal trials: developing a register of published reports of controlled trials. Control Clin Trials 1986;7:306–24.
45. Cochrane Neonatal Group. Available at: http://neonatal.cochrane.org/.
46. Normand SL. Meta-analysis: formulating, evaluating, combining, and reporting. Stat Med 1999;18:321–59.
47. Chou R, Helfand M. Challenges in systematic reviews that assess treatment harms. Ann Intern Med 2005;142:1090–9.
48. Subhedar NV, Shaw NJ. Dopamine versus dobutamine for hypotensive preterm infants. Cochrane Database Syst Rev 2003;(3):CD001242.
49. Ohlsson A, Walia R, Shah SS. Ibuprofen for the treatment of patent ductus arteriosus in preterm and/or low birth weight infants. Cochrane Database Syst Rev 2013;(4):CD003481.
50. Crowley P. Prophylactic corticosteroids for preterm birth. Cochrane Database Syst Rev 2006;(2):CD000065.
51. Stroup DF, Berlin JA, Morton SC, et al. Meta-analysis of observational studies in epidemiology: a proposal for reporting. meta-analysis of observational studies in epidemiology (MOOSE) group. JAMA 2000;283:2008–12.
52. Cox E, Martin BC, Van Staa T, et al. Good research practices for comparative effectiveness research: approaches to mitigate bias and confounding in the design of nonrandomized studies of treatment effects using secondary data sources: the international society for pharmacoeconomics and outcomes research good research practices for retrospective database analysis task force report—part II. Value Health 2009;12:1053–61.

53. Helfand M, Tunis S, Whitlock EP, et al. A CTSA agenda to advance methods for comparative effectiveness research. Clin Transl Sci 2011;4:188–98.

54. Dreyer NA, Tunis SR, Berger M, et al. Why observational studies should be among the tools used in comparative effectiveness research. Health Aff (Millwood) 2010;29:1818–25.

55. Cotten CM, Taylor S, Stoll B, et al. Prolonged duration of initial empirical antibiotic treatment is associated with increased rates of necrotizing enterocolitis and death for extremely low birth weight infants. Pediatrics 2009;123:58–66.

56. Greenberg RG, Benjamin DK Jr, Gantz MG, et al. Empiric antifungal therapy and outcomes in extremely low birth weight infants with invasive candidiasis. J Pediatr 2012;161:264–9.e2.

57. Lee BH, Stoll BJ, McDonald SA, et al. Neurodevelopmental outcomes of extremely low birth weight infants exposed prenatally to dexamethasone versus betamethasone. Pediatrics 2008;121:289–96.

58. Azzopardi D, Strohm B, Edwards AD, et al. Treatment of asphyxiated newborns with moderate hypothermia in routine clinical practice: how cooling is managed in the UK outside a clinical trial. Arch Dis Child Fetal Neonatal Ed 2009;94: F260–4.

59. Batton B, Li L, Newman NS, et al. Use of antihypotensive therapies in extremely preterm infants. Pediatrics 2013;131:e1865–73.

60. Blumenthal D, Tavenner M. The "meaningful use" regulation for electronic health records. N Engl J Med 2010;363:501–4.

61. Narus SP, Srivastava R, Gouripeddi R, et al. Federating clinical data from six pediatric hospitals: process and initial results from the PHIS+ Consortium. AMIA Annu Symp Proc 2011;2011:994–1003.

62. Eichenwald EC, Zupancic JA, Mao WY, et al. Variation in diagnosis of apnea in moderately preterm infants predicts length of stay. Pediatrics 2011;127:e53–8.

63. Pallotto EK, Hunt PG, Dykes FD, et al. Topics in neonatal informatics: infants and data in the electronic health record era. Neoreviews 2013;14:e57–62.

64. Berger ML, Mamdani M, Atkins D, et al. Good research practices for comparative effectiveness research: defining, reporting and interpreting nonrandomized studies of treatment effects using secondary data sources: the ISPOR good research practices for retrospective database analysis task force report—part I. Value Health 2009;12:1044–52.

65. Spitzer AR, Ellsbury DL, Handler D, et al. The Pediatrix baby steps data warehouse and the Pediatrix quality steps improvement project system–tools for "meaningful use" in continuous quality improvement. Clin Perinatol 2010;37: 49–70.

66. Clark RH, Bloom BT, Spitzer AR, et al. Empiric use of ampicillin and cefotaxime, compared with ampicillin and gentamicin, for neonates at risk for sepsis is associated with an increased risk of neonatal death. Pediatrics 2006;117:67–74.

67. Pallotto EK, Hunt PG, Reber K, et al. Topics in neonatal informatics: standardizing diagnoses in neonatology: bronchopulmonary dysplasia and beyond. Neoreviews 2012;13:e577–82.

68. Gould JB. The role of regional collaboratives: the California perinatal quality care collaborative model. Clin Perinatol 2010;37:71–86.

69. Escobar GJ, Fischer A, Kremers R, et al. Rapid retrieval of neonatal outcomes data: the Kaiser Permanente neonatal minimum data set. Qual Manag Health Care 1997;5:19–33.

70. Aschner JL, Poland RL. Sodium bicarbonate: basically useless therapy. Pediatrics 2008;122:831–5.

71. Stevens TP, Finer NN, Carlo WA, et al. Respiratory outcomes of the surfactant positive pressure and oximetry randomized trial (SUPPORT). J Pediatr 2014; 165(2):240–9.e4.
72. Jobe AH, Bancalari E. Bronchopulmonary dysplasia. Am J Respir Crit Care Med 2001;163:1723–9.
73. Hanley B, Truesdale A, King A, et al. Involving consumers in designing, conducting, and interpreting randomised controlled trials: questionnaire survey. BMJ 2001;322:519–23.
74. Evans BA, Bedson E, Bell P, et al. Involving service users in trials: developing a standard operating procedure. Trials 2013;14:219.
75. Janvier A, Farlow B, Wilfond BS. The experience of families with children with trisomy 13 and 18 in social networks. Pediatrics 2012;130(2):293–8.
76. Partridge JC, Martinez AM, Nishida H, et al. International comparison of care for very low birth weight infants: parents' perceptions of counseling and decision-making. Pediatrics 2005;116:e263–71.
77. Hack M, Taylor HG, Drotar D, et al. Poor predictive validity of the Bayley scales of infant development for cognitive function of extremely low birth weight children at school age. Pediatrics 2005;116:333–41.
78. Saigal S, Stoskopf B, Pinelli J, et al. Self-perceived health-related quality of life of former extremely low birth weight infants at young adulthood. Pediatrics 2006; 118:1140–8.
79. Boss RD, Kinsman HI, Donohue PK. Health-related quality of life for infants in the neonatal intensive care unit. J Perinatol 2012;32:901–6.
80. Varni JW, Limbers CA, Neighbors K, et al. The PedsQL infant scales: feasibility, internal consistency reliability, and validity in healthy and ill infants. Qual Life Res 2011;20:45–55.
81. Varni JW, Sherman SA, Burwinkle TM, et al. The PedsQL family impact module: preliminary reliability and validity. Health Qual Life Outcomes 2004;2:55.
82. PROMIS: Dynamic Tools to Measure Health Outcomes from the Patient Perspective. Available at: http://www.nihpromis.org/.
83. Wu AW, Kharrazi H, Boulware LE, et al. Measure once, cut twice—adding patient-reported outcome measures to the electronic health record for comparative effectiveness research. J Clin Epidemiol 2013;66:S12–20.

Conquering Racial Disparities in Perinatal Outcomes

Earnestine Willis, MD, MPH[a],*, Patricia McManus, PhD, RN[b],
Norma Magallanes, BSc[a], Sheri Johnson, PhD[a], Amber Majnik, PhD[c]

KEYWORDS

- African American infant mortality • Racial and ethnic disparities
- Adverse birth outcomes • Preterm births • Low birth weight
- Social determinants of health • Life course • Resiliency

KEY POINTS

- Staggering disparities in infant mortality exist between racial/ethnic and socioeconomically disadvantaged groups in the United States and other industrialized countries.
- Environmental epigenetics provides a biological mechanism for the cumulative impact of environmental exposures through the life course that may cross multiple generations and contribute to the understanding of racial/ethnic disparities in adverse birth outcomes.
- For communities of color, discriminatory policies and practices that affect their developmental trajectory should be examined and modified to design culturally tailored action plans, with the goal of eliminating the influence of racism that permeates service systems such as education, health care, housing, justice, and labor.
- Early childhood programs such as supplemental nutrition, parenting support, and quality early childhood education programs are important components of a long-term strategy to ameliorate disparities in birth outcomes for current and future generations.

INFANT MORTALITY RANKING WITH A FOCUS ON THE RACIAL/ETHNIC WIDENING GAP IN THE UNITED STATES

Infant mortality rate (IMR) is defined as the death of an infant per 1,000 live births, before their first birthday.[1] In this article, African Americans and blacks are used interchangeably, unless otherwise specified. Despite the best efforts by medical and public health communities, black infants are twice as likely to die as white infants. In 1960, the

Disclosures: None.
[a] Department of Pediatrics, Center for the Advancement of Underserved Children, Medical College of Wisconsin, 8701 West Watertown Plank Road, Milwaukee, WI 53226, USA; [b] Black Health Coalition of Wisconsin, Inc., 3020 West Vliet Street, Milwaukee, WI 53208-2461, USA; [c] Department of Pediatrics, Division of Neonatology, Medical College of Wisconsin, 8701 West Watertown Plank Road, Milwaukee, WI 53226, USA
* Corresponding author.
E-mail address: ewillis@mcw.edu

Clin Perinatol 41 (2014) 847–875
http://dx.doi.org/10.1016/j.clp.2014.08.008
0095-5108/14/$ – see front matter © 2014 Elsevier Inc. All rights reserved.
perinatology.theclinics.com

average US IMR (26 infant deaths per 1,000 live births) was lower than the average IMR (40.4 infant deaths per 1,000 live births) reported for other industrialized countries who are members of the Organization for Economic Cooperation and Development (OECD).[2] IMR in the United States has been declining since 1960 to a rate of 6.1 reported in 2011, as shown in **Fig. 1**.[2–5] In the United States, advances in medical technology and public health have significantly contributed to the reduction in IMRs.[1] However, the widening racial gaps in IMR observed between black and white birth outcomes over this same period is disappointing.[3,6] From 1960 to 1971, the IMR for black infants declined at a faster rate (14 deaths/1,000 live births) compared with white infants (5.8 deaths/1,000 live births), leading to a narrowing of the infant mortality ratio from 1.9 in 1960 to 1.8 reported in 1971, as reflected in **Fig. 2**.[3–5] However, after 1971, this trend reversed, and by 1988, the ratio in the United States was 2.1, remaining relatively unchanged based on the ratio of 2.2 reported in 2011 (see **Fig. 2**).[3,5] Moreover, in 1960, the United States ranked favorably among 34 OECD countries with the 12th lowest IMR.[2] For that year, countries with the highest IMRs were Turkey (189.5) and Chile (120.3).[2] Recent available data (2009–2011 average) show remarkable progress for decreasing IMRs in Turkey (8.6), and Chile (7.7), which is rapidly converging to the 34 OECD country average of 4.2 deaths per 1,000 live births, as shown in **Fig. 3**.[2,7] Conversely, reduction of IMRs in the United States has been slower than the aforementioned countries.[7] The average IMR (6.2) from 2009 to 2011 in the United States was 32.3% higher than the collective average for the 34 OECD countries of 4.2 and is ranked as 31st among these countries, as shown in **Fig. 3**.[2,7] Despite substantial progress to reduce IMRs in the United States, the downward trend obscures persistent racial/ethnic and geographic disparities.[1]

The primary reason for higher IMRs in the United States compared with European countries can be explained by higher percentages of preterm births (infants born before 37 weeks of gestation are completed).[8] Shorter gestation periods are closely linked with low-birth-weight (LBW) infants (weighing <2,500 g), and those infants

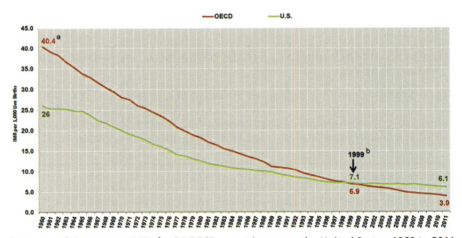

Fig. 1. Trends in average IMRs for 34 OECD countries versus the United States, 1960 to 2011. Death rates are expressed as deaths per 1,000 live births. [a] In 1960, the IMR in the United States (26) was lower than the average OECD IMR (40.4). [b] Since 1999, the IMR in the United States has been higher (7.1) than the average OECD IMR (6.9), and in subsequent years, the United States IMR reduction has slowed when compared with the average IMR among other industrialized countries. (*Data from* Refs.[2–5])

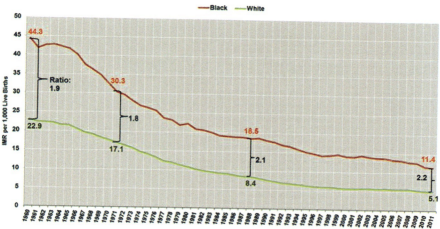

Fig. 2. IMR gaps between blacks and whites in the United States from 1960 to 2011. (*Data from Refs.*[3–5])

have a greater risk of death and associated morbidities of serious long-term, physical, mental, and emotional disabilities.[6,9,10] The United States and Turkey report the highest preterm births (12%) among industrialized nations, as shown in **Fig. 4**, and consequently hold a poor IMR ranking of 6.2 in the United States and 8.6 in Turkey, as shown in **Figs. 4**.[2,8,9,11] Conversely, OECD countries with the lowest percentages of preterm birth are closely paralleled with the lowest IMRs. Countries showing this parallel are Finland (5.5% of preterm birth outcomes; IMR of 2.4), followed by Sweden (5.9%; 2.4, respectively) and Japan (5.9%; 2.3, respectively), and then Iceland (6.5%:1.6, respectively) as shown in **Figs. 3** and **4**.[2,8,9]

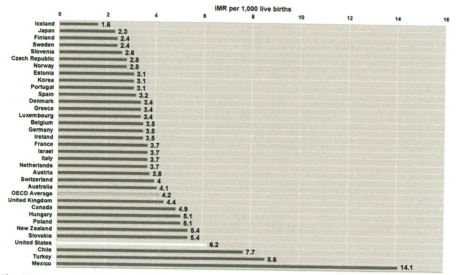

Fig. 3. Average IMRs for 34 OECD countries, 2009 to 2011. (*Data from* OECD. Health status: material and infant mortality. Organization for Economic Cooperation and Development stat extracts. 2013. p. 36–7. Available at: http://stats.oecd.org/. Accessed February 27, 2014.)

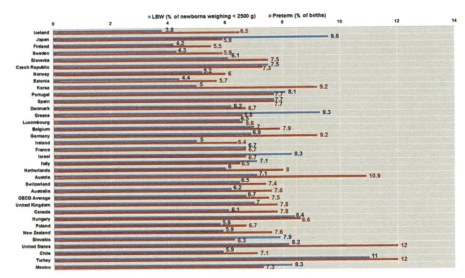

Fig. 4. LBW (2008-2010) and preterm births (2010) (rate per 1,000 live births) among OECD countries. (*Data on LBW from* OECD. Lafortune G, van Gool K, Biondi K. Infant health: low birth weight. Organization for Economic Cooperation and Development stat extracts 2013. p. 38–9. Available at: http://stats.oecd.org/. Accessed February 28, 2014. *Data on preterm birth from* March of Dimes, PMNCH, Save the Children, WHO. Born too soon: the global action report on preterm birth. In: Howson CP, Kinney MV, Lawn JE, editors. White Plains, New York: World Health Organization; 2012. Available at: http://www.marchofdimes.com/mission/global-preterm.aspx. Accessed on March 4, 2014.)

REGIONAL DIFFERENCES IN INFANT MORTALITY RATE IN THE UNITED STATES

Available linked infant birth/death datasets from 2010 reported wide and persistent disparities in IMRs by race and geography.[12] Across the United States, IMRs are higher in southern states and midwestern states compared with the overall IMR of 6.1 in the United States, as shown in **Fig. 5**.[12] From 2008 to 2010, states and jurisdictions with the highest IMRs were the state of Mississippi (9.9) followed by the District of Columbia (9.7), Alabama (8.8), Louisiana (8.5), and Tennessee (8.5), as shown in **Fig. 5**.[12]

For 2007 to 2009, available data reported that excess infant mortality occurred in regions IV and VI (see **Fig. 5**).[3,13] Furthermore, ecological studies show that southern states finish at the bottom tier for the poorest economic factors, such as poverty, lower high-school graduation, and high unemployment rates, influencing health-related outcomes.[14] These states are disproportionately populated with higher black births to account for 59% of the regional disparity, and much of the remainder regional disparity is caused by white births (37%), when compared with births in the rest of the country.[13]

PROFILE OF INFANT DEATH DISPARITIES AND CAUSES

Differences in IMRs between white and black infants can be examined by determining the relative conditions leading to the causes of death.[3] The 4 leading causes of infant deaths are profiled by ranking in 2000 and 2010 in **Table 1**.[12,15] These data reflect persistent racial/ethnic disparities and little change between the 2000 and 2010 generations. Again, the greatest underlying contributor to racial disparities in infant

IMR per 1,000 live births

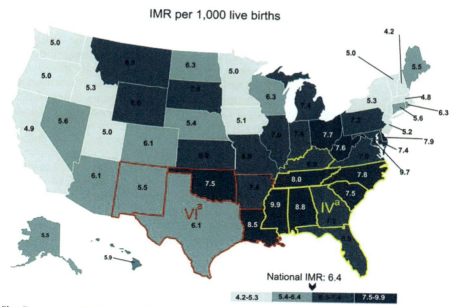

National IMR: 6.4

| 4.2-5.3 | 5.4-6.4 | 6.5-7.4 | 7.5-9.9 |

Fig. 5. Averaged IMR per 1,000 live births by states, 2008 to 2010. [a] Region VI and IV labels reference data from 2007 to 2009 to show regional differences in IMR. (*Data from* Mathews TJ, MacDorman MF. Infant mortality statistics from the 2010 period linked birth/infant death data set. Natl Vital Stat Rep 2013;62(8):1–26; and [region VI and IV] Hirai AH, Sappenfield WM, Kogan MD, et al. Contributors to excess infant mortality in the US south. Am J Prev Med 2014;46(3):219–27.)

mortality seems to be related to shorter gestational periods and LBW rates. Although the leading cause of death for white infants was congenital malformations, these conditions were the only causes of deaths that were comparable for both black and white infants, as shown in **Table 1**.[12,15] **Figs. 6** and **7** show a close correlation of trends in IMR and preterm-related infant deaths for blacks, Puerto Ricans, and American Indians or Alaska Native women.[12]

DIFFERENTIAL INTERGENERATIONAL BIRTH OUTCOMES

In the past, investigators attributed the racial/ethnic disparities in birth outcomes to genetic differences after controlling for socioeconomic factors.[6] Subsequently, with advancements in population genetics variations, researchers have argued against the genetic or race causality.[6] In 1997, David and Collins compared singleton birth weights of infants born in Illinois to 3 groups of women: US-born blacks, African-born blacks, and US-born whites. These investigators predicted that if specific alleles underlie the observed differences in birth weights between blacks and whites in the United States, women of the purest African ancestry would be expected to deliver infants with the lowest birth weights. US-born black women with higher European ancestry would be expected to deliver infants of intermediate birth weights, between African-born black women and US-born white women.[6,16] However, investigators found that the mean birth weight distributions of infants born to African-born black women (3,333 g) and US-born white women (3,446 g) were nearly identical.[16] Regardless of socioeconomic status, Collins and David's epidemiologic research showed that US-born black infants weighed less than African-born black infants, as shown in Fig. 8.[6,16] Furthermore, an analysis for race-specific birth weight distribution across 3 generations of female descendants (US-born white; European-born white; US-born black and African-born black women) showed differential intergenerational trends. For both white groups (generation 1) who grew up in the United States, there was a shift toward a higher birth weight by generation 2 and 3 for female descendants.[17] For US-born black female descendants, there was a smaller degree (17 g) of birth weight gain by generation 3. The opposite intergenerational trend was observed among female descendants (generation 3) from African-immigrants mothers living in the United States (generation 1), showing a birth weight of 57 g less than their mothers (generation 2). Further evidence shows that among Illinois US-born Mexican-American women, descendants have a greater LBW rate when compared with Mexican-born women. However, higher generations of US-born Mexican-American women approximate birth weights of Mexican-born women.[18] These findings by Collins and colleagues[6,17,18] suggest that women of color's social status and exposures to intergenerational factors are closely linked to the racial disparity in IMRs, refuting the genetic concept of race as the major contributor to differential birth weights. Extensive literature suggests that acculturation to the US lifestyle is a risk factor in addition to perceived or real discriminatory practices as contributors for adverse birth outcomes among racial/ethnic groups.

Epigenetic Tools Addressing Racial Disparities in Perinatal Outcomes

The engine that drives racial differences in infant mortality and preterm birth has yet to emerge from the tunnel. Genetic differences alone fail to explain the disparity.[16,19] Similarly, differences persist even when specific environmental influences are considered. The literature suggests that the gap is independent of maternal education,[20] prenatal care use,[21,22] and upward socioeconomic mobility.[23] Likely, the mechanism is one that encompasses both genetic and multiple environmental influences throughout a lifetime. Epigenetics exists at the intersection between genetics and the environment.

It is believed that environmental factors rely on epigenetics to induce biological change and adaptation. The study of how the environment affects phenotype is environmental epigenetics. Environmental exposures over a lifetime result in multifactorial risk factors for adverse birth outcomes. This concept is the life course model.[24] Epigenetics provides a biological mechanism for the appearance of the accumulation of environmental exposures throughout a lifetime.

A cell holds many epigenetic tools to modify its gene expression in response to environmental exposures. Some of these tools include methylation, histone modifications, and noncoding RNA. Although it is likely to be of great importance, the role of noncoding RNA in epigenetics is just beginning to be understood. The role of histones in epigenetics is better understood. Histones are proteins that package and order DNA. Histones have N-terminal tails that are subject to covalent modifications. These modifications are critical for the modulation and expression of DNA. Methylation is the most studied epigenetic change.

Methylation involves the addition of a methyl group to a substrate, such as DNA. DNA CpG methylation can change gene expression. DNA CpG methylation can be influenced by nutrients and vitamins in diet, such as folate. Folate is a major source of the 1 carbon group used to methylate DNA. Controlled feeding studies show that folate-deficient diets result in decreased global methylation levels, whereas methylation levels increase on a folate supplemented diet.[25] This finding highlights the

Table 1
Four leading causes of infant deaths among non-Hispanic black and non-Hispanic white infants: United States, 2000, 2010

Causes of Death	Non-Hispanic Black Ranking 2000	Rates 2000	Non-Hispanic White Ranking 2000	Rates 2000	Ratio 2000	Non-Hispanic Black Ranking 2010	Rates 2010	Non-Hispanic White Ranking 2010	Rates 2010	Ratio 2010
All causes		13.5		6	2.3		11.5		5.2	2.2
Congenital malformations (Q00-Q99)	2	1.7	1	1.4	1.2	2	1.6	1	1.2	1.3
Disorders related to short gestation and LBW (P07)	1	2.9	2	0.7	4.1	1	2.6	2	0.7	3.7
Sudden infant death syndrome (R95)	3	1.2	3	0.5	2.4	3	1	3	0.5	2
Newborn affected by maternal pregnancy complications (P01)	4	0.8	4	0.3	2.7	4	0.8	4	0.3	2.7

Comparison of the causes of infant deaths for the years 2000 and 2010 for Non-Hispanic Black and Non-Hispanic Whites based on mother's racial/ethnic background. Codes in parentheses are from the International Classification of Diseases, 10th Revision. In Mathews TJ, MacDorman MF, Menacker F. Infant mortality statistics from the 2000 period linked birth/infant death data set. Natl Vital Stat Rep; vol 50 no 12. Hyattsville, Maryland: National Center for Health Statistics. 2002; and Mathews TJ, MacDorman MF, Division of Vital Statistics. Infant Mortality Statistics from the 2010 Period Linked Birth/Infant Death Data Set. National Center for Health Statistics 2013; Vol. 62, No 8.

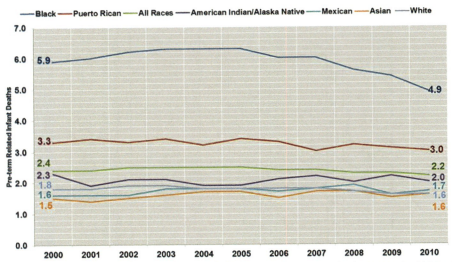

Fig. 6. Preterm-related infant deaths per 1,000 live births by racial/ethnic group, 2000 to 2010. (*From* Mathews TJ, MacDorman MF. Infant mortality statistics from the 2010 period linked birth/infant death data set. Natl Vital Stat Rep 2013;62(8):1–26.)

impact of dietary folate. Dietary folate in pregnant women may have even more consequential effects.

Nutritional environment affects birth outcomes and may contribute to racial disparities. Insufficient maternal folate is associated with LBW, intrauterine growth restriction, and preterm birth.[26] A study investigating folate intake[27] reported that white women were more likely to have increased folic acid supplementation before and

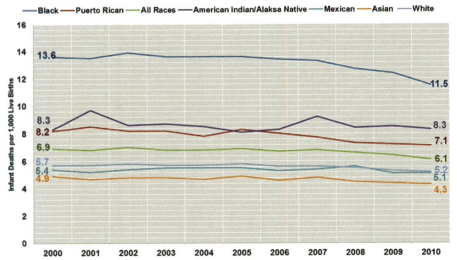

Fig. 7. IMRs per 1,000 live births by racial/ethnic group, 2000 to 2010. (*From* Mathews TJ, MacDorman MF. Infant mortality statistics from the 2010 period linked birth/infant death data set. Natl Vital Stat Rep 2013;62(8):1–26.)

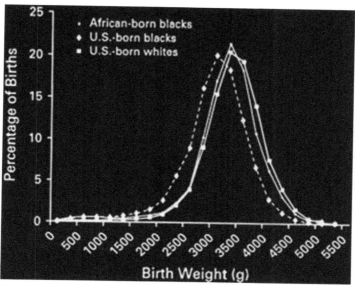

Fig. 8. Birth weight distribution of three Illinois subpopulations, 1980 to 1995. (*Data from* David R, Collins J. Differing birth weight among infants of US-born Blacks, African-born blacks, and US-born Whites. N Engl J Med 1997;337:1211.)

during pregnancy compared with black women. Similarly, folic acid and multivitamin supplementation may decrease the risk of preterm birth and increase birth weight, especially in blacks.[26,28,29] Differences in dietary folate intake can alter epigenetics and may thereby contribute to racial disparities in adverse birth outcomes.

Human studies have begun to show an association between epigenetic changes and adverse birth outcomes, including those that contribute to racial disparities. Haggarty and colleagues[30] investigated the association between birth weight, length, placental weight, and duration of gestation and 4 DNA methylation gene variants as well as methylation of LINE1 and 3 imprinted genes. These investigators found that DNMT3L allele in the infant was associated with higher birth weights, birth lengths, placental weights, and reduced risks of requiring neonatal care. Although the DNMT3B allele in the mother was associated with an increased risk of prematurity, birth weight was also associated with LINE1 and IGF2 methylation. Another study assessed methylation at the ZAC1 gene, which is important for fetal growth and meta-bolism.[31] The degree of methylation was found to correlate with fetal weight at 32 weeks' gestation, at birth, and at 1 year of age. Maternal intake of alcohol and vitamin B_2 also positively correlated with ZAC1 methylation, indicating the importance of the maternal environment.[31]

The maternal environment influences multiple generations, compounding the effects of racial disparities. Recent evidence suggests that environmental influences on epigenetics are not limited to the person with direct exposure but may be trans-mitted to subsequent generations as well. This transmission may occur through expo-sure of a pregnant mother, as well as the developing fetus and the developing germ cells inside the fetus that form the F2 generation. Three generations can therefore be directly affected. Environmental contributions to racial disparities in birth outcomes of multiple generations may be particularly true for African Americans, who have endured environments of discrimination and chronic stress for generations.[32–35]

Transgenerational effects of chronic stress can infiltrate multiple generations, contributing to racial disparities in birth outcomes. Collins and colleagues[36] investigated the transgenerational effect of neighborhood poverty on infant birth weight among blacks. These investigators determined that LBW rates increased as a maternal grandmother's residential environment during pregnancy deteriorated. This change in birth weights was independent of the mother's residential environment during pregnancy. This important study suggests that the maternal grandmother's exposure to neighborhood poverty during pregnancy is a risk factor for LBW across multiple generations of blacks. Similarly, a maternal grandmother's place of birth decreases the birth weight of the third-generation black women.[17,19] This finding may be the result of maternal lifelong minority status and corresponding stressors.

Animal studies lay the foundation for our understanding of environmental influences in epigenetics across multiple generations. During early and postnatal development, the stress of chronic unpredictable maternal separation in mice leads to depressive-like behavior and alters the methylation profile in the promoter of candidate genes in the germ line and brain of affected males, as well as in the germ line of their offspring.[37] Maternal care, modeled by the licking and grooming behavior of rats, has also been shown to be associated with epigenetic changes and inheritance.[38] Mouse studies have also shown that maternal exposure to high-fat diet results in increased body size and reduced sensitivity to insulin through 2 generations via both the maternal and paternal lineages.[39] This effect is manifested in females into the third generation via the paternal lineage.[40] This transgenerational epigenetic inheritance of diet is associated with imprinted gene patterns and changes in methylation. Diet and stress are important predictors of birth outcomes. Epigenetic changes induced by differential exposures to diet and stress can influence racial disparities in birth outcomes.

Understanding the mechanisms that promote racial disparities is critical to derailing their subsequent adverse birth outcomes. Maternal environments, including neighborhood location, and nutritional milieu both contribute to the epigenetic state of multiple generations. The goal is to use epigenetics to anticipate health outcomes in individuals and, more importantly, within populations and across generations.

Improving Perinatal Outcomes Through Community Action: Two Case Studies

Case study 1: the Milwaukee Healthy Beginnings Project
The Black Health Coalition of Wisconsin (BHCW) developed the Milwaukee Healthy Beginnings Project (MHBP) in March, 1998 as part of the Federal Healthy Start Initiative Phase II. The overall goal of MHBP is to decrease infant mortality by reducing preterm births for high-risk mothers in the Milwaukee areas. The targeted population is African American (black) women of childbearing age along with their infants and family who reside in 7 zip codes in the central city of Milwaukee. Targeted zip codes are 53206, 53208, 53209, 53210, 53212, 53216, and 53218. Targeted zip codes are located in the most economically depressed and racially segregated area of the city. Stakeholders include the following participants: community residents; community-based organizations, such as fatherhood programs, job development agencies, homeless projects, and antipoverty agencies; federally qualified community health centers; local and state health department officials; academic institutions; and health care systems. The strength of the MHBP model is that it maximizes the assets, skills, and expertise of various stakeholders in the community to foster partnerships aimed at reducing adverse birth outcomes. There is much in the literature, especially in the maternal and child health (MCH) journals, highlighting the need to look beyond the standard medical and public health models for improving perinatal outcomes. From the

beginning of MHBP, principles such as life course, social determinants of health, resiliency, cultural dynamics, community empowerment, and inclusion of populations most affected have been used to coordinate systems of services for Milwaukee's most at-risk pregnancies and interconceptional women. Unpublished work by Edair and McManus in 1995 reported that resilient inner city African American families shared the following characteristics: (1) strong family ties, whether there was a male in the home or not; (2) shared resources across family households; (3) spiritual anchors; (4) self-efficacy and hope toward the future; (5) belief in strong discipline; (6) recognition of their children as resources; (7) their own means of transportation; and (8) referral to their families as the first line of assistance instead of community agencies. MHBP included these factors in the development of its family and community interventions. MHBP is a unique collaboration that includes: (1) identification of pregnant women and their infants; (2) recruitment of families into early or consistent prenatal care; (3) improvement of the birth outcomes of high-risk infants; (4) capacity building through bidirectional knowledge exchange; and (5) development of participants' leadership skills in health policy issues at both the local and state levels. MHBP provides (1) targeted case management, which recognizes social determinants of health in the Milwaukee area affecting birth outcomes, (ie, object poverty, housing segregation, racism), and (2) a Milwaukee African American Infant Mortality Task Force, which is community controlled and designed to advocate for improvement in the quality of life for African Americans in Milwaukee.

Since 2000, MHBP has recognized the need to provide services to higher at-risk groups. More specifically, these groups include pregnant women in the Milwaukee County Jail, and since 2006, pregnant women who had children in out-of-home placement. Both of these higher-risk groups in the black community are compared with other case management/home visiting programs. Instead of just providing basic health education and referrals for resources, MHBP increases support and advocacy services for women and infant participants. The expanded services include MHBP staff attending court hearings, family team meetings of the Bureau of Milwaukee Child Welfare, prenatal health care provider visits, and home visiting infant health encounters with the parents/caregivers. Moreover, MHBP staff accompany parents to school meetings, especially in relation to the establishment of individual educational plans for their children. Case management services are strategies and tactics critical to accomplishing stress reduction. Participants benefitting from MHBP services expressed their appreciation of having staff available to assist them in many different situations that required them to interact with established service systems. Staff have documented the following observations: (1) beginning to advocate for themselves and (2) participants taking personal control of their situations. MHBP staff have found it to be vital to document effective strategies and tactics to improving social circumstances that result from identified stressors and ameliorate adverse birth outcomes. In 2012, a local evaluator conducted an analysis of longitudinal trends in birth certificate data of prenatal care and birth outcomes in participating pregnant women and infants in MHBP. From 2004 to 2011, the evaluator compared trends for all births in the MHBP project area to the MHBP participants. The overall design of the evaluation was a comparison analysis, consisting of a quasi-experimental review of the study cohort; the targeted population (all MHBP participants who gave birth during each year of study) versus a comparison population, comprising all women residing in the project area who gave birth during these same years. The analysis focused on indicators for prenatal care, infant birth weights, and preterm birth. To conduct more focused analyses across different sociodemographic groups, data were stratified by categories of race/ethnicity, age, and educational attainment. This report is based on data from birth certificates, provided by the Department of Public Health of the city of Milwaukee for the years 2004 to 2011. Birth certificates were linked to MHBP prenatal and post-partum participants for each year. For each year, aggregate data from birth certificates was provided for the MHBP project area. Variables extracted from birth certificates for analysis included: LBW (1500–2499 g) rates, very LBW (VLBW) (<1500 g) rates, pre-term birth rates (23–36 weeks' gestation), early initiation of prenatal care (first trimester), and late initiation (≥third trimester) or no prenatal care.

Analysis design Aggregate annual data for mothers or infants who were positive for a given outcome indicator were subtracted from the total number of live births or the number of live births within race/ethnic groups (blacks), ages (<20 years old and ≥20 years old), and educational attainment groups (less than high school completion, completed high school, and some college). These outcome data were then weighted to create disaggregated indicator variables for birth outcomes or prenatal care out-comes for each calendar year. To estimate the significance of longitudinal trends (ie, the association between outcomes and years) within either the MHBP participants or women in the comparison project area population, outcome variables were entered into a series of logistic regressions. Another logistic regression was conducted after estimating the longitudinal change in outcomes between MHBP participants and the project area population, as a whole, to test the association between outcomes by years and populations. Data analysis first examined longitudinal trends for all indi-cators, comparing the total MHBP participants with project area populations. These analyses were then repeated for black participant subgroups. For each outcome variable, an average annual percentage was calculated to represent the overall trends among aggregate MHBP participants and project area populations.

Comparisons of infant mortality rate–related indicators in project area births versus Milwaukee Healthy Beginnings Project births, 2004 to 2011 Comparisons of births to mothers in MHBP cohorts and the project area from 2004 to 2011 on all 5 variables are presented in **Table 2**. The 8-year LBW data show that changes in births for infants in the project area were statistically significant ($P<.001$), whereas variations in LBW for MHBP participants were not statistically significant. In addition, there were not signif-icant differences in the rates of LBW between the MHBP cohort and the project area. Rates for VLBW reflected virtually no change in the project area, and only a modest (0.1%) decrease in prevalence among MHBP participants. Average rates of preterm births have increased annually in the project area (0.2%) and in the MHBP cohort (0.1%); however, since 2009, both groups have reversed their trends. Over the 8-year period, the average annual trend for the percent of women who initiated prenatal care in the first semester decreased by 3.4% in the project area, which was statisti-cally significant ($P<.001$). MHBP participants dramatically increased the prevalence of early prenatal care between 2009 and 2011, although not significantly from the low point in 2008. The difference between the rates of initiation of prenatal care in the first trimester for the project area and MHBP cohort was significant ($P<.03$). Trend data for late (third trimester) or no prenatal care showed a statistically significant in-crease ($P<.001$) across average annual rates among project area populations. For the same indicator, among the MHBP cohort, there was an average annual decrease, although not statistically significant. Comparative analyses indicated that differences between these 2 groups of women were significant ($P<.05$).

Comparisons of infant mortality rate–related indicators in project area births versus Milwaukee Healthy Beginnings Project births among black mothers, 2004 to 2011 Comparisons of births for black mothers from 2004 to 2011 on all 5 indicators are presented in **Table 3**. The average annual prevalence of LBW among black infants in the project area population increased significantly (*P*<.01). Over the same period, MHBP black infants showed an average annual decrease in LBW, which was also statistically significant (*P*<.03). Comparative analysis did not indicate significant differences in trends between the MHBP cohort and project area population. Longitudinal trends for VLBW indicated virtually no change in the project area, whereas MHBP black infants showed a modest average annual decrease. However, logistic regression analysis did not show any statistical significance between trends for any comparison groups. Preterm birth rates increased slightly and were statistically significant (*P*<.01) for project area black infants. MHBP black infants showed an average annual decrease in rates of preterm births, although not statistically significant, and comparative analysis was not significant between groups. Prevalence of early prenatal care showed an average annual decrease among project area black women and was statistically significant (*P*<.001). MHBP black women showed a statistically significant (*P*<.01) average annual increase in the prevalence of early prenatal care. Results for late (third trimester) or no prenatal care showed a statistically significant (*P*<.001) increase among project area black women, whereas MHBP black women showed a decrease, which was not significant. Comparative analysis of the 2 populations showed that the trends were not significantly different.

Implications In interpreting the statistical findings, several limitations of the research design and data analysis need to be acknowledged. Examination of indicators of infant mortality and morbidity among mothers and infants in the overall project area afforded a comparative standard against which progress of MHBP participants could be assessed. Project coordinators were unable to conduct a true experiment with randomized assignment to treatment and control groups, or even a quasiexperiment with matched samples by enrolled participants. To control for population differences in our study, coordinators performed limited population analyses by subgroups stratified by race, age, and education attainment. Thus, various confounding factors and possible competing explanations for statistical analysis results cannot be completely accounted for. Such confounders might include the exposure of some project area mothers to limited doses of MHBP interventions (eg, information from ≥1 media campaigns, local health fairs), or the exposure of pregnant women in either or both populations to health information or access to services that did not originate with MHBP. Also, although the use of aggregate data allowed some insight into the larger impact (ie, both direct and indirect) of all elements of MHBP interventions, a drawback of this approach is the loss of sensitivity for assessing the specific effects of various components within the model for different groups of mothers and their infants.

Although our initial design intended to compare African American, Hispanic, and white race/ethnicity groups, changes over time to both the size and location of the MHBP project area resulted in unacceptably small numbers of Hispanic and white race/ethnicity participants. Therefore, the analysis was conducted in subgroups exclusively for African American project area and Healthy Start participants. Despite these limitations, data indicate that considerable progress was made from 2004 to 2011 with respect to key risk factors for adverse birth outcomes. At a minimum, data suggest that the incidence of VLBW decreased among infants born to the MHBP cohort. The largest changes in the VLBW rates within the MHBP cohort seem to have occurred among the greatest at-risk subgroups: black, younger than 20 years, and less-educated mothers. During the period investigated, LBW rates remained static or increased slightly, with 1 exception: LBW births decreased significantly among black MHBP mothers. From 2004 to 2011, there was a reduction in

Table 2
LBW, preterm births, early and late/no prenatal care from 2004 to 2011: all MHBP project area births versus all MHBP participants

	2004	2005	2006	2007	2008	2009	2010	2011	Average Annual Change
Total Births									
MHBP project area	7637	7714	7922	7455	7867	5956	4210	4088	
MHBP participants	199	242	160	184	133	141	99	84	
LBW (1500–2499 g)									
MHBP project area	605	651	657	665	665	595	431	414	
% of total births	7.9	8.4	8.3	8.9	8.5	10.0	10.2	10.1	0.3[a]
MHBP participants	18	22	22	20	12	20	6	4	
% of total births	9.0	9.1	13.8	10.9	9.0	14.2	6.1	4.8	−0.6
VLBW (<1500 g)									
MHBP project area	208	229	199	165	191	153	118	122	
% of total births	2.7	3.0	2.5	2.2	2.4	2.6	2.8	3.0	0.0
MHBP participants	6	3	1	3	0	2	2	2	
% of total births	3.0	1.2	0.6	1.6	0.0	1.4	2.0	2.4	−0.1
Preterm Births (23–36 wk gestation)									
MHBP project area	876	931	904	802	855	690	494	529	
% of total births	11.5	12.1	11.4	10.8	10.9	11.6	11.7	12.9	0.2
MHBP participants	29	36	20	21	13	30	9	13	
% of total births	14.6	14.9	12.5	11.4	9.8	21.3	9.1	15.5	0.1

Initiated Prenatal Care in First Trimester									
MHBP project area	5789	5743	5880	5522	5595	4444	3134	2116	
% of total births	75.8	74.4	74.2	74.1	71.1	74.6	74.4	51.8	−3.4[a,b]
MHBP participants	138	175	104	121	79	93	63	63	
% of total births	69.3	72.3	65.0	65.8	59.4	66.0	63.6	75.0	0.8[b]
Late or No Prenatal Care									
MHBP project area	358	382	432	417	463	321	247	328	
% of total births	4.7	5.0	5.5	5.6	5.9	5.4	5.9	8.0	0.5[a,b]
MHBP participants	18	15	14	16	11	13	10	5	
% of total births	9.0	6.2	8.8	8.7	8.3	9.2	10.1	6.0	−0.4[b]

The following indicators are reported for years 2004–2011.

LBW (1,500–2,499 g) births increased from 7.9% in 2004 to 10.1% in 2011 for infants within the project area, this trend was significant ($P<.001$). The LBW rate among MHBP participants decreased from 9% in 2004 to 4.8% in 2011, an average of −0.6% per year. However, this trend was not statistically significant, and the regression analysis did not find a significant difference in the rates of change between project area population and MHBP participants.

For VLBW infants (VLBW-<1,500 g), data showed virtually no change in rates in the project area, and only a modest (−0.1%) decrease in the prevalence of VLBW births among MHBP participants. Regression analysis found that neither of the population trends between years or between populations was statistically significant.

Rates of preterm births both in the project area and among MHBP participants had been trending downward between 2004 and 2011; however, in both cases, these trends have reversed since 2009. For the entire 8-year period of study, the average rates of premature births for the project area and MHBP participants increased annually by 0.2% and 0.1%, respectively, although neither of these trends was statistically significant.

The percent of project area women who initiated prenatal care in the first trimester was fairly consistent throughout most of the study period; but it decreased by more than 20% in 2011, and the average annual trend was −3.4% over the 8-year period. This trend was significant ($P<.001$). On the other hand, among MHBP participants, the prevalence of early prenatal care increased dramatically from 2009 to 2011 after a low point of 59.4% in 2008, for an average annual rate of +0.8%). Although the statistical trend among MHBP participants was not significant, the difference in the rates of change between the project area and MHBP participants was significant ($P<.03$).

With respect to trends on late (third trimester) or no prenatal care, the data showed an average annual increase of 0.5% in the prevalence of late/no prenatal care among the project area population, and this increase was statistically significant ($P<.001$). Among MHBP participants, the rate of late/no prenatal care showed an overall average decrease of −0.4%, although the trend was not consistent and was not statistically significant. However, analysis did indicate that the difference in the trends between project area women and MHBP participants was significant ($P<.05$).

[a] Indicates a statistically significant trend in the change for an outcome between 2004 and 2011 within either the MHBP project area or among MHBP clients.
[b] Indicates a statistically significant difference in rate of change from 2004 and 2011 between the MHBP project area and MHBP clients.

Table 3
LBW, preterm births, early and late/no prenatal care from 2004 to 2011 among black mothers in the MHBP project area versus black MHBP participants

	2004	2005	2006	2007	2008	2009	2010	2011	Average Annual Change
Total Births									
MHBP project area	4256	4375	4439	4181	4415	4009	3312	3050	
MHBP black participants	143	147	120	124	100	109	87	67	
LBW (1500–2499 g)									
MHBP project area	440	453	465	469	464	483	380	352	
% of total births	10.3	10.4	10.5	11.2	10.5	12.0	11.5	11.5	0.2[b]
MHBP black participants	16	14	19	15	10	17	6	3	
% of total births	11.2	9.5	15.8	12.1	10.0	15.6	6.9	4.5	−1.0[b]
VLBW (<1500 g)									
MHBP project area	157	161	147	123	134	123	109	106	
% of total births	3.7	3.7	3.3	2.9	3.0	3.1	3.3	3.5	0.0
MHBP black participants	6	2	0	2	0	2	2	2	
% of total births	4.2	1.4	0.0	1.6	0.0	1.8	2.3	3.0	−0.2
Preterm Births (23–36 wk gestation)									
MHBP project area	598	624	607	531	565	523	428	441	
% of total births	14.1	14.3	13.7	12.7	12.8	13.0	12.9	14.5	0.1[b]
MHBP black participants	25	24	13	15	10	24	9	11	
% of total births	17.5	16.3	10.8	12.1	10.0	22.0	10.3	16.4	−0.2

Initiated Prenatal Care in First Trimester

MHBP project area	3253	3335	3325	3109	3072	3109	2439	1514	
% of total births	76.4	76.2	74.9	74.4	69.6	77.6	73.6	49.6	–3.8[a,b]
MHBP black participants	101	110	76	85	64	71	56	51	
% of total births	70.6	74.8	63.3	68.5	64.0	65.1	64.4	76.1	0.8[a]
Late or No Prenatal Care									
MHBP project area	202	214	249	260	324	260	221	270	
% of total births	4.7	4.9	5.6	6.2	7.3	6.5	6.7	8.9	0.6[b]
MHBP black participants	13	10	10	9	8	9	9	3	
% of total births	9.1	6.8	8.3	7.3	8.0	8.3	10.3	4.5	–0.7

The following indicators are reported for years 2004–2011.

The prevalence of LBW births among black women in the project area population increased significantly ($P<.01$), at an average annual rate of 0.2% between 2004 and 2011. During the same period, black MHBP participants showed an average annual decrease of –1% in rates of LBW births, and this trend was statistically significant ($P<.03$). Comparative analysis did not indicate a significant difference in the trends between MHBP participants and the project area population.

Longitudinal trends in VLBW (<1,500 g) infants indicated virtually no change within the overall project area, whereas the data showed a modest (–0.2%) average annual decrease in the VLBW rate among MHBP participants. However, logistic regression analysis did not show any statistically significant trends in this indicator.

Rates of preterm births among black women in the project area increased slightly (0.1%), and this trend was statistically significant ($P<.01$). The rate of premature births delivered to black MHBP participants showed an average annual decrease of –0.2%; however, the trend was inconsistent from year to year, and not statistically significant. Comparative analysis did not show a significant difference between the populations.

Prevalence of early prenatal care appeared to be fairly stable among project area black women, until it decreased more than 20% in 2011. The overall trend was –3.8% and was statistically significant ($P<.001$). Among black MHBP participants, trend data showed an average annual increase of 0.8%, and the difference in the rates of change between MHBP participants and the project area population was significant ($P<.01$).

Results for late (third trimester) or no prenatal care showed an average annual increase of 0.6% among black women in the project area, and the regression analysis confirmed that this trend was significant at $P<.001$. Among MHBP black participants, the data indicated a no significant decrease in trend of late/no prenatal care of –0.7%. Comparative analysis of the 2 populations showed that the trends were not significantly different.

a Indicates a statistically significant difference in the rate of change from 2004 and 20 between the MHBP project area and MHBP clients.
b Indicates a statistically significant trend in the change for an outcome between 2004 and 2011 within either the MHBP project area or among MHBP clients.

the incidence of preterm births of MHBP black infants, which can be considered a success of the partnership's collective efforts. In this MHBP cohort (black mothers), premature births decreased by 6.3% over the 8-year period. Other subpopulations of MHBP participants who experienced significant improvement for this indicator were mothers (≥20 years old) and those with at least high-school diplomas. Among all MHBP cohorts, the patterns for early prenatal care increased to statistically significant levels, whereas the pattern for late/no prenatal care decreased, although that latter trend was not statistically significant. Over the past 5 years, data have shown a significant downturn in rates of early (first trimester) prenatal care in the project area, as well as increases in the prevalence of late (third trimester) or no prenatal care. These findings suggest that culturally appropriate and targeted case management, addressing both social and health-related stressors for at-risk populations, promotes improved birth outcomes. Therefore, more research, including assessments for population-specific resiliencies, and resources need to be considered as essential factors for future approaches to eliminating health disparities.

Case study 2: the Milwaukee Lifecourse Initiative for Healthy Families community action plan

The Lifecourse Initiative for Healthy Families (LIHF) community action plan was launched in 2009, with the Planning Council of Greater Milwaukee being designated to serve as the convening agency for the Milwaukee LIHF Project by the University of Wisconsin School of Medicine and Public Health. Since the fall of 2010 to spring of 2012, a group of concerned Milwaukeeans (frontline workers, professionals, practitioners, academics, everyday citizens, and experts, both black and white) came together to learn about the city's black-white infant mortality gap to draft a culturally focused plan to address this specific disparity. Established leaders from the community and academic sectors agreed to serve, because of their commitment to inclusion of the community voice in every aspect of the planning process. Objections to evening meetings and deferring to the black community preferences were challenged throughout this collaborative planning process. Despite these challenges, most of the involved stakeholders agreed with the need for visible signs of true community collaboration. The following are just 2 examples of ensuring that the community voice, culture, and assets were included in the final community action plan (Milwaukee LIHF, unpublished plan, 2012);

A. Development of an African American community task force (AACTF), consisting of only African Americans, who had final approval of strategies advanced in the action plan. There were 3 taskforces fashioned to align with the 12-point life course plan proposed by Dr Lu. These domains were: (1) strengthening African American families; (2) increasing health care access; and (3) social determinants of health (**Box 1**). Each taskforce was named after the 3 domains and they had representation of agencies and persons from the African American community. The AACTF adapted guiding principles from the BHCW, which were used to vet strategies developed by the 3 domain taskforces. These guiding principles were as follows:
   a. Be culturally-appropriate
   b. Be community-driven
   c. Be family-centered
   d. Recognize the unique role of black organizations
   e. Address racism
   f. Integrate the concept of life course
   g. Work toward fulfilling the project vision of reducing stress and improving birth outcomes

---

Box 1
Community action plan for social determinants of health

1. Addressing increased access to quality care

   Interconception care

   Preconception care

   Prenatal care

   Expand health care access throughout the life course

2. Strengthening the family and community systems

   Promote fatherhood engagement with attention to economic opportunities

   Elimination of fragmentation in the health care system

   Ensure community infrastructure

   Foster civic engagement for positive population health

3. Addressing social determinants of health

   Closing the education gap

   Reducing poverty

   Providing safe and affordable housing

   Ensuring quality schools

   Ensuring safe neighborhoods

   Providing accessible parks and recreation

   Ensuring clean air and water

   Supporting working mothers through paid leaves for women with a newborn

   Securing breastfeeding in the workplace

Adapted from Lu MC, Kotelchuck M, Hogan V. Closing the black-white gap in birth outcomes: a life-course approach. Ethn Dis 2010;20(2):62–76.

B. The AACTF vetted recommendations for each domain taskforce and then decided which strategies would be in the final community action plan. In addition, the AACTF recommended that 60% of funding be used for fatherhood programs and policy strategies. These recommendations were approved by the steering committee.

At the end of the planning process, the stakeholders voted to have the AACTF serve on the steering committee to ensure that community input occurred at the highest levels. However, AACTF retained its ability to meet separately to discuss issues related to the black community as a whole and bring recommendations to the LIHF collaborative. This collaborative is an example of a community convening to develop a plan that was truly inclusive and highly directed by the targeted community, in which disagreements were resolved to achieve mutual satisfaction.

Program and Policy Opportunities to Reduce Disparities in Adverse Birth Outcomes

Early childhood, a highly sensitive developmental phase, focuses on gaining capacities necessary for future health and reproductive capacity, and warrants the heightened although not exclusive attention of population health practitioners.[41,42] For example, Hanson and colleagues[43] reported that brain growth trajectories for infants and toddlers from low-income families were slower than trajectories for children in higher-income family environments, and total gray matter in the frontal and parietal lobe of the brain was significantly affected by exposure to poverty. The life course health development perspective recognizes that biological, social, and environmental factors across the life span contribute to adverse birth outcomes.[41,44] Life course theory posits that the timing, intensity, and type of environmental exposures affect health development.[41] Socioeconomic disadvantages result in differences in language acquisition and academic achievement. By age 3 years, a 30-million-word gap exists between children who grow up in poverty compared with children in higher socioeconomic family environments.[45]

Historical and contemporary inequities between racial/ethnic groups drive disparities in adverse birth outcomes. Although no evidence for race as a genetic marker for health outcomes exists, race as a social marker for exposure to adversity and cumulative socioeconomic disadvantage is well documented.[16,46–48] Natural experiments show that integration of blacks into the hospitals systems and increased access to medical technology in Mississippi during the civil rights era resulted in dramatic improvements in birth outcomes.[49] Conversely, stress exposures over the life span, including the stress of perceived racial discrimination, have been associated with LBW for black women.[50] Conquering racial/ethnic disparities in health outcomes requires ensuring equitable access to goods, services, and opportunities in society.[51] The following sections focus on 3 targets for investment to avert poor birth outcomes: nutrition, parenting, and early childhood education.

Nutrition

Systematic differences in social and economic environments associated with poor nutrition exist in the United States.[52] Exposure to inadequate nutrition in the intrauterine environment is associated with poor proximal outcomes such as LBW and with distal adverse health impacts, including impaired endocrine and metabolic functioning.[53,54] Using the developmental origins of adult health and disease framework, Kuzawa and Sweet[55] summarized research to show how maternal experiences and health affect fetal biological systems, resulting in a higher risk of developing cardiovascular disease in adulthood. Prenatal undernourishment in 1 generation can result in changed glucose metabolism, blood pressure regulation, and fat deposition associated with adult hypertension and diabetes.[55] Thus, programs that ensure adequate nutrition for expectant mothers, such as the Women Infants and Children (WIC) supplemental nutrition program are well positioned to buffer against adverse birth outcomes during pregnancy.[56] However, all eligible pregnant women, infants, and children in the United States do not yet benefit from WIC, despite evidence of significant benefits garnered from participating in this program, specifically, the associated reduction in black-white birth disparities.[57] The reversal of nutritional deprivation in 1 generation may undo the cascade of gene-environment interactions hypothesized to affect metabolic pathways that lead to the adult onset of diseases in subsequent generations.[41]

Parenting and healthy relationship programs

Child caregivers' capacities to create safe, stable, and nurturing environments are critical to promoting child health.[42] Research documenting differential impacts of family stability on children's well-being suggests that parental resources, parental mental health, quality adult-child relationships, quality of parenting, and father involvement represent key pathways for optimal childhood development. Children growing up in unstable versus stable family systems are more at risk for poor developmental and health outcomes.[58] Thus, interventions aimed at strengthening the coparenting alliance have increased.[59] However, mixed results from healthy relationship programs targeting low-income black and Latino parents are inconclusive and disappointing. This finding indicates that further investigation of coparenting interventions, with a focus on cultural fit and attention to family resiliency, are warranted.[60-62] Although the controversy over how to best strengthen families and stabilize environments for children is unresolved, agreement regarding the positive outcomes associated with quality relationships between early caregivers and youth health-related behaviors is well documented.[63]

Early childhood education

Scientific evidence exists regarding the positive impact of early childhood education on multiple measures of adult well-being, including educational attainment, employment status, income levels, and physical and mental health.[64,65] Educational advantages during childhood have been associated with greater likelihood of productivity in the workforce into adulthood. This positive association is especially pronounced for black women, who tend to have the highest predicted probability of health-induced limitations by midlife.[66] This research amplifies the importance of equitable investment in early childhood education, as a long-term, cross-generational solution to redressing disparities in adverse birth outcomes.

According to Karoly and colleagues,[67] 19 early childhood interventions for children from disadvantaged environments between birth and age 5 years had favorable outcomes in physical, social, emotional, and cognitive development. Moreover, 6 programs, which incorporated home visiting, parent education, or early childhood education, have undergone benefit-cost analysis, which involves measurement of the benefits and costs for society. Outcomes (benefits) are valued in dollars and compared with costs. Results of short-term and long-term follow-up studies yielded benefit/cost ratios of up to 16.1:1.[67,68] Using a matched comparison sample design, Reynolds and colleagues[69] reported that participation in the Chicago Child-Parent Early Education Program yielded a $10.83 return for every dollar invested. Overall societal benefits included increased earnings, tax revenue, and reduced criminal justice costs. The Perry Preschool Project followed participants to age 40 years and reported increasing benefit/cost ratios.[70,71]

Children of color in the United States who are poor have less access to high-quality early childhood education programs.[72] Yet, high-quality early childhood education programs increase the chances that children from disadvantaged backgrounds have cognitive, social, emotional, and academic capacity necessary to thrive in society. Magnuson and Waldfogel[72] estimated that school readiness gaps between black, white, and Hispanic children can be narrowed substantially by both increasing enrollment of low-income children and increasing the quality of early childhood education programs. Critical periods for rapid development in executive function skills (ie, self-control, goal setting, and problem solving) occur between ages 3 and 5 years, and again, in adolescence and young adulthood. Thus, 2-generational interventions that simultaneously build capacities among adult caregivers and their children should be tested.[73]

Embedding of historical, social, and environmental experiences that result in alteration of biological processes may span generations and be an important part of explaining persistent population differences in adverse birth outcomes.[74] Early childhood programs, such as supplemental nutrition, parenting support, and quality early childhood education programs, are important components of a long-term strategy to ameliorate disparities in birth outcomes for current and future generations.

Discussion of Adverse Perinatal Outcomes in Context

Observed trends to reduce the IMRs among developed countries show that the United States has made positive progress along with the other 33 industrialized countries of the OECD. However, in the United States, IMR disparities among racial/ethnic groups have not realized the same benefits of social and medical advances to the degree that whites have, especially for black infants. IMRs from communities of color skew the higher IMR ranking of the United States on the international stage. Evidence that the origin of many adult health conditions begins with adversities experienced in the early years of life has been well documented. Experts have established that toxic environmental exposures early in life result in biological modifications to weaken physiologic systems and produce latent vulnerabilities or health problems in later adult years.[75] The widening racial/ethnic perinatal gap (eg, 1.9 black/white ratio in 1960 to a 2.2 black/white ratio in 2011) suggests that higher priority should be given to the elimination of this persistent disparity as a prevention pathway to adulthood vulnerabilities.

Experts have accepted that shorter gestation periods provide less time for infants to acquire healthy birth weights and are amendable to policy interventions.[76] Interventions must incorporate historical context, social status, access to societal resources throughout the life course, and political will to address population-specific reductions to adverse perinatal outcomes. Given that black women are at a disproportionately higher risk for adverse birth outcomes, much of this article focuses on this population.

WEATHERING HYPOTHESIS, LIFE COURSE PERSPECTIVE, AND RESILIENCY

Researchers have shown that maternal aging is associated with cumulative impact of experiences and socioeconomic factors, including education, income, and access to health care; this phenomenon is referred to as the weathering hypothesis.[77–79] However, investigators have reported that these factors tend to disproportionately influence black women more than other racial/ethnic groups. Lu and colleagues[80] suggest that closing the black-white infant mortality gap requires more than improving access to prenatal care for black women. According to Lu and colleagues,[80] the life course perspective conceptualizes birth outcomes as the end product of not only the 9 months of pregnancy but the entire life course of mothers before pregnancy, synthesizing early programming and cumulative pathways to perinatal outcomes. These investigators proposed a 12-point plan as an ecological approach to improving perinatal outcomes, which longitudinally integrates services for women and families. Altogether, this plan indicates that the life course influences perinatal outcomes and that perinatal outcomes affect the life course perspectives for generations to come. It will take political will in the United States to intervene using a life course approach by addressing early life disadvantages and alleviating the cumulative impact, or the allostatic load, of early life exposures influencing future reproductive potentials.

Resiliency is an asset-based approach that explores factors associated with positive outcomes. It does not ignore risk factors, and it includes values, beliefs, attitudes, and behaviors. For blacks, it seems that cultural resources shape and influence coping strategies, thereby facilitating adaptive responses during times of stress and adversity. The ability to resist or recover from stressors should be examined not only from the perspective of individual context but should also be inclusive of family, community, and systems dynamics. Understanding the process of resilience may be helpful toward identifying how different confounders may result in positive or negative perinatal outcomes. With this understanding, the goal of improved birth outcomes should explore ways to enhance parents' and families' resiliency.

POLITICAL HISTORY AND ORIGINS OF ADVERSE BIRTH OUTCOMES

Only during the last 49 years, since the Civil Rights Act of 1965, have blacks been recognized as citizens. Those 49 years represent only approximately 12% of the history of blacks in the United States, and health consequences from the previous 346 years have persisted over generations, as summarized in **Table 4**.[81,82] Social stratification leading to poor health outcomes is rooted in history and social ecology, which includes racism, perceived acts of racism, poverty, social-environment degradation, and violence, leading to ecological pathways of adverse birth outcomes.[81] Thus, when examining the cumulative effects of adverse exposures on perinatal outcomes between blacks and whites, historical context and unequal starting points must be considered.[81] Similar health disparities in infant mortality occur in other racial/ethnic populations residing in the United States, including African-born blacks, Puerto Ricans, Native Americans, and Mexican-Americans. Therefore, understanding the health impact of persistent inequities and not oversimplifying

Table 4
African American citizenship status and health experience from 1619 to 2014

Time Span	Citizenship Status	Citizenship Status[a]	Citizenship Status[b]	Health and Health System Experience
1619–1865	Chattel slavery	246	62	Disparate/inequitable treatment Poor health status and outcomes Slave health deficit and Slave health subsystem in effect
1865–1965	Virtually no citizenship rights	100	25	Absent or inferior treatment and facilities De jure segregation/discrimination in south, de facto throughout most of health system Slave health deficit uncorrected
1965–2014	Most citizenship rights: United States struggles to transition from segregation and discrimination to integration of African Americans	49	12	Southern medical school desegregation (1948) Imhotep Hospital Integration Conference (1957–1964) Hospital desegregation in federal court (1964) Disparate health status, outcomes, and services with apartheid, discrimination, institutional racism and bias in effect
1619–2014	Struggles for humanity and equality	395	100	Health disparities/inequities

[a] Citizenship status reflected as number of years in the United States.
[b] Citizenship status reflected as percent of time in the United States.
  Adapted from Byrd WM, Clayton LA. An American health dilemma. A medical history of African Americans and the problem of race: beginnings to 1900, vol. 1. New York: Routledge; 2000. p. 3; with permission.

solutions is the challenge that the United States must face to adequately address adverse perinatal outcomes. The weathering hypothesis, life course perspective, and epigenetic pathways need to clearly identify the most critical periods and duration of exposures (inclusive of historical inequalities, stress exposures, and adaptive resilience) in health trajectories for specific populations to avert poor perinatal adverse outcomes.

IMPLICATIONS OF COMMUNITY INTERVENTIONS AND PUBLIC POLICIES

Consistent with the life course perspective, a community action plan must be inclusive and engaging of all aspects of health and environmental exposures to facilitate the connectedness of factors that affect the reproductive capital. This goal can be accomplished by following the key domains of the 12-point plan within a life course perspective, as shown in **Box 1**.[80] For communities of color, institutionalized racism permeates service systems, such as education, health care, housing, justice, and labor, and influences their developmental health trajectory. Any intervention targeting the most vulnerable populations must address these barriers to reach the goal of eliminating health disparities. Hogan and colleagues[81] recognized the social context that black women must navigate, including food insecurity; job loss; lack of practical and emotional support; incarceration of a partner; domestic, social, or political violence; housing insecurity; illiteracy; and disproportional exposures to environmental toxins. If the home, social, and work environments do not support women to optimize their reproductive capacities, any intervention is incomplete, because only part of any intervention happens in the clinical or public health settings. The cultural and social context of black women and families plays a major role in the educational and intervention effectiveness. Epigenetic research suggests that environmental-related experiences and social status contribute to health disparities and have proven transgenerational effects on health. To understand the roles and mechanisms of environmental stressors and confront early childhood origins of disparities in physical and mental health, a substantial amount of evidence-based research and innovative interventions remain to conquer challenges in disparities in infant mortality. A promising starting point to conquering this challenge is through the implementation of quality early childhood education programs for greater returns on investments.

Minimizing future disparities in health is contingent on addressing inequality in the current environment to reverse stress-induced epigenetic modifications and to identify positive effects of environmental enrichment. Successful interventions to eliminate the IMR disparities across racial/ethnic groups must be multidisciplinary, multilevel, and multilayered. For example, multidisciplinary includes the most affected populations, researchers, practitioners, and public policymakers; multilevel considers historical, psychosocial, health access, and environmental experiences; and multilayered addresses family stability, neighborhoods, and workplace exposures. Investments in quality early child care, parenting, and safe and stable supporting living conditions early in the life for children paired with community-engaged research in partnership with the populations most affected can produce measurable benefits in later education achievement, economic productivity, and responsible citizenship. Family stability has been recognized as a protective factor that allows communities of color to thrive, despite the unique adversities that they face. Therefore, research should focus on identifying and recognizing resiliency factors as an avenue to strengthening families of color and for reducing infant mortality disparities.

REFERENCES

1. Barfield W, D'Angelo D, Moon R, et al. CDC grand rounds: public health approaches to reducing US infant mortality. MMWR Morb Mortal Wkly Rep 2013;62(31):625–8.
2. OECD. Health status: material and infant mortality. Organization for Economic Cooperation and Development stat extracts. 2012. Available at: http://stats.oecd.org/index.aspx?DataSetCode=HEALTH_STAT. Accessed February 27, 2014.
3. MacDorman MF, Rosenberg HM. Trends in infant mortality by cause of death and other characteristics, 1960-1988. Natl Vital Stat Rep 1993;20(20):1–49.
4. Murphy SL, Xu JQ, Kochanek KD. Deaths: final data for 2010. Natl Vital Stat Rep 2013;61(4):1–117 Hyattsville (MD): National Center for Health Statistics.
5. Hoyert DL, Xu JQ. Deaths: preliminary data for 2011. Natl Vital Stat Rep 2012; 61(6):1–51 Hyattsville (MD): National Center for Health Statistics.
6. Collins JW, David R. Racial disparity. Racial disparity in low birth weight and infant mortality. Clin Perinatol 2009;36:63–73.
7. Lafortune G, van Gool K, Biondi K. Health Status: Maternal and infant mortality. Organization for Econoic Cooperation and Development stat extracts 2013;36–7. Available at: http://stats.oecd.org/. Accessed February 27, 2014.
8. MacDorman MF, Mathews TJ. Behind international rankings of infant mortality: how the United States compares with Europe. Hyattsville (MD): National Center for Health Statistics; 2009. NCHS data brief, no 23.
9. March of Dimes, PMNCH, Save the Children, WHO. Born too soon: the global action report on preterm birth. In: Howson CP, Kinney MV, Lawn JE, editors. White Plains, New York: World Health Organization; 2012. Available at: http://www.marchofdimes.com/mission/global-preterm.aspx. Accessed March 4, 2014.
10. Lafortune G, van Gool K, Biondi K. Infant health: low birth weight. Organization for Economic Cooperation and Development stat extracts 2013;38–9. Available at: http://stats.oecd.org/. Accessed February 28, 2014.
11. OECD. Health status: infant health. Organization for Economic Cooperation and Development stat extracts. 2012. Available at: http://stats.oecd.org/index.aspx?DataSetCode=HEALTH_STAT. Accessed February 27, 2014.
12. Mathews TJ, MacDorman MF. Infant mortality statistics from the 2010 period linked birth/infant death data set. Natl Vital Stat Rep 2013;62(8):1–26.
13. Hirai AH, Sappenfield WM, Kogan MD, et al. Contributors to excess infant mortality in the US south. Am J Prev Med 2014;46(3):219–27.
14. Menfield CE, Dawson J. Infant mortality in southern states: a bureaucratic nightmare. J Health Hum Serv Adm 2008;31(3):385–402.
15. Mathews TJ, MacDorman MF, Menacker F. Infant mortality statistics from the 2000 period linked birth/infant death data set. Natl Vital Stat Rep 2002;50(12): 1–28 Hyattsville (MD): National Center for Health Statistics.
16. David RJ, Collins JW. Differing birth weight among infants of US-born blacks, African-born blacks, and US-born whites. N Engl J Med 1997;337(17):1209–14.
17. Collins JW Jr, Wu SY, David RJ. Differing intergenerational birth weights among the descendants of US-born and foreign-born Whites and African Americans in Illinois. Am J Epidemiol 2002;155(3):210–6.
18. Collins JW Jr, David RJ. Pregnancy outcome of Mexican-American women: the effect of generational residence in the United States. Ethn Dis 2004;14(2): 317–21.
19. David R, Collins J Jr. Disparities in infant mortality: what's genetics got to do with it? Am J Public Health 2007;97(7):1191–7.

20. Schoendorf KC, Hogue CJ, Kleinman JC, et al. Mortality among infants of black as compared with white college-educated parents. N Engl J Med 1992;326(23): 1522–6.

21. Murray JL, Bernfield M. The differential effect of prenatal care on the incidence of low birth weight among blacks and whites in a prepaid health care plan. N Engl J Med 1988;319(21):1385–91.

22. Barfield WD, Wise PH, Rust FP, et al. Racial disparities in outcomes of military and civilian births in California. Arch Pediatr Adolesc Med 1996;150(10):1062–7.

23. Colen CG, Geronimus AT, Bound J, et al. Maternal upward socioeconomic mobility and black-white disparities in infant birthweight. Am J Public Health 2006;96(11):2032–9.

24. Lu MC, Halfon N. Racial and ethnic disparities in birth outcomes: a life-course perspective. Matern Child Health J 2003;7(1):13–30.

25. Jacob RA, Gretz DM, Taylor PC, et al. Moderate folate depletion increases plasma homocysteine and decreases lymphocyte DNA methylation in postmenopausal women. J Nutr 1998;128(7):1204–12.

26. Scholl TO, Johnson WG. Folic acid: influence on the outcome of pregnancy. Am J Clin Nutr 2000;71(Suppl 5):1295s–303s.

27. Hoyo C, Murtha A, Schildkraut J, et al. Folic acid supplementation before and during pregnancy in the Newborn Epigenetics STudy (NEST). BMC Public Health 2011;11(1):46.

28. Catov JM, Bodnar LM, Ness RB, et al. Association of periconceptional multivitamin use and risk of preterm or small-for-gestational-age births. Am J Epidemiol 2007; 166(3):296–303.

29. Burris HH, Mitchell AA, Werler MM. Periconceptional multivitamin use and infant birth weight disparities. Ann Epidemiol 2010;20(3):233–40.

30. Haggarty P, Hoad G, Horgan GW, et al. DNA methyltransferase candidate polymorphisms, imprinting methylation, and birth outcome. PLoS One 2013; 8(7):e68896.

31. Azzi S, Sas TC, Koudou Y, et al. Degree of methylation of ZAC1 (PLAGL1) is associated with prenatal and post-natal growth in healthy infants of the EDEN mother child cohort. Epigenetics 2013;9(3):338–45.

32. Hughes D, Chen L. When and what parents tell children about race: an examination of race-related socialization among African American families. Appl Dev Sci 1997;1(4):200–14.

33. White-Johnson RL, Ford KR, Sellers RM. Parental racial socialization profiles: association with demographic factors, racial discrimination, childhood socialization, and racial identity. Cultur Divers Ethnic Minor Phycol 2010;16(2):237–47.

34. Geronimus AT. Understanding and eliminating racial inequalities in women's health in the United States: the role of the weathering conceptual framework. J Am Med Womens Assoc 2001;56(4):133–6, 149-50.

35. Clark R, Anderson NB, Clark VR, et al. Racism as a stressor for African Americans. A biopsychosocial model. Am Psychol 1999;54(10):805–16.

36. Collins JW Jr, David RJ, Rankin KM, et al. Transgenerational effect of neighborhood poverty on low birth weight among African Americans in Cook County, Illinois. Am J Epidemiol 2009;169(6):712–7.

37. Franklin TB, Russig H, Weiss IC, et al. Epigenetic transmission of the impact of early stress across generations. Biol Psychiatry 2010;68(5):408–15.

38. Pena CJ, Neugut YD, Champagne FA. Developmental timing of the effects of maternal care on gene expression and epigenetic regulation of hormone receptor levels in female rats. Endocrinology 2013;154(11):4340–51.

39. Dunn GA, Bale TL. Maternal high-fat diet promotes body length increases and insulin insensitivity in second-generation mice. Endocrinology 2009;150(11): 4999–5009.

40. Dunn GA, Bale TL. Maternal high-fat diet effects on third-generation female body size via the paternal lineage. Endocrinology 2011;152(6):2228–36.

41. Halfon N, Larson K, Lu M, et al. Lifecourse health development: past, present and future. Matern Child Health J 2014;18:344–65.

42. Shonkoff JP, Richter L, van der Gaag J, et al. An integrated scientific framework for child survival and early childhood development. Pediatrics 2012;129(2): e460–72.

43. Hanson JL, Hair N, Shen DG, et al. Family poverty affect the rate of human infant brain growth. PLoS One 2013;8(12):e80954.

44. Garner AS, Shonkoff JP, Siegel BS, et al, Committee on Psychosocial Aspects of Child and Family Health, Committee on Early Childhood, Adoption, and Dependent Care, Section on Developmental and Behavioral Pediatrics. Early childhood adversity, toxic stress, and the role of the pediatrician: translating developmental science into lifelong health. Pediatrics 2012;129(1):e224–31.

45. Hart B, Risley TR. The early catastrophe: the 30 million word gap by age 3. American Educator 2003;27(1):4–9.

46. Kaplan JB, Bennett T. Use of race and ethnicity in biomedical publication. JAMA 2003;289(20):2709–16.

47. Lorusso L. The justification of race in biological explanation. J Med Ethics 2011; 37:535–9.

48. Acevedo-Garcia D, Soobader M, Berkman L. The differential effect of foreign born status on low birth weight by race/ethnicity and education. Pediatrics 2005;115:e20.

49. Almond DV, Chay KY, Greenstone M. Civil rights, the war on poverty, and black-white convergence in infant mortality in Mississippi. Berkeley (CA): Center for Labor Economics, University of California; 2001.

50. Dominguez TP, Dunkel-Schetter C, Glynn LM, et al. Racial differences in birth outcomes: the role of general, pregnancy and racism stress. Health Psychol 2008;27(2):194–203.

51. Jones CP. Levels of racism: a theoretic framework and a gardener's tale. Am J Public Health 2000;90(8):1212–5.

52. Hilmers A, Hilmers DC, Dave J. Neighborhood disparities in access to healthy foods and their effects on environmental justice. Am J Public Health 2012; 102(9):1644–54.

53. Barker D. Mothers, babies and disease in later life. London: British Medical Journal; 1994.

54. Kuzawa C. Developmental origins of life history: growth, productivity and reproduction. Am J Human Biol 2007;19:654–61.

55. Kuzawa C, Sweet E. Epigenetics and the embodiment of race: developmental origins of US racial disparities in cardiovascular health. Am J Human Biol 2009;21(1):2–15.

56. Kowaleski-Jones L, Duncan GJ. Effects of participation in the WIC Program on birthweight: evidence from the national longitudinal survey of youth. Am J Public Health 2002;92(5):799–804.

57. Khanani I, Elam AS, Hearn R, et al. The impact of prenatal WIC participation on infant mortality and racial disparities. Am J Public Health 2010;100:S204–9.

58. Waldfogel J, Craigie T, Brooks-Gunn J. Fragile families and child well being. Future Child 2010;20(2):113–31.

59. McHale J, Waller MR, Pearson J. Coparenting interventions for fragile families: what do we know and where do we need to go next? Fam Process 2012; 51(3):284–306.
60. Johnson MD. Healthy marriage initiatives: on the need for empiricism in policy implementation. Am Psychol 2012;67(4):296–308.
61. Hawkins AJ, Stanley SM, Cowan PA, et al. A more optimistic perspective on government-supported marriage and relationship education programs for lower income couples. Am Psychol 2013;68(2):110–1.
62. Johnson MD. Optimistic or quixotic? More data on marriage and relationship education programs for lower income couples. Am Psychol 2013;68(2): 111–2.
63. Hillis SD, Anda RA, Dube SR, et al. The protective effect of family strengths in childhood against adolescent pregnancy and its long-term psychosocial consequences. Perm J 2010;14(3):18–27.
64. National Research Council and Institute of Medicine. From neurons to neighborhoods: the science of early childhood development. In: Committee on Integrating the Science of Early Childhood Development, Shonkoff JP, Phillips DA, editors. Board on Children, Youth and Families, Commission on Behavioral and Social Sciences and Education. Washington, DC: National Academy Press; 2000.
65. Campbell F, Conti G, Heckman J, et al. Early childhood investments substantially boost adult health. Science 2014;343(6178):1478–85.
66. Walsemann K, Geronimus AT, Gee G. Accumulating disadvantage over the life course: evidence from a longitudinal study investigating the relationship between educational advantage in youth and health in middle age. Res Aging 2008;30:169–99. http://dx.doi.org/10.1177/0164027507311149.
67. Karoly LA, Kilburn M, Cannon J. Early childhood interventions: proven results, Future Promise. Santa Monica (CA): RAND; 2005. Available at: http://www.rand.org/pubs/monographs/MG341.
68. National Academy of Sciences, Committee on Early Childhood Care and Education Workforce, Board on Children, Youth and Families, Institute of Medicine and National Research Council of the National Academies. The early childhood care and education workforce: challenges and opportunities: a workshop report. Washington, DC: The National Academies Press; 2012.
69. Reynolds AJ, Temple JA, White BA, et al. Age 26 cost-benefit analysis of the child-parent center early education program. Child Dev 2011;82(1):379–404.
70. Karoly LA. Toward standardization of benefit-cost analyses of early childhood interventions. Santa Monica (CA): RAND; 2011.
71. Karoly LA. Using benefit-cost analysis to inform early childhood care and education policy. Presented at The Early Childhood Care and Education Workforce: A Workshop. Washington, DC, February 28 and March 1, 2011.
72. Magnuson KA, Waldfogel J. Early childhood care and education: effects on ethnic and racial gaps in school readiness. Future Child 2005;15(1):169–88.
73. Shonkoff JP, Fisher PA. Rethinking evidence-based practice and two-generation programs to create the future of early childhood policy. Dev Psychopathol 2013; 25(4 Pt 2):1635–53.
74. Hertzman C, Boyce T. How experience gets under the skin to create gradients in developmental health. Annu Rev Public Health 2010;31:329–47.
75. Shonkoff JP, Boyce TW, McEwen BS. Neuroscience, molecular biology, and the childhood roots of health disparities. Building a framework for health promotion and disease prevention. JAMA 2009;301(21):2252–9.

76. Heisler EJ. The US infant mortality rate: international comparisons, underlying factors, and federal programs. Federation of American Scientists; 2012. Available at: https://www.fas.org/sgp/crs/misc/R41378.pdf. Accessed on March 13, 2014.
77. Geronimus AT. The weathering hypothesis and the health of African American women and infants: evidence and speculations. Ethn Dis 1992;2:207–21.
78. Giscombe CL, Lobel M. Explaining disproportionately high rates of adverse birth outcomes among African Americans: the impact of stress, racism and related factors in pregnancy. Psychol Bull 2005;131:662–83.
79. Wightkin J, Magnus JH, Farley TA, et al. Psychosocial predictors of being an underweight infant differ by racial group: a prospective study of Louisiana WIC program participants. Matern Child Health J 2007;11:49–55.
80. Lu MC, Kotelchuck M, Hogan V. Closing the black-white gap in birth outcomes: a life-course approach. Ethn Dis 2010;20(2):62–76.
81. Hogan VK, Rowley D, Bennett T, et al. Life course, social determinants, and health inequities: toward a national plan for achieving health equity for African American infants–a concept paper. Matern Child Health J 2012;16:1143–50.
82. Byrd WM, Clayton LA. An American health dilemma. A medical history of African Americans and the problem of race: beginnings to 1900, vol. 1. New York: Routledge; 2000. p. 3.

It's Not Your Mother's Marijuana

Effects on Maternal-Fetal Health and the Developing Child

Tamara D. Warner, PhD[a], Dikea Roussos-Ross, MD[b],*,
Marylou Behnke, MD[a]

KEYWORDS

- Pregnancy • Marijuana • Cannabis • Prenatal exposure • Substance use
- Perinatal outcomes • Fetal effects • Developmental effects

KEY POINTS

- Pro-marijuana advocacy may result in an increase in the prevalence of marijuana use during pregnancy, particularly among young adolescents who already report the highest use among all pregnant women.
- Today's marijuana is 6 to 7 times more potent than in the 1970s; average marijuana consumption may be higher owing to growing popularity of blunts compared with joints.
- Adverse fetal outcomes related to marijuana use during pregnancy remain unclear. However, prenatal use has been associated with infertility, placental complications, and fetal growth restriction.
- Long-term effects of prenatal marijuana use on exposed offspring include poorer executive functioning skills and attention, increased conduct and behavior problems, and poorer school achievement.
- Intersecting political forces and medical issues mandate that physicians be knowledgeable marijuana use by their patients and be prepared to counsel their patients about the effects of prenatal marijuana use on fertility, pregnancy, and the exposed offspring.

INTRODUCTION

Societal attitudes toward marijuana use in the United States are undergoing an historical shift. In the 1960s, a generation of young people embraced marijuana for personal

The authors have no conflicts of interest or affiliations with companies that have direct financial interests in the subject matter of this article.
[a] Department of Pediatrics, University of Florida, PO Box 100296, Gainesville, FL 32610-0296, USA; [b] Department of Obstetrics and Gynecology, University of Florida, PO Box 100294, Gainesville, FL 32610-0294, USA
* Corresponding author.
E-mail address: kroussos@ufl.edu

recreational use. Today, "medical" marijuana (*cannabis sativa*) has been approved for use in 22 states and the District of Columbia either by legislation or by popular vote in statewide referenda or ballot initiatives; 15 of the 22 legal actions were passed in the last decade (since 2004).[1] As of May, 2014, another 7 states have pending legislation or ballot measures to legalize medical marijuana.[2] In addition, 2 states—Colorado and Washington state—have legalized marijuana for recreational use. The attitudinal shift is apparent not just among adults but among teens as well. The most recent annual survey of adolescent drug use indicates that the annual prevalence of marijuana use has been trending upward since 2008 for 8th, 10th, and 12th graders; perhaps more important, the perceived risk of regular marijuana use has declined sharply in recent years, a trend that started in 2005.[3,*]

Epidemiology of Marijuana Use Among Pregnant Women

Marijuana is the most commonly used illicit drug during pregnancy. **Table 1** shows the 2011 through 2012 combined annual prevalence rates based on past-month use for illicit drugs, alcohol, and cigarettes by pregnant women in the United States.[4] The rate for marijuana and hashish was 5.2%, which translates to 115,000 pregnant women using marijuana annually. Still, the prevalence rates for marijuana are significantly lower than the rates for alcohol (8.5%) and cigarette (15.9%) use during pregnancy. **Table 1** also shows the prevalence rates by age and trimester for marijuana, cigarette, and alcohol use by pregnant women. Young adolescents (ages 15–17) have the highest rate of marijuana use during pregnancy (16.5%), which is more than double the rate for 18- to 25-year-olds (7.5%).[4] Marijuana use during pregnancy is highest during the first trimester (10.7%), then declines significantly during the second trimester (2.8%) and third trimester (2.3%).[4] After childbirth, marijuana use rebounds quickly.[5] **Box 1** outlines some of the sociodemographic characteristics that are common among women who use illicit drugs during pregnancy and some that may be unique to women who use marijuana during pregnancy.[6]

Potential Impact of Medical Marijuana

The legal status of medical marijuana is under debate. Marijuana is a Schedule I drug under the Controlled Substance Act, a federal law that preempts actions taken by individual states to legalize its use, cultivation, and distribution.[7] Legal scholars have argued that when used for medicinal purposes, marijuana should be considered a pharmaceutical agent governed by the Food, Drug and Cosmetic Act with regulatory oversight, including evaluation of its safety and efficacy, provided by the Food and Drug Administration.[7]

There is emerging evidence that states with legalized medical marijuana have higher rates of marijuana use, depending on specific aspects of laws and policies.[8] In states that allow home cultivation and legal dispensaries, higher levels of recreational use and higher levels of heavy use are found. By contrast, states that restrict broad access to medical marijuana by requiring annual registration of patients have lower prevalence rates and treatment admissions compared with those that do not.[9]

---

* As used herein, *marijuana* refers to the crude drug derived from *Cannabis sativa*, specifically dried preparations of the floral and foliar material from outdoor-grown pollinated female plants commonly called *herbal cannabis* in Europe. *Sinsemilla* is used to refer to indoor-grown unfertilized female plants (known as *skunk* in the United Kingdom). Our use of the term *marijuana* excludes *hashish* preparations (*resin* in Europe) and hash oil. *Cannabis* is used as the umbrella term to refer to 2 or more preparations of the plant.

Table 1

Percentage substance use in the past month among women ages 15 to 44 by pregnancy status, age group and trimester

Drug	Total Sample	Pregnancy Status		Pregnancy Age Group			Trimester Use		
		Nonpregnant Women	Pregnant Women	15-17	18-25	26-44	First	Second	Third
Illicit drugs[a]	10.5	10.7	5.9	18.3	9.0	3.4	11.6	4.0	2.3
Marijuana and Hashish	8.2	8.3	5.2	16.5	7.5	3.3	10.7	2.8	2.3
Cigarettes	24.2	24.6	15.9	[b]	20.9	12.5	23.2	13.6	11.1
Alcohol	53.8	55.5	8.5	13.4	7.3	9.0	17.9	4.2	3.7

[a] Illicit drugs include marijuana/hashish, cocaine (including crack), heroin, hallucinogens, inhalants, or prescription-type psychotherapeutics used nonmedically.

[b] Low precision; no estimate reported.

Data from Substance Abuse and Mental Health Services Administration (SAMHSA), Center for behavioral health statistics and quality, national survey on drug use and health, 2011–2012 (Miscellaneous Tables 6.71B, 6.73B, 6.74B, 6.75B and 6.76B). Available at: http://www.samhsa.gov/data/NSDUH/2012SummNatFind DetTables/DetTabs/NSDUH-DetTabsTOC2012.htm.

> **Box 1**
> **Sociodemographic characteristics of illicit drug-using pregnant women**
>
> *Common Among Women Who Use Illicit Drugs During Pregnancy*
> - Prepregnancy body mass index scores in the underweight range
> - Folic acid supplementation lacking in the periconceptional period
> - Alcohol use and cigarette smoking during pregnancy
> - Partners are illicit drug users
> - Intimate partner violence
> - Lower levels of education and income
> - Higher rates of unemployment
>
> *May Be Unique to Women Who Use Marijuana During Pregnancy[a]*
> - Excessive weight gain during pregnancy
> - More likely to be nulliparous
> - More likely to have had an induced abortion in the past
>
> [a] Data is from a population-based study using the National Birth Defects Prevention Study with a relatively small sample of marijuana users (n = 189).

Growing pro-marijuana advocacy efforts may increase marijuana use among pregnant women. In the absence of public health messages about the potential risks, marijuana may be perceived as "safe" to use during pregnancy compared with other illicit drugs and in comparison with alcohol and cigarettes. Medical marijuana laws that involve the use of dispensaries have been shown to drive down prices,[10,11] which will likely increase use among certain groups.[9] In a recent study, urban, low-income, primarily African-American postpartum women reported perceptions of relatively lower risk of marijuana compared with licit drugs as well as roughly equivalent costs of marijuana and cigarettes.[12]

Increasing Potency and Consumption of Marijuana

The potency of marijuana has increased markedly during the past 40 years in the United States, and elsewhere (review by McLaren and colleagues[13]). From the 1970s to the 2000s, there has been an estimated 6- to 7-fold increase in the potency of cannabis seized in the United States as measured by the percentage of Δ^9-tetrahydrocannabinol (THC), the most psychoactive of the 70 cannabinoids found in cannabis.[14] Between 1993 and 2008, the mean concentration of THC rose from 3.4% to 8.8%.[15]

In addition to concerns about potency, the amount of marijuana consumed, on average, seems to be increasing among younger adults, particularly minorities owing to the growing popularity of blunts (marijuana-filled cigars) compared with joints and pipes. One study found that blunts contain significantly greater amounts of marijuana—up to 1.5 times more than joints and 2.5 times more than pipes.[16]

ISSUES RELATED TO MARIJUANA USE DURING PREGNANCY
Screening Pregnant Women for Marijuana Use

Box 2 summarizes some of the recommendations made by the American College of Obstetrics and Gynecology[17–19] and the American Society of Addiction Medicine[20]

> **Box 2**
> **Professional organizations' recommendations related to drug use during pregnancy**
>
> *American College of Obstetrics and Gynecology[1]*
> - Universal screening for drug use in females of reproductive age
> - Screening at the first prenatal or intake visit and at least once per trimester thereafter
> - Consider drug testing (with patient consent) when screening tests are positive
> - Refer for substance abuse treatment for all pregnant women who have evidence of drug use in pregnancy
> - Protect the physician–patient relationship
>
> *American Society of Addiction Medicine[2]*
> - Prenatal education about all drugs for all pregnant women
> - Universal screening to identify "at risk" women including repeated follow-up assessments
> - Culturally competent public prevention programs to educate the public about realistic dangers of drug use in pregnancy
> - Education of health care providers in the care and management of women with evidence of drug use before, during, and after pregnancy
> - Women who are pregnant should receive priority admission to substance treatment facilities
>
> *Data from* ProCon.org. 22 legal medical marijuana states and dc: laws, fees, and possession limits - I summary chart. Available at: http://medicalmarijuana.procon.org/view.resource.php?resourceID=000881. Accessed May 30, 2014; and ProCon.org. 4 states with pending legislation to legalize medical marijuana (as of May 29, 2014). Available at: http://medicalmarijuana.procon.org/view.resource.php?resourceID=002481. Accessed May 30, 2014.

related to drug use during pregnancy. The American College of Obstetrics and Gynecology recommends that screening for substance abuse be part of complete obstetric care and be performed routinely throughout pregnancy because women may be more willing to disclose substance abuse as they develop rapport with their provider.[19] Additionally, it is recommended that providers become knowledgeable on brief intervention techniques and referral services for treatment. The American Society of Addiction Medicine also advocates universal screening for drug use among pregnant women and appropriate referral for substance treatment when patients who require services are identified.[20]

Screening should be performed with the consent of the pregnant woman and can be conducted with standardized questionnaires such as the 4 Ps or the CRAFFT Interview[18] (CRAFFT is available for download in 13 languages at http://www.ceasar-boston.org/CRAFFT/screenCRAFFT.php). Another evidence-based and readily available screening tool is the 5 Ps,[21] an adaptation of the 4 Ps that includes a question about peers (friends); an "integrated" version also asks about intimate partner violence, emotional health (worry, anxiety, depression, or sadness), and cigarette use.[22] Drug testing can be performed with the woman's permission. The 3 most commonly used specimens to establish drug use during the prenatal and perinatal periods are urine, meconium, and hair.[23] Of these, urine is used most frequently owing to the ease of collection.[23] In regular marijuana users, urine testing can be positive up to 10 days after use; for chronic or heavy users, urine can be positive for up to 30 days after last use. Meconium is easily collected in the newborn nursery. It reveals exposure to marijuana in the second and third trimesters because this is when meconium is formed in the fetus.[23] Hair sampling has not been found to be as useful for detection of marijuana.

When considering drug testing in pregnancy, it is important for the clinician to be familiar with the reporting laws of the state in which he or she practices. States vary about whether evidence of drug exposure to a fetus or newborn mandates reporting the case to the child welfare system with possible removal of children and/or incarceration of the mother.[18] As of May 2014, there are 17 states that consider substance abuse during pregnancy to be child abuse under civil child welfare statutes; 3 states consider it grounds for involuntary commitment to a mental health or substance abuse treatment facility (**Table 2**).[24] These laws have been found to hinder the physician–patient relationship, decrease compliance with prenatal care, and increase the risk of perinatal mortality.[17,18,25] Owing to fears of incarceration or the loss of one's children, pregnant women may not be willing to disclose their use. For this reason, it is imperative to preserve the physician–patient relationship, which will allow women to feel safer discussing drug use with their provider. Pregnant women who are identified as using drugs should be counseled and referred for substance abuse treatment. Early detection of drug use allows for timely implementation of harm reduction strategies during pregnancy.[26]

Aside from the legal implications, there are additional barriers that obstetricians face when deciding whether to screen and/or test patients for substance use. Two such barriers are concerns about having the time to screen patients appropriately and a lack of local substance use treatment resources, particularly for pregnant women. The time barrier could be reduced if reimbursement was provided to physicians for screening pregnant patients for substance use, similar to the reimbursement for tobacco use screening. Local substance abuse treatment facilities can be located through the online Behavioral Health Treatment Services Locator, available from the Substance Abuse and Mental Health Services Administration at http://findtreatment.samhsa.gov/locator/home.

Effects of Prenatal Marijuana Use

A list of the possible pregnancy-related effects of prenatal marijuana use can be found in **Box 3**. Marijuana easily passes through the maternal circulation, into the placenta, and then fetus. It is also found in breast milk. Marijuana can be detected in umbilical cord blood, neonatal urine, and meconium.

Preclinical studies are important because they can (1) provide a level of control for confounding variables not achievable in clinical studies, (2) offer a framework for developing hypotheses for further study in human populations, and (3) help to identify the pathologic changes that underlie the medical and behavioral changes observed in clinical studies. A full discussion of the preclinical literature is beyond the scope of this review and the reader is referred to pertinent studies and reviews available in the extant literature.[27–30]

Research into the effects of THC in humans began in the late 1800s with 2 major advances occurring when the main psychoactive compound in marijuana, THC, was identified by Gaoni and Mechoulam in 1964[31] and when the existence of cannabinoid receptors, called the endocannabinoid system, was confirmed by Devane and colleagues[32] in 1988.

Cannabinoid receptors are found in various tissues throughout the human body, including the brain and uterine decidua. Thus, the physiologic functions of the endocannabinoid system are important to both early embryonic development and synaptic brain plasticity. However, exposure to exogenous cannabinoids could result in pathophysiologic changes secondary to the longer binding of THC to the receptors compared with naturally occurring endocannabinoids.

With regard to early embryonic development, it is possible that exogenous cannabinoids could significantly disrupt regulation of blastocyst maturation, oviductal transport, implantation, and pregnancy maintenance. In addition, THC acts as an in vivo weak competitor of the estrogen receptor, producing a primary estrogen effect in male and female rats,[33] stifles trophoblast cell proliferation, and inhibits successful placentation, possibly producing other pregnancy-related complications.[34,35]

In the brain, cannabinoids alter executive functions in the prefrontal cortex, including working memory, attention, and cognitive flexibility. Additionally, the release of neurotransmitters such as dopamine, serotonin, and acetylcholine, each of which affects cognitive functions in the prefrontal cortex, as well as behavior and mood, has been shown to be altered in the face of cannabinoid exposure.

Marijuana and Infertility

Human studies on male subjects have shown disruptions in the hypothalamic–pituitary–testicular axis with decreased luteinizing hormone, decreased testosterone, oligospermia, and decreased sperm motility, thus possibly affecting male infertility.[36] Likewise, in women, chronic marijuana exposure has been associated with suppressed ovulation, altered prolactin, follicle-stimulating hormone, luteinizing hormone, and estrogen.[37,38]

Pregnancy-Related Complications

The endocannabinoid system is present in the uterine decidua, thus suggesting possible involvement in pregnancy complications such as miscarriage, preeclampsia, growth restriction and preterm labor.[35] Additionally, first trimester placentas express cannabinoid receptors, further implicating the role that alterations in the endocannabinoid system may play in pregnancy complications. Marijuana use during pregnancy has been shown to be associated with an increased fetal pulsatility index and resistance index of the uterine artery,[39] suggestive of increased placental resistance.[40] These findings may provide a partial explanation for intrauterine growth restriction.[41]

Fetal Growth and Birth Outcomes

Available data to this point do not reveal marijuana-associated fetal teratogenicity. Studies on the effects of prenatal maternal marijuana use on fetal growth and birth outcomes have yielded inconsistent results. A 2013 review of studies on prenatal marijuana exposure by Huizink[41] specifically examined fetal growth, birth outcomes and early infant development using data from several sources including 3 prospective longitudinal studies: (1) The Ottawa Prenatal Prospective Study (OPPS), which began in 1978 and enrolled a predominantly middle-class, low-risk, Caucasian sample from Ottawa, Canada,[42] (2) the Maternal Health Practice and Child Development Study (MHPCD), which started in 1982 and enrolled a high-risk, low socioeconomic status mixed Caucasian and African-American sample from Pittsburgh, Pennsylvania,[43] and (3) the Generation R study, which started in 2010 and recruited a multi-ethnic population-based cohort in Rotterdam, The Netherlands.[44] Of the 3 cohorts, only the Generation R study has examined fetal growth through ultrasound assessments several times during pregnancy.

Fetal growth

A study using elective mid-gestation aborted fetuses (17–22 weeks) who were exposed to marijuana, tobacco, and alcohol demonstrated decreased weight and decreased foot length that was associated with marijuana exposure after controlling for other drug exposures.[45] No association was found between prenatal marijuana

Table 2
State policies on substance abuse during pregnancy

State	Substance Abuse During Pregnancy Considered		When Abuse Suspected, State Requires		Targeted Program Created	Drug Treatment for Pregnant Women	
	Child Abuse	Grounds for Civil Commitment	Reporting	Testing		Pregnant Women Given Priority Access in General Programs	Pregnant Women Protected from Discrimination in Publicly Funded Programs
Alaska			X				
Arizona			X			X	
Arkansas	X				X		
California					X		
Colorado	X				X		
Connecticut					X		
Florida	X				X		
Georgia						X	
Illinois	X		X		X		
Indiana	X						
Iowa	X		X	X			X
Kansas						X	X
Kentucky				X	X		
Louisiana	X		X		X		
Maryland			X		X	X	
Massachusetts			X				
Michigan			X				

State							
Minnesota	X						
Missouri	X		X			X[a]	
Montana			X				X
Nebraska	X				X[b]		
Nevada	X						
New York							
North Carolina							
North Dakota			X	X			
Ohio							
Oklahoma	X		X			X	X
Oregon				X	X[c]		
Pennsylvania					X		
Rhode Island	X		X		X		
South Carolina	X[d]						
South Dakota	X						
Tennessee	X					X	
Texas	X					X	
Utah			X				
Virginia	X		X		X		
Washington				X	X		
Wisconsin	X		X			X	
TOTAL	*17*	*3*	*15*	*4*	*18*	*10*	*4*

[a] Priority applies to pregnant women referred for treatment.
[b] Applies only to women and newborns eligible for Medicaid.
[c] Establishes requirements for health care providers to encourage and facilitate drug counseling.
[d] The South Carolina Supreme Court held that a viable fetus is a "person" under the state's criminal child endangerment statute and that "maternal acts endangering or likely to endanger the life, comfort, or health of a viable fetus" constitute criminal child abuse.

Data from Guttmacher Institute. State policies in brief: substance abuse during pregnancy (as of May 2014). New York: Guttmacher Institute; 2014.

> **Box 3**
> **Possible pregnancy-related effects of prenatal marijuana use**
>
> - Decreased male fertility
> - Decreased ovulation
> - Altered hormones (prolactin, follicle-stimulating hormone, luteinizing hormone, estrogen)
> - Altered oviductal transport, embryo implantation, and maintenance of pregnancy
> - Altered placental blood flow
> - Intrauterine growth restriction
> - Decreased gestational age
> - Decreased birth weight

exposure and body length or head circumference after controlling for covariates.[45] Results from the Generation R study have shown reduced fetal growth from the second trimester onward, particularly for mothers who used early marijuana during pregnancy or throughout the entire pregnancy.[46]

Birth outcomes

Results have differed between the 3 longitudinal cohorts described, with the OPPS reporting reduced gestational age but no differences in birth weight,[47] the MPHCD reporting reduced birth length after first trimester exposure and unexpectedly, increased birth weight after third trimester exposure,[48] and Generation R reporting lower birth weight.[46]

Studies drawn from other sources yield conflicting results. A recent study by Hayatbakhsh and colleagues[49] reported lower birth weight, by an average of 375 g, lower gestational age, shorter body length, and an increase in neonatal intensive care unit admissions owing to marijuana exposure after adjusting for tobacco, alcohol, and other illicit drug exposures. However, studies reporting no association between marijuana use and fetal growth include the Maternal Lifestyle Study,[50] a multicenter, prospective study of 8600 women (which also included cocaine use)[51] and the Avon Longitudinal Study of Pregnancy cohort of more than 12,000 pregnant women.[52] A population-based study using data from the National Birth Defects Prevention Study also found no associations between marijuana use during pregnancy and mean birth weight, gestational age, low birth weight, or preterm delivery.[6]

Maternal Marijuana Use and Lactation

There is a paucity of data regarding the effects of maternal marijuana use on breastfeeding and infant outcomes. Small to moderate amounts of THC are secreted into breast milk after maternal use with significant absorption by the infant. However, identification of side effects in the lactation-exposed infant are inconsistent,[53,54] and no long-term outcome studies are available. As noted in the previous section, studies of the endocannabinoid system from both the animal and human literature indicate there are neurobehavioral complications after marijuana exposure during pregnancy, raising the possibility of complications after exposure during lactation as well. More detailed information is available in recent reviews by Rowe and colleagues[55] and Hill and Reed.[25] At the present time, the American Academy of Pediatrics recommends that women who are using street drugs, including marijuana, not breastfeed their infants.[56]

DEVELOPMENTAL OUTCOMES OF PRENATAL MARIJUANA EXPOSURE: NEONATAL PERIOD TO EARLY ADULTHOOD

As outlined previously, several prospective, longitudinal cohort studies have evaluated the effects of prenatal marijuana exposure on offspring. However, the OPPS and the MHPCD are the only cohorts that have been followed into adolescence and early adulthood. Despite the demographic differences between these 2 cohorts, when the results overlap, they are remarkably consistent.

Neonatal Withdrawal and Neurobehavior

Withdrawal
Neonatal withdrawal from marijuana exposure has not been reported in any of the prospective, longitudinal studies.

Neurobehavior
Evidence of altered state regulation, manifested as increased startles and tremors, was identified in the OPPS sample during the first week of life[57] using the Neonatal Behavioral Assessment Scale[58] with similar results found again at 9 and 30 days[59] using the Prechtl[60] neurologic examination. Poorer visual habituation and responses were also noted during the first week of life,[57] but these problems were not seen again at 9 or 30 days.[59] No effects were reported from the MHPCD on newborn behavior using the Neonatal Behavioral Assessment Scale.[43] However, exposed newborns demonstrated altered sleep patterns with a decrease in quiet sleep and increased sleep motility, suggesting increased activity in the noradrenergic system.[61] Other newborn studies have demonstrated abnormal newborn cry,[62] also suggestive of increased arousal. Other investigators have found no abnormalities in infant behavior.[63,64]

Prenatal Marijuana Exposure and Outcomes from Late Infancy to Young Adulthood

This section focuses on the areas of development where prenatal marijuana exposure seems to have a significant impact: Executive function, attention, achievement, and behavior. Findings in other areas of development can be summarized as follows, with details found in **Box 4**.

Executive function and attention
Of importance, both cohorts have reported a negative effect of prenatal marijuana exposure on specific areas of cognition related to executive function at age 3 years,[70] 4 years,[66] and 6 years.[80] Findings in both cohorts include poorer scores on memory and verbal measures. At 6 years, Fried and colleagues[81] reported a negative effect of prenatal marijuana exposure on the attentiveness of subjects using a vigilance task. This finding is consistent with that from the MHPCD at 6 years, which showed increased impulsivity on a vigilance task.[82] Children ages 9 to 12 in both the OPPS

Box 4
Finding in areas of development in prenatal marijuana exposure

1. Minimal, inconsistent effect on general cognition[65–70]
2. Altered sleep patterns[71]
3. No effect on language[65–67,72]
4. Minimal effect on motor development[54,65,69,73,74]
5. Minimal effects on growth and pubertal development[47,75–79]

and the MHPCD showed poorer abstract/visual reasoning, impulse control, hypothesis testing, and visual problem solving.[83–85] At age 10, marijuana-exposed youth in the MHPCD were more likely to exhibit hyperactivity, impulsivity, and inattention, according to maternal report.[86] Finally, 2 studies from the OPPS when subjects were 13 to 16 years old documented continued problems with executive function and attention. Adolescents with prenatal marijuana exposure demonstrated decreased attentional stability as evidenced by a decreasing consistency in reaction time as the test progressed and by an increase in errors of omission.[87] The exposed adolescents also had poorer scores on 2 measures indicative of problems with visual memory, analysis, and integration.[68] Several additional studies from the Ottawa sample have used functional magnetic resonance imaging to evaluate the subjects between 18 and 22 years. While performing a response inhibition task, changes in neural activity were noted on functional magnetic resonance imaging when compared with nonexposed subjects.[88] Although the exposed subjects committed more errors of commission, all were able to finish the task with 85% accuracy or more. While performing a visuospatial working memory task, the exposed subjects showed changes in neural activity on functional magnetic resonance imaging when compared with the nonexposed subjects, although there were no group differences in performance.[89,90]

Academic achievement
Using tests, studies from the OPPS at ages 6 to 9 years[91] and 13 to 16 years[92] showed no effect of prenatal marijuana exposure on standardized academic achievement test scores. This is in contrast to the findings from the MHPCD. Again, using standardized achievement tests, prenatally exposed children had lower reading, spelling, and reading comprehension scores at age 10.[93] Similar results were found at age 14 with lower global achievement and reading scores in the prenatally exposed adolescents.[94]

Behavior problems
Parental reports for subjects in the OPPS showed increased conduct disorders in children from 6 to 9 years old.[91] Parental and teacher reports obtained at age 10 for subjects in the MHPCD revealed increased delinquency and externalizing behaviors.[86] Also, an increase in self-reported depressive symptoms was identified at age 10 for exposed subjects in the MHPCD.[95] At age 14, the age of onset and frequency of the youth's marijuana use was predicted by their prenatal exposure.[96] This finding was also seen in 16- to 21-year-olds from the OPPS.[97] In this study, subjects who were prenatally exposed to marijuana were at greater risk for initiating cigarette smoking and daily use and for initiating marijuana use.

SUMMARY

Evidence about the effects of marijuana use during pregnancy- and fetal-related complications and child development is inconclusive. Data from preclinical studies is suggestive of negative outcomes based on disruptive effects on the endocannabinoid system. The results from longitudinal, prospective studies that started in the late 1970s and early 1980s indicate subtle effects on attention, executive functions, and behavior, particularly as marijuana-exposed youth develop into adolescence and early adulthood. Given that today's marijuana is 6 to 7 times more potent and more likely to be consumed in greater average amounts by younger users, continued surveillance is warranted and may reveal more significant short-term and long-term harms. The practice of medicine for physicians who care for marijuana-using pregnant women is being shaped by shifting societal pressures. Increasingly, marijuana is being thought of as "medicine" by the general public as evidenced by "medical" marijuana laws. Pro-marijuana advocacy efforts may lead to perceptions about marijuana as being relatively "safe" and result in increased use by several groups, including pregnant women. At the same time, pregnant women who use illicit drugs and controlled substances such as prescription opioid analgesics are being criminalized and charged with child abuse and other felonies, despite efforts from scientists and medical professionals. Nationwide educational efforts are imperative to ensure women are not misled into believing that marijuana use in pregnancy is without possible danger to the developing fetus. Further research is critical to ascertain the specific risks to the developing fetus both in utero and beyond.

REFERENCES

1. ProCon.org. 22 legal medical marijuana states and dc: laws, fees, and possession limits - I Summary chart. Available at: http://medicalmarijuana.procon.org/view.resource.php?resourceID=000881. Accessed May 30, 2014.
2. ProCon.org. 4 states with pending legislation to legalize medical marijuana (as of May 29, 2014). Available at: http://medicalmarijuana.procon.org/view.resource.php?resourceID=002481. Accessed May 30, 2014.
3. Johnston LD, Miech RA, Bachman JG, et al. Monitoring the future national survey results on drug use: 1975-2013: overview, key findings on adolescent drug use. Ann Arbor (MI): Institute for Social Research, The University of Michigan; 2014.
4. Substance Abuse And Mental Health Services Administration. Results from the 2012 national survey on drug use and health: summary of national findings, NSDUH series H-46, HHS publication no. (SMA) 13-4798. Rockville (MD): US Department of Health and Human Services, Substance Abuse And Mental Health Services Administration, Center for Behavioral Health Statistics and Quality; 2013.
5. Substance Abuse and Mental Health Services Administration Office of Applied Studies. The NSDUH report: substance use among women during pregnancy and following childbirth. Rockville (MD): Office of Applied Studies, Substance Abuse and Mental Health Services Administration (SAMHSA); 2009.
6. Van Gelder MM, Reefhuis J, Caton AR, et al. Characteristics of pregnant illicit drug users and associations between cannabis use and perinatal outcome in a population-based study. Drug Alcohol Depend 2010;109(1–3):243–7.
7. Cohen PJ. Medical marijuana: the conflict between scientific evidence and political ideology part one of two. J Pain Palliat Care Pharmacother 2009;23(1): 120–40.
8. Cerdá M, Wall M, Keyes KM, et al. Medical marijuana laws in 50 states: investigating the relationship between state legalization of medical marijuana and marijuana use, abuse and dependence. Drug Alcohol Depend 2012;120(1–3):22–7.
9. Pacula RL, Sevigny EL. Marijuana liberalization policies: why we can't learn much from policy still in motion. J Policy Anal Manage 2014;33(1):212–21.
10. Anderson DM, Hansen B, Rees DI. Medical marijuana laws and teen marijuana use. IZA discussion papers, no 6592 [rev]. Bonn (Germany): Institute for the Study of Labor (IZA); 2012.
11. Sevigny EL, Pacula RL, Heaton P. The effects of medical marijuana laws on potency. Int J Drug Policy 2014;25(2):308–19.
12. Beatty JR, Svikis DS, Ondersma SJ. Prevalence and perceived financial costs of marijuana versus tobacco use among urban low-income pregnant women. J Addict Res Ther 2013;3(4):1–12.

13. McLaren J, Swift W, Dillon P, et al. Cannabis potency and contamination: a review of the literature. Addiction 2008;103(7):1100–9.
14. Sevigny EL. Is today's marijuana more potent simply because it's fresher? Drug Test Anal 2013;5(1):62–7.
15. Mehmedic Z, Chandra S, Slade D, et al. Potency trends of Δ^9-THC and other cannabinoids in confiscated cannabis preparations from 1993 to 2008. J Forensic Sci 2010;55(5):1209–17.
16. Mariani JJ, Brooks D, Haney M, et al. Quantification and comparison of marijuana smoking practices: blunts, joints, and pipes. Drug Alcohol Depend 2011;113(2–3):249–51.
17. American College of Obstetricians and Gynecologists. ACOG Committee opinion No. 422: at-risk drinking and illicit drug use: ethical issues in obstetric and gynecologic practice. Obstet Gynecol 2008;2008(422):1449–60.
18. American College of Obstetricians and Gynecologists Committee on Health Care for Underserved Women. ACOG Committee opinion No. 473: substance abuse reporting and pregnancy: the role of the obstetrician-gynecologist. Obstet Gynecol 2011;117(1):200–1.
19. American College of Obstetricians and Gynecologists Committee on Health Care for Underserved Women and the American Society of Addiction Medicine. ACOG committee opinion no. 524: opioid abuse, dependence, and addition in pregnancy. Obstet Gynecol 2012;119(5):1070–6.
20. American Society of Addiction Medicine. Public policy statement on women, alcohol and other drugs, and pregnancy. Chevy Chase (MD): American Society of Addiction Medicine; 2011.
21. Kennedy C, Finkelstein N, Hutchins E, et al. Improving screening for alcohol use during pregnancy: the Massachusetts asap program. Matern Child Health J 2004;8(3):137–47.
22. Institute for Health and Recovery. Integrated 5 P's screening tool. Watertown (MA): Massachusetts Health Quality Partners; 2005.
23. Behnke M, Smith VC. Prenatal substance abuse: short- and long-term effects on the exposed fetus. Pediatrics 2013;131(3):e1009–24.
24. Guttmacher Institute. State policies in brief: substance abuse during pregnancy (as of may 2014). New York: Guttmacher Institute; 2014.
25. Hill M, Reed K. Pregnancy, breast-feeding, and marijuana: a review article. Obstet Gynecol Surv 2013;68(10):710–8.
26. Jaques SC, Kingsbury A, Henshcke P, et al. Cannabis, the pregnant woman and her child: weeding out the myths. J Perinatol 2014;34(6):417–24.
27. Egerton A, Allison C, Brett RR, et al. Cannabinoids and prefrontal cortical function: insights from preclinical studies. Neurosci Biobehav Rev 2006;30(5):680–95.
28. Trezza V, Cuomo V, Vanderschuren LJ. Cannabis and the developing brain: insights from behavior. Eur J Pharmacol 2008;585(2–3):441–52.
29. Jutras-Aswad D, DiNieri JA, Harkany T, et al. Neurobiological consequences of maternal cannabis on human fetal development and its neuropsychiatric outcome. Eur Arch Psychiatry Clin Neurosci 2009;259(7):395–412.
30. Campolongo P, Trezza V, Palmery M, et al. Developmental exposure to cannabinoids causes subtle and enduring neurofunctional alterations. Int Rev Neurobiol 2009;85:117–33.
31. Gaoni Y, Mechoulam R. Isolation, structure, and partial synthesis of an active constituent of hashish. J Am Chem Soc 1964;86(8):1646–7.
32. Devane W, Dysarz F, Johnson M, et al. Determination and characterization of a cannabinoid receptor in rat brain. Mol Pharmacol 1988;34(5):605–13.

33. Rawitch A, Schultz G, Ebner K, et al. Competition of delta 9-tetrahydrocannabinol with estrogen in rat uterine estrogen receptor binding. Science 1977;197(4309):1189–91.
34. Sun X, Xie H, Yang J, et al. Endocannabinoid signaling directs differentiation of trophoblast cell lineages and placentation. Proc Natl Acad Sci U S A 2010;107(39):16887–92.
35. Fonseca BM, Correia-da-Silva G, Almada M, et al. The endocannabinoid system in the postimplantation period: a role during decidualization and placentation. Int J Endocrinol 2013;2013:510540.
36. Fronczak CM, Kim ED, Barqawi AB. The insults of illicit drug use on male fertility. J Androl 2012;33(4):515–28.
37. Lee SY, Oh SM, Chung KH. Estrogenic effects of marijuana smoke condensate and cannabinoid compounds. Toxicol Appl Pharmacol 2006;214(3):270–8.
38. Brown TT, Dobs AS. Endocrine effects of marijuana. J Clin Pharmacol 2002;42(S1):90S–6S.
39. El Marroun H, Tiemeier H, Steegers EA, et al. A prospective study on intrauterine cannabis exposure and fetal blood flow. Early Hum Dev 2010;86(4):231–6.
40. Boito S, Struijk PC, Ursem NT, et al. Umbilical venous volume flow in the normally developing and growth-restricted human fetus. Ultrasound Obstet Gynecol 2002;19(4):344–9.
41. Huizink A. Prenatal cannabis exposure and infant outcomes: overview of studies. Prog Neuropsychopharmacol Biol Psychiatry 2013;52:45–52.
42. Fried PA. The Ottawa Prenatal Prospective Study (OPPS): methodological issues and findings — it's easy to throw the baby out with the bath water. Life Sci 1995;56(23–24):2159–68.
43. Richardson GA, Day NL, Taylor PM. The effect of prenatal alcohol, marijuana, and tobacco exposure on neonatal behavior. Infant Behav Dev 1989;12(2):199–209.
44. Jaddoe VW, Mackenbach JP, Moll HA, et al. The generation R study: design and cohort profile. Eur J Epidemiol 2006;21(6):475–84.
45. Hurd YL, Wang X, Anderson V, et al. Marijuana impairs growth in mid-gestation fetuses. Neurotoxicol Teratol 2005;27(2):221–9.
46. El Marroun H, Tiemeier H, Steegers EA, et al. Intrauterine cannabis exposure affects fetal growth trajectories: the generation r study. J Am Acad Child Adolesc Psychiatry 2009;48(12):1173–81.
47. Fried PA, O'Connell CM. A comparison of the effects of prenatal exposure to tobacco, alcohol, cannabis and caffeine on birth size and subsequent growth. Neurotoxicol Teratol 1987;9(2):79–85.
48. Day N, Sambamoorthi U, Taylor P, et al. Prenatal marijuana use and neonatal outcome. Neurotoxicol Teratol 1991;13(3):329–34.
49. Hayatbakhsh MR, Flenady VJ, Gibbons KS, et al. Birth outcomes associated with cannabis use before and during pregnancy. Pediatr Res 2012;71(2):215–9.
50. Lester BM, Tronick EZ, LaGasse L, et al. The maternal lifestyle study: effects of substance exposure during pregnancy on neurodevelopmental outcome in 1-month-old infants. Pediatrics 2002;110(6):1182–92.
51. Bada HS, Das A, Bauer CR, et al. Low birth weight and preterm births: etiologic fraction attributable to prenatal drug exposure. J Perinatol 2005;25(10):631–7.
52. Fergusson DM, Horwood LJ, Northstone K. Maternal use of cannabis and pregnancy outcome. BJOG 2002;109(1):21–7.
53. Tennes K, Avitable N, Blackard C, et al. Marijuana: prenatal and postnatal exposure in the human. NIDA Res Monogr 1985;59:48–60.

54. Astley SJ, Little RE. Maternal marijuana use during lactation and infant development at one year. Neurotoxicol Teratol 1990;12(2):161–8.
55. Rowe H, Baker T, Hale TW. Maternal medication, drug use, and breastfeeding. Pediatr Clin North Am 2013;60(1):275–94.
56. American Academy of Pediatrics Section on Breastfeeding. Breastfeeding and the use of human milk. Pediatrics 2012;129(3):e827–41.
57. Fried PA, Makin JE. Neonatal behavioural correlates of prenatal exposure to marihuana, cigarettes and alcohol in a low risk population. Neurotoxicol Teratol 1987;9(1):1–7.
58. Brazelton T. Neonatal behavioral assessment scale. Clinics in developmental medicine no. 50. London, UK: Spastics International Medical Publications in association with Heinemann Medical Books and Philadelphia: Lippincott; 1973.
59. Fried P, Watkinson B, Dillon F, et al. Neonatal neurologic status in a low-risk population after prenatal exposure to cigarettes, marijuana, and alcohol. J Dev Behav Pediatr 1987;8(6):318–26.
60. Prechtl HF. The neurological examination of the full term newborn infant: 2nd Edition. Clinics in developmental medicine no. 63. London, UK: Spastics International Medical Publications in association with Heinemann Medical Books and Philadelphia: Lippincott; 1977.
61. Scher MS, Richardson GA, Coble PA, et al. The effects of prenatal alcohol and marijuana exposure: disturbances in neonatal sleep cycling and arousal. Pediatr Res 1988;24(1):101–5.
62. Lester BM, Dreher M. Effects of marijuana use during pregnancy on newborn cry. Child Dev 1989;60(4):765–71.
63. Hayes JS, Dreher MC, Nugent JK. Newborn outcomes with maternal marihuana use in Jamaican women. Pediatr Nurs 1988;14(2):107–10.
64. Dreher MC, Nugent K, Hudgins R. Prenatal marijuana exposure and neonatal outcomes in Jamaica: an ethnographic study. Pediatrics 1994;93(2):254–60.
65. Fried PA, Watkinson B. 12- and 24-month neurobehavioural follow-up of children prenatally exposed to marihuana, cigarettes and alcohol. Neurotoxicol Teratol 1988;10(4):305–13.
66. Fried P, Watkinson B. 36- and 48-month neurobehavioral follow-up of children prenatally exposed to marijuana, cigarettes and alcohol. J Dev Behav Pediatr 1990;11(2):49–58.
67. Fried P, O'Connell C, Watkinson B. 60- and 72-month follow-up of children prenatally exposed to marijuana, cigarettes and alcohol: cognitive and language assessment. J Dev Behav Pediatr 1992;13:383–91.
68. Fried PA, Watkinson B, Gray R. Differential effects on cognitive functioning in 13- to 16-year-olds prenatally exposed to cigarettes and marihuana. Neurotoxicol Teratol 2003;25(4):427–36.
69. Richardson GA, Day NL, Goldschmidt L. Prenatal alcohol, marijuana, and tobacco use: infant mental and motor development. Neurotoxicol Teratol 1995;17(4):479–87.
70. Day NL, Richardson GA, Goldschmidt L, et al. Effect of prenatal marijuana exposure on the cognitive development of offspring at age three. Neurotoxicol Teratol 1994;16(2):169–75.
71. Dahl RE. A longitudinal study of prenatal marijuana use. Arch Pediatr Adolesc Med 1995;149(2):145.
72. Fried PA, Watkinson B, Siegel LS. Reading and language in 9- to 12-year olds prenatally exposed to cigarettes and marijuana. Neurotoxicol Teratol 1997;19(3):171–83.

73. Chandler LS, Richardson GA, Gallagher JD, et al. Prenatal exposure to alcohol and marijuana: effects on motor development of preschool children. Alcohol Clin Exp Res 1996;20(3):455–61.
74. Willford JA, Chandler LS, Goldschmidt L, et al. Effects of prenatal tobacco, alcohol and marijuana exposure on processing speed, visual-motor coordination, and interhemispheric transfer. Neurotoxicol Teratol 2010;32(6):580–8.
75. Fried PA, Watkinson B, Gray R. Growth from birth to early adolescence in offspring prenatally exposed to cigarettes and marijuana. Neurotoxicol Teratol 1999;21(5):513–25.
76. Fried PA, James DS, Watkinson B. Growth and pubertal milestones during adolescence in offspring prenatally exposed to cigarettes and marihuana. Neurotoxicol Teratol 2001;23(5):431–6.
77. Day N, Cornelius M, Goldschmidt L, et al. The effects of prenatal tobacco and marijuana use on offspring growth from birth through 3 years of age. Neurotoxicol Teratol 1992;14(6):407–14.
78. Day NL, Richardson GA, Geva D, et al. Alcohol, marijuana, and tobacco: effects of prenatal exposure on offspring growth and morphology at age six. Alcohol Clin Exp Res 1994;18(4):786–94.
79. Cornelius MD, Goldschmidt L, Day NL, et al. Alcohol, tobacco and marijuana use among pregnant teenagers: 6-year follow-up of offspring growth effects. Neurotoxicol Teratol 2002;24(6):703–10.
80. Goldschmidt L, Richardson GA, Willford J, et al. Prenatal marijuana exposure and intelligence test performance at age 6. J Am Acad Child Adolesc Psychiatry 2008;47(3):254–63.
81. Fried PA, Watkinson B, Gray R. A follow-up study of attentional behavior in 6-year-old children exposed prenatally to marihuana, cigarettes, and alcohol. Neurotoxicol Teratol 1992;14(5):299–311.
82. Leech SL, Richardson GA, Goldschmidt L, et al. Prenatal substance exposure: effects on attention and impulsivity of 6-year-olds. Neurotoxicol Teratol 1999;21(2):109–18.
83. Fried PA, Watkinson B, Gray R. Differential effects on cognitive functioning 9- to 12-year olds prenatally exposed to cigarettes and marihuana. Neurotoxicol Teratol 1998;20(3):293–306.
84. Fried PA, Watkinson B. Visuoperceptual functioning differs in 9- to 12-year olds prenatally exposed to cigarettes and marihuana. Neurotoxicol Teratol 2000;22(1):11–20.
85. Richardson G. Prenatal alcohol and marijuana exposure: effects on neuropsychological outcomes at 10 years. Neurotoxicol Teratol 2002;24(3):309–20.
86. Goldschmidt L, Day NL, Richardson GA. Effects of prenatal marijuana exposure on child behavior problems at age 10. Neurotoxicol Teratol 2000;22(3):325–36.
87. Fried P, Watkinson B. Differential effects on facets of attention in adolescents prenatally exposed to cigarettes and marihuana. Neurotoxicol Teratol 2001;23(5):421–30.
88. Smith AM, Fried PA, Hogan MJ, et al. Effects of prenatal marijuana on response inhibition: an fMRI study of young adults. Neurotoxicol Teratol 2004;26(4):533–42.
89. Smith AM, Fried PA, Hogan MJ, et al. Effects of prenatal marijuana on visuospatial working memory: an fMRI study in young adults. Neurotoxicol Teratol 2006;28(2):286–95.
90. Smith AM, Longo CA, Fried PA, et al. Effects of marijuana on visuospatial working memory: an fMRI study in young adults. Psychopharmacology (Berl) 2010;210(3):429–38.

91. O'Connell CM, Fried PA. Prenatal exposure to cannabis: a preliminary report of postnatal consequences in school-age children. Neurotoxicol Teratol 1991; 13(6):631–9.
92. Fried PA. Behavioral outcomes in preschool and school-age children exposed prenatally to marijuana: a review and speculative interpretation. NIDA Res Monogr 1996;164:242–60.
93. Goldschmidt L, Richardson GA, Cornelius MD, et al. Prenatal marijuana and alcohol exposure and academic achievement at age 10. Neurotoxicol Teratol 2004;26(4):521–32.
94. Goldschmidt L, Richardson GA, Willford JA, et al. School achievement in 14-year-old youths prenatally exposed to marijuana. Neurotoxicol Teratol 2012;34(1): 161–7.
95. Gray KA, Day NL, Leech S, et al. Prenatal marijuana exposure: effect on child depressive symptoms at ten years of age. Neurotoxicol Teratol 2005;27(3):439–48.
96. Day NL, Goldschmidt L, Thomas CA. Prenatal marijuana exposure contributes to the prediction of marijuana use at age 14. Addiction 2006;101(9):1313–22.
97. Porath AJ, Fried PA. Effects of prenatal cigarette and marijuana exposure on drug use among offspring. Neurotoxicol Teratol 2005;27(2):267–77.

Pain Management in Newborns

Richard W. Hall, MD[a], Kanwaljeet J. S. Anand, MBBS, D.Phil., FRCPCH[b],*

KEYWORDS

- Analgesia • Sedation • Pain • Stress • NICU • Infant-newborn

KEY POINTS

- Neonatal pain should be assessed routinely every 4-6 hours or if clinically indicated using context-specific, validated, and objective pain assessment methods.
- Nonpharmacologic and environmental measures are effective for nonspecific distress or acute procedural pain, or can be used as adjunctive therapies for severe ongoing pain.
- Moderate or severe pain requires local/topical anesthetic agents, acetaminophen, NSAIDs, morphine, fentanyl, ketamine, or dexmedetomidine, singly or in combination to avoid side effects or tolerance/withdrawal.
- Evidence-based guidelines for pain management in the Neonatal Intensive Care Unit can be implemented and modified collaboratively using a Quality Improvement approach that is outlined.

INTRODUCTION
Historical Perspective

Routine assessment and management of neonatal pain has evolved to become an important therapeutic goal in the twenty-first century. During the twentieth century, however, most procedures and clinical practices established in neonatal intensive care units (NICUs) uniformly denied or disregarded the occurrence of neonatal pain. One unfortunate consequence was that infant surgery was conducted routinely with minimal or no anesthesia until the late 1980s.[1,2] Robust responses to painful stimuli were often dismissed as physiologic or behavioral reflexes and not related to the conscious experience of pain.[3] A recent historical analysis suggests that 4 related

Disclosure: None.
The authors would like to acknowledge the NIGMS IDeA Program award P30 GM110702 (R.W. Hall), the European Economic Commission – FP7 Programme, and the Oxnard Foundation (K.J.S. Anand) for research funding during the preparation of this article.
^a Department of Pediatrics/Neonatology, University of Arkansas Hospital, 4305 West Markham Street, Little Rock, AR 72205, USA; ^b Department of Pediatrics/Critical Care Medicine, Le Bonheur Children's Hospital, University of Tennessee Health Science Center, 50 North Dunlap Street, Room 352R, Memphis, TN 38103, USA
* Corresponding author.
E-mail address: kanand@uthsc.edu

causes contributed to a widely prevalent denial of infant pain[4]: (1) a Darwinian view that held newborns as less evolved human beings; (2) extreme caution and skepticism in interpreting scientific data that suggested infant pain; (3) a reductionistic approach whereby mechanistic behaviorism became the dominant model human psychology in the earlier half of the twentieth century (following J. B. Watson's[5] Behaviorist Manifesto in 1913); and as the behaviorist movement waned, it was followed by (4) an era placing undue emphasis on the structural development of the brain and its responses.[6–8]

This popular precept was challenged by accumulating data on hormonal-metabolic responses to surgical procedures performed under minimal anesthesia,[9,10] which were effectively reduced by giving potent anesthesia,[11–13] the identification of a pain system and initial data on its early development, as well as detailed observations on crying activity and other behaviors of newborns subjected to painful stimuli in the NICU—all of which contributed to a scientific rationale for neonatal pain perception and its clinical implications.[3] Once the existence of neonatal pain was acknowledged and methods for clinical assessment had been validated,[14,15] the stage was set for advances in neonatal pain management.

Importance of Neonatal Pain

The American Academy of Pediatrics (AAP) and the Canadian Pediatric Society (CPS) updated their guidelines in 2006,[16] recommending that each health care facility treating newborns should establish a neonatal pain control program that includes

- Performing routine assessments to detect neonatal pain
- Reducing the number of painful procedures
- Preventing or treating acute pain from bedside invasive procedures
- Anticipating and treating postoperative pain after surgical procedures
- Avoiding prolonged or repetitive pain/stress during NICU care

Numerous clinical studies have demonstrated that failure to treat pain leads to short-term complications and long-term physiologic, behavioral, and cognitive sequelae, including altered pain processing, attention-deficit disorder, impaired visual-perceptual ability or visual-motor integration,[17–19] and impaired executive functions.[20,21] Conversely, other studies showed needless analgesic therapy prolongs the need for mechanical ventilation, delays feeding, or leads to other sequelae, including impaired brain growth, poor socialization skills, and impaired performance in short-term memory tasks.[17,18] About 460,000 neonates in the United States require care in NICUs each year and are exposed to acute pain from invasive procedures or prolonged pain from surgery or inflammation.[22–24] Assessing neonatal pain is difficult to teach, time and labor intensive, often open to subjective interpretation, and a source of conflict in NICU care.[25–27]

PAIN ASSESSMENT

Current practice requires the nursing staff to make a global pain assessment of neonates or apply validated pain scoring methods before taking appropriate actions to ameliorate newborn pain or discomfort.[24,28,29] The current nursing workload in the NICU does not allow bedside nurses to assess neonatal pain accurately. Many pain scales lump together behavioral, physiologic, and other variables; but these variables may not respond to neonatal pain in similar or specific ways. The interrater reliability and subjectivity of human assessments are further limiting factors in their prevalent use.[27,30–32]

The use of qualitative or subjective methods,[27,32] rather than quantifiable data for neonatal pain assessment, results in inconsistencies and variability in analgesic therapy. Because of a large pharmacokinetic variability of analgesic drugs in neonates, their pain management is often of poor quality and inconsistent from shift to shift.[33] Adopting an objective pain assessment method greatly enhances the quality of pain management in NICUs and elsewhere by avoiding untreated pain or excessive analgesia. Pain assessment methods should be designed to reduce the nursing workload; the side effects of underdosing or overdosing analgesics; the clinical practice variability within and across different NICUs; and complications like tolerance, withdrawal, or delayed recovery from analgesia/sedation.[34–36]

Pain Assessment Methods

Currently available methods for neonatal pain assessment may be unidimensional (one parameter) or multidimensional (physiologic, behavioral, or other parameters).[31,37,38] Several multidimensional assessment tools with demonstrated validity, reliability, and clinical utility are used in the NICU.[15,39,40] These tools are based on indicators readily assessed at the bedside, such as changes in heart rate, respiratory pattern, blood pressure, or oxygen saturation. Behavioral responses include crying, changes in facial expressions, and body movements.[41,42] For example, total facial activity and a cluster of specific facial findings (brow bulge, eye squeeze, nasolabial furrow, open mouth) were associated with acute and postoperative pain.[43,44]

The tools most commonly used in the NICU for acute pain assessment include the Premature Infant Pain Profile (PIPP),[39] Neonatal Pain Agitation and Sedation Scale (N-PASS),[45,46] Neonatal Infant Pain Scale (NIPS),[47] and the CRIES scale (Crying, Requires Oxygen Saturation, Increased Vital Signs, Expression, Sleeplessness).[15] Premature infants, the most likely group to undergo painful procedures, are less likely to consistently demonstrate the responses to pain selected by these assessment tools.[41,48–50] These scales have been evaluated for acute pain and some for postoperative pain, but none of these methods assess persistent or chronic pain in neonates.[32,51] Two multicenter studies reported a wide range of pain assessment methods used in NICUs: 12 sites evaluated by the 2002 Neonatal Intensive Care Quality Improvement Collaborative used 5 different assessment tools,[28] whereas 10 sites in the Child Health Accountability Initiative used 8 different assessment tools.[24]

Limitations of these pain assessment methods include:

- Most methods were developed from and validated for neonates undergoing acute pain (eg, venipuncture, heelstick).
- Many of the signs used in these assessment tools require subjective evaluations by observers. As a result, there is significant interobserver variability in the evaluation of behavioral responses.[52]
- Some parameters like heart rate variability or palmar skin conductance require specialized equipment that is not routinely available at the bedside.
- Other measures like salivary cortisol or other biomarkers are not available in real time to be clinically useful.
- Behavioral pain responses may be altered in neurologically impaired neonates and absent in those who receive neuromuscular blockade.

Methods for the assessment of persistent or prolonged pain in neonates (for major surgery, osteomyelitis, necrotizing enterocolitis) have not been developed or validated.[32,51,53] During episodes of persistent pain, newborns exhibit a passive state, with limited or no body movements, expressionless facies, reduced physiologic variability, and decreased oxygen consumption. Also, behavioral responses depend on the subjective judgments of rotating care providers,[32] leading to significant interobserver variability. Clinicians must also recognize potentially important relationships between the infant's pain response and the sensitivity and receptivity of the infant's care providers.[54]

Current efforts to improve the accuracy of pain assessment tools include the use of neuroimaging and neurophysiologic techniques that measure brain activity in order to validate neonatal pain scales.[32,55] Their goal is to provide clinicians at the bedside reliable and accurate methods to detect pain and quantify its intensity.

MANAGEMENT OF PAIN
Nonpharmacologic Approaches

Nonpharmacologic approaches to pain relief are underappreciated, underutilized, and understudied.[56] These methods of pain relief have demonstrated effectiveness in NICU care in certain situations, and modern NICUs should use these methods when appropriate. Although opinions differ on the use of complementary and alternative medicine, up to half of the population of the developed countries use this form of therapy[57]; 13.7% of the US population seeks advice from alternative therapists and doctors annually.[58] Opinions range from "Research on alternative medicine is frequently of low quality and methodologically flawed, which might cause these results to be exaggerated" (Report on Complementary & Alternative Medicine in the United States, Institute of Medicine, 2005) and "clothe naked quackery and legitimise pseudoscience"[59] to being "less dangerous and as effective as pharmacologic therapy."[60]

Reduction of painful events

Perhaps the most effective method to eliminate neonatal pain is to reduce the number of procedures performed and episodes of patient handling. NICUs and newborn nurseries should develop policies that limit handling and invasive procedures, without compromising the care of the infants. With forethought and planning, clustered care can reduce the number of bedside disruptions; but it may increase pain responses.[61,62] Other approaches include

1. Decrease bedside disruptions by timing routine medical interventions (daily physical examinations) with other care procedures (diaper change or suctioning).
2. Anticipate laboratory testing to minimize the frequency of blood sampling.
3. Use handheld devices that can perform several analyses (pH, Pao_2, $Paco_2$, electrolytes, calcium, bilirubin, lactate) from a single small blood sample, thereby reducing the number of heelsticks required for laboratory testing.
4. Place peripheral arterial or central venous catheters in patients who need more than 3 to 4 heelsticks per day. These procedures should be performed with adequate analgesia.
5. If clinically appropriate, use noninvasive monitoring, such as transcutaneous Pao_2, $Paco_2$, oxygen saturations, glucose or bilirubin levels, or near infrared spectroscopy, to avoid the need for blood sampling.
6. Consider the use of noninvasive therapeutic approaches for providing analgesia in newborns (eg, transdermal patches, iontophoresis, compressed air injectors).

Kangaroo care and facilitated tucking

Kangaroo care (KC) is defined as skin-to-skin contact, most commonly instituted shortly after birth. KC has been used in developing countries for warmth and bonding, while decreasing morbidity and mortality, especially in preterm neonates.[63] In developed countries, many health care workers are unaware of the benefits of KC. During heelsticks, KC decreases crying time, improves pain scores, and decreases stress in preterm neonates, similar to facilitated tucking.[64,65] The mechanism of action of KC is unclear. Possibilities include the ability of the newborn to hear the maternal heartbeat, less maternal stress, and enhanced self-regulation.[66,67] KC is safe in preterm neonates who are stable and weigh more than 1000 g. However, 2 hours of KC daily was not effective in reducing stress levels in preterm neonates as measured by salivary cortisol.[68] During holding, KC decreases adverse cardiorespiratory events.[69]

Facilitated tucking is defined as placing a hand on the baby's hands or feet and positioning the baby to provide support yet allow them to control their own body movements and is similar to providing KC. It has been used to alleviate pain during endotracheal suctioning and heelsticks.[70] However, it may not be as effective as oral sucrose for repeated painful procedures.[71]

Non-nutritive sucking, sucrose and other sweeteners

Pain relief has been provided by non-nutritive sucking, with and without sucrose, glucose, and breast feeding. Non-nutritive sucking and sweeteners seem to work by increasing endogenous endorphins, as naloxone seems to blunt the response; however, the mechanism is not completely understood.[72] Sweeteners seem to augment the antinociceptive response to pain compared with non-nutritive sucking.[73] Both sucrose and glucose enhance its effectiveness; they both decrease crying time and improve pain scores after acute mild pain, such as from heelsticks.[74,75] A recent meta-analysis revealed that glucose is an acceptable alternative to sucrose, decreasing PIPP scores and crying times associated with venipuncture and heelstick.[76] Sucrose is efficacious in reducing the pain from single events, such as retinopathy of prematurity screening,[77] oral gastric tube insertion,[78] and heelsticks.[71] However, sucrose is controversial when given repeatedly, possibly leading to adverse long-term outcomes.[79] Optimal dosing of sucrose is not known, and a recent Cochrane Review raised concerns about repeated dosing or use in extremely preterm or ill neonates.[80] Breast feeding, especially when accompanied by skin-to-skin contact, is more efficacious than either alone in reducing pain associated with heelstick; however, there is a limited number of studies in the preterm population.[81]

Massage therapy

Massage therapy involves hands-on and skin-to-skin manipulation of the soft tissue that includes gentle effleurage (rhythmic, gliding strokes confirming to the contours of the body), light petrissage (lifting, rolling, kneading strokes done slowly), and compression (light compression of selected areas) and nerve stroke (very light brushing of the skin). It is thought to work by enhancing vagal activity, modulating insulin and insulin-like growth factor 1, as well as decreasing levels of cortisol and epinephrine.[82] Massage therapy has demonstrated effectiveness in randomized trials. Massage decreased NIPS scores in 13 infants receiving heelsticks preceded by a 2 minute-massage in the ipsilateral leg,[83] increased weight gain via vagal stimulation,[84] and improved neurodevelopmental outcomes in very low birth weight neonates.[85] It does not induce sleep in stable preterm neonates, limiting its usefulness as a sedative (Yates CC, personal communication, 2014).

Acupuncture

Acupuncture is the stimulation of acupuncture points by mechanical or electrical means[86] to elicit pain relief. It works by stimulation of the endorphin or non-opioidergic analgesic systems. Despite its use in China for thousands of years and its frequent use by patients in developed countries, it has not gained widespread acceptance in conventional Western medicine.

In conclusion, nonpharmacologic therapies are safe and effective for minor pain and as an adjunct for moderate or severe pain. KC is effective for pain relief during the holding period; it is safe in clinically stable term and preterm neonates weighing more than 1000 g and has beneficial effects on growth, mother-infant bonding, and long-term neurodevelopmental outcomes. Facilitated tucking can provide some pain relief for endotracheal suctioning but is not as effective as sucrose for skin-breaking procedures. Sucrose, glucose, breast milk, and other sweeteners with or without non-nutritive sucking have specific analgesic effects for most skin-breaking procedures, although the safety of repeated use has not been established. Massage therapy decreases pain scores and promotes weight gain in preterm neonates, whereas acupuncture has been inadequately studied in neonates. The use of non-pharmacologic therapies is often recommended as the first step in neonatal pain management, particularly because of their favorable side-effect profile, their ability to diminish acute pain from invasive or noninvasive procedures, and their beneficial long-term effects as compared with the systemic analgesics.

Local Anesthetics

Lidocaine infiltration

Lidocaine inhibits axonal transmission by blocking sodium ion channels. Lidocaine infiltration is commonly used for various penile blocks for circumcision. In this circumstance, its use has demonstrated effectiveness in decreasing the pain response to immunizations as long as 4 months after circumcision compared with neonates who received placebo.[87] Compared with a dorsal penile root block or eutectic mixture of local anesthetics (lidocaine and prilocaine combination [Eutectic Mixture of Local Anesthetic (EMLA)]) cream, the ring block has been shown to be the most effective means of pain relief for circumcision.[88]

Topical anesthetics

Topical anesthetics are effective for certain types of procedural pain, such as venous cannulation,[89] lumbar puncture,[90] or venipuncture.[91] One study reported combining sucrose with topical analgesia, which resulted in lower Douleur Aigue Nouveau-ne (DAN) scores.[92] Another study demonstrated increased success with venipuncture in young infants and children if the cream was left in place for 2 hours or more.[93] EMLA cream was studied in preterm neonates subjected to venipuncture. N-PASS scores were significantly lower in the treated group compared with placebo, leading the investigators to recommend this method of analgesia.[94] Tetracaine is also used topically, with varying success. When combined with sucrose, one study found no benefit of this formulation,[95] whereas another review found similar efficacy but with a more rapid onset of action as compared with EMLA cream, making it attractive for clinical use.[96]

Complications of the topical creams include methemoglobinemia and transient skin rashes.[97] Concerns for methemoglobinemia are exaggerated in preterm neonates because of a thinner epidermis, high dermal permeability, and limited circulating antioxidants. However, when used properly (as recommended by the Food and Drug Administration), very few neonates develop toxic methemoglobinemia even after repeated EMLA use.[98–101] Newer topical anesthetics include 4% tetracaine and 4% liposomal lidocaine, with a shorter onset of action; but they are not more effective.

Unfortunately, topical anesthetics have not been effective in providing pain relief for heelsticks, one of the most common skin-breaking procedures,[102] although they may reduce hyperalgesia following the tissue injury associated with heelsticks.[103]

Opioid Therapy

Opioids provide the most effective therapy for moderate to severe pain in patients of all ages. They produce both analgesia and sedation, have a wide therapeutic window, and also attenuate the physiologic stress responses of neonates. Morphine and fentanyl are the most commonly used opioids, although some NICUs report the use of more potent (eg, sufentanil),[104] shorter-acting (eg, alfentanil,[105,106] remifentanil[107,108]), or mixed opioids (eg, tramadol[109]).

Morphine

Morphine is the most commonly used opioid for neonatal analgesia, often used as a continuous infusion in ventilated or postoperative infants or intermittently to reduce the acute pain associated with invasive procedures. Its effectiveness and safety for these indications has not been established but remains under active investigation.

Morphine improves ventilator synchrony in ventilated neonates,[110,111] although recent multicenter trials have questioned the benefit of routine morphine infusions in ventilated preterm infants. The Neurologic Outcomes and Pre-emptive Analgesia in Neonates (NEOPAIN) multicenter trial evaluated 898 ventilated preterm infants (23–32 weeks' gestation) randomly assigned to morphine or placebo infusions.[112] Open-label morphine was given for additional analgesia based on the clinical judgment of clinicians in each of the NICUs. There were no differences in the rates of mortality, severe intraventricular hemorrhage (IVH), or periventricular leukomalacia (PVL) between the two groups, even though neonates in the morphine group seemed to have lower PIPP scores and smaller increases in heart rate and respiratory rate.[112] These differences were small but reached statistical significance because of the large sample size. Infants treated with morphine were more likely to develop hypotension,[113] required a longer duration of mechanical ventilation, and took longer to tolerate enteral feeds.[112,114]

Another trial that randomized 150 ventilated term and preterm neonates in 2 Dutch centers found no differences in the analgesic effects of morphine versus placebo using multiple measures of pain assessment. A lower incidence of IVH occurred in the morphine group, but no differences in poor neurologic outcome occurred between the two groups.[115] A systematic review selected 13 randomized controlled trials (RCTs) on the use of opioids in ventilated infants. Pooled data from 4 studies using PIPP scores showed reduced pain in the patients who received morphine versus placebo (weighted mean difference −1.71, 95% confidence interval −3.18 to −0.24).[116] Additional analyses demonstrated no differences in mortality rates (5 RCTs), duration of mechanical ventilation (10 RCTs), or neurodevelopment outcomes evaluated at 5 to 6 years of age (2 RCTs) and no differences in secondary outcomes (rates of necrotizing enterocolitis (NEC), bronchopulmonary dysplasia (BPD), IVH, PVL, and hypotension), except that preterm infants in the morphine groups took longer to tolerate full enteral feeds.[116]

Morphine analgesia is associated with significant side effects in preterm infants, but it may or may not alter their long-term cognitive or behavioral outcomes.[17,18,116–119] A retrospective study of 52 term neonates with hypoxic-ischemic insults following birth asphyxia showed less brain injury on MRI and improved neurodevelopmental outcomes in infants who received morphine in the first week after birth compared with those who did not receive opioid therapy.[120] The routine use of morphine infusions is not recommended for ventilated preterm neonates but may be beneficial for term neonates following birth asphyxia.

Morphine analgesia may not be associated with the same risk profile in ventilated term infants but may still increase the duration of ventilation. A retrospective study of 62 ventilated term newborns found that postoperative morphine infusions prolonged the need for mechanical ventilation but was not associated with apnea, hypotension, or other complications.[121] A series of RCTs comparing intermittent versus continuous morphine infusions found that morphine is safe and effective for postoperative pain in term neonates and older infants.[122–128] Currently, however, there are no RCTs that have investigated the safety and efficacy of postoperative morphine analgesia in preterm neonates.

The analgesic effects of morphine in reducing acute procedural pain are controversial.[115,129,130] During CVL placement, one RCT found that ventilated neonates receiving morphine alone and morphine plus tetracaine had lower pain scores than the no treatment or tetracaine alone groups. However, patients who received morphine required greater ventilatory support in the 12 hours following the procedure.[130] In contrast, the NEOPAIN and Dutch morphine trials evaluated the responses to heelstick or tracheal suctioning, respectively, in preterm infants randomized to continuous morphine or placebo infusions and found no difference in pain scores between the two groups.[115,129,131] Morphine pharmacodynamics studies in ventilated preterm neonates also found no relationship between plasma morphine levels and responses to tracheal suctioning.[131,132] Of note, the preparation of morphine infusions in the NICU from regular morphine vials involves the manual dilution of small volumes, leading to significant inaccuracies in the concentrations delivered to neonates.[133]

Fentanyl

As a highly lipophilic drug, fentanyl provides rapid analgesia with minimal hemodynamic effects in term and preterm newborns, although its popular use is not supported with evidence from large multicenter RCTs. Smaller trials reported that fentanyl reduces stress hormone levels, episodes of hypoxia, and behavioral stress scores in ventilated infants as compared with placebo controls.[134–136] Although infants who received fentanyl required greater ventilatory support, no differences occurred in clinical outcomes between the fentanyl- and placebo-treated groups.[135,136] Another RCT reported that behavioral pain scores and cytokine release following heel sticks were reduced to a greater extent with fentanyl (1–2 mcg/kg) as compared with facilitated tucking.[137]

Fentanyl[138–141] or its shorter-acting derivatives (eg, alfentanil,[105] remifentanil[142,143]) are often used for analgesia before procedures in preterm and term newborns. A randomized trial in 20 preterm newborns found that overall intubating conditions were significantly improved in those receiving remifentanil versus morphine. However, no complications occurred following either intravenous (IV) morphine or remifentanil.[143]

Although the AAP/CPS guidelines do not recommend the routine use of continuous fentanyl infusions in ventilated preterm neonates, this occurs frequently in many NICUs.[144,145] In a multicenter RCT in 131 mechanically ventilated preterm infants (23–32 weeks' gestation), fentanyl infusions reduced acute pain (PIPP) scores; no differences occurred in the prolonged pain Échelle Douleur Inconfort Nouveau-Né (EDIN) scores between the two groups, although fewer neonates showed EDIN scores greater than 6 in the fentanyl (6.8%) versus placebo groups (10.6%).[146] Those receiving fentanyl infusions had a longer duration of mechanical ventilation and delayed passage of meconium.[146]

Fentanyl analgesia is associated with less sedative or hypotensive effects, reduced effects on gastrointestinal motility or urinary retention, but greater opioid tolerance and withdrawal as compared with morphine.[146–149] A single-center RCT compared infusions of fentanyl (1.5 mcg/kg/h) versus morphine (20 mcg/kg/h) in 163 ventilated neonates and reported similar pain scores, catecholamine responses, and vital signs in both groups. There were no adverse respiratory effects or difficulties in weaning from ventilation in either group, but decreased beta-endorphin levels and gastrointestinal dysmotility occurred in the fentanyl group.[149] In another double-blind RCT, single doses of fentanyl (3 mcg/kg) reduced physiologic and behavioral indicators of pain, improved postoperative comfort scores, and increased growth hormone levels in ventilated preterm neonates.[134] Among postoperative preterm infants, fentanyl and tramadol provided equally effective analgesia, with no differences between the two groups for the duration of mechanical ventilation or the time to reach enteral feeds.[109]

Fentanyl should be used when a rapidly acting opioid is required for analgesia in a controlled setting, where any associated side effects (bradycardia, hypotension, laryngospasm, and chest wall rigidity[150]) can be addressed rapidly and adequately. Other indications include fentanyl analgesia for postoperative pain (following cardiac surgery)[151,152] or for patients with pulmonary hypertension (primary or secondary).[153,154] A single-center RCT using continuous fentanyl infusions following cardiac surgery found significant differences in postoperative complications and mortality compared with intermittent doses of morphine and diazepam,[13] although it is unclear whether these clinical outcomes were related to anesthetic management or postoperative analgesia. Further studies of fentanyl analgesia for ventilated preterm neonates, and for term and preterm neonates exposed to postoperative pain, are required to evaluate its safety and efficacy in these patients.

Based on current evidence and clinical experience, the routine use of fentanyl infusions in ventilated preterm infants cannot be recommended at this time,[116] except for neonates undergoing tracheal intubation, central line placement, or surgery. Morphine analgesia may be used in ventilated term neonates following surgery or birth asphyxia or in those requiring moderately invasive procedures, such as central venous catheterization, tracheal intubation, or chest tube placement. Exercise extreme caution if using opioid analgesia for preterm neonates at 22 to 26 weeks' gestation or in those with preexisting hypotension because of the increased risk for adverse events, including hypotension, bradycardia, severe IVH, impaired gut motility, and worse neurodevelopmental outcomes.[113]

Remifentanil, alfentanil, sufentanil

Remifentanil has a chemical structure similar to that of fentanyl but has twice its analgesic potency with an ultrashort duration of action (3–15 minutes). It is metabolized by plasma esterases in erythrocytes and tissue fluids, thus its excretion is independent of liver and renal function.[155] Remifentanil is used for pain relief during brief procedures, such as central line placement[142] or tracheal intubation.[143] Alfentanil is more potent than morphine but has approximately one-third the potency of fentanyl and has a short duration of action (20–30 minutes).[105,156] These drugs have been used successfully for tracheal intubation and other brief invasive procedures in neonates, but detailed safety and efficacy data are lacking.[157]

For a summary of the opiates see **Table 1**.

Nonopioid Therapies

Benzodiazepines

Benzodiazepines activate gamma aminobutyric acid A (GABA$_A$) receptors[158] and are commonly used in NICUs, but they have no analgesic effects. These drugs provide sedation and muscle relaxation, making them useful for noninvasive procedures, such as imaging studies and as an adjunct for motion control in invasive procedures. Their adverse effects include myoclonic jerking, excessive sedation, respiratory depression, and occasional hypotension.

Table 1
Opioids

Drug	Advantages	Disadvantages
Morphine	Potent pain relief Better ventilator synchrony Sedation Hypnosis Muscle relaxation Inexpensive	Respiratory depression Arterial hypotension Constipation, nausea Urinary retention Central nervous system depression Tolerance, dependence Long-term outcomes not studied Prolonged ventilator use
Fentanyl	Fast acting Less hypotension	Respiratory depression Short half-life Quick tolerance and dependence Chest wall rigidity Inadequately studied
Remifentanil	Fast acting Degraded in the plasma Unaffected by liver metabolism	—

Midazolam Midazolam is the most commonly used benzodiazepine in the NICU, although concerns regarding its usage have been raised. Although there are relatively few studies to support the use of midazolam in neonates, it is common practice to use this drug for mechanical ventilation or procedural pain.[159] One recent review found no apparent clinical benefit of midazolam compared with opiates in mechanically ventilated neonates.[160] There are some concerns regarding the use of midazolam in neonates. One study reported an increased incidence of adverse short-term effects (intraventricular hemorrhage, periventricular leukomalacia, or death) and a longer hospital stay associated with midazolam compared with morphine.[161] Midazolam has also been associated with benzyl alcohol exposure.[162] A recent Cochrane Review found insufficient data to promote the use of IV midazolam as a sedative in the NICU, in addition to "concerns about the safety of midazolam in neonates."[163] It is also used for noninvasive procedures, such as computed tomography (CT) scans[164] and less invasive procedural sedation.[165] One recent study found a significant effect of midazolam on pain scores after surgery.[166] There have been no long-term studies describing a benefit or harm with midazolam. In summary, midazolam seems to provide sedative effects in mechanically ventilated neonates; but it should be used with caution because of reported adverse effects, particularly when used alone. The decreased number of GABA$_A$ receptors in neonates compared with adults may contribute to the neonates' risk of neuroexcitability and myoclonic activity that resembles and, in some cases, may progress to seizure activity.[167]

A starting dose of 100 mcg/kg with a maintenance dosage of 50 to 100 mcg/kg/h can be used in neonates to provide sedation.[168] Oral midazolam is also effective, with 50% bioavailability compared with the IV preparation.[169,170] Finally, intranasal midazolam was effective for fundoscopic examinations in older children; but this mode of delivery has not been tested in neonates.[171] Metabolism of these drugs occurs through glucuronidation in the liver; there is potential for decreased bilirubin metabolism, especially in asphyxiated or preterm newborns. Its half-life is only 30 to 60 minutes, which is prolonged in preterm and sick neonates. Recent pharmacokinetic data reveal a significant effect of maturation and body weight on the clearance of midazolam, which has elucidated the ability to predict levels in this age group.[172]

However, it adheres to the tubing in patients on extracorporeal membrane oxygenation (ECMO), increasing their dosing requirements by 50%.[173]

Lorazepam Lorazepam has also been used in the NICU, albeit not as routinely as midazolam. It is a longer-acting drug than midazolam, with a duration of action 6 to 12 hours, so it does not have to be given as an infusion. It has been used successfully for seizure control in neonates who are refractory to phenobarbital and phenytoin despite its potential for neuronal toxicity.[174] Its use has also been associated with propylene glycol exposure.[162] For a summary of the benzodiazepines see **Table 2**.

Other sedatives

Phenobarbital Phenobarbital is usually considered as the drug of choice for seizure control. There is sparse evidence for the antinociceptive effects of phenobarbital in animals,[175] but it has no significant analgesic effects in humans. It was used in conjunction with opioids for sedation,[161] although there is little recent evidence that it is effective. Classically, it has been used for neonatal abstinence syndrome; but recent work by Ebner and others[176] has demonstrated that opiates shorten the time required for treatment. However, because of its anticonvulsant effects, phenobarbital is an attractive agent for patients with seizures.

Propofol Propofol has become popular as an anesthetic agent for young children, but it has not been studied extensively in neonates.[177] One study compared propofol with morphine, atropine, and suxamethonium for intubation and found that propofol led to shorter intubation times, higher oxygen saturations, and less trauma than the combination regimen in neonates; but these effects were not significantly different.[178,179] However, propofol should be used with caution in young infants because its clearance and potential for neurotoxicity are inversely related to neonatal and postmenstrual age. There is significant interindividual variability in the pharmacokinetics of propofol in preterm neonates[180]; its use can lead to severe hypotension, with transient decreases in heart rate and oxygen saturations.[181]

Table 2
Benzodiazepines

Drug	Advantages	Disadvantages
Benzodiazepines	Better ventilator synchrony Antianxiety Sedation Hypnosis Muscle relaxation Amnesia Anticonvulsant	No pain relief Arterial hypotension Respiratory depression Constipation, nausea Urinary retention Myoclonus Seizures Central nervous system depression Tolerance, dependence Alters bilirubin metabolism Propylene glycol and benzyl alcohol exposure
Midazolam	Most studied benzodiazepine Quickly metabolized	Short acting Benzyl alcohol exposure
Lorazepam	Longer acting Better anticonvulsant	More myoclonus reported Propylene glycol exposure
Diazepam	—	Not recommended in the neonate

Ketamine Ketamine is a dissociative anesthetic that provides analgesia, amnesia, and sedation. Although ketamine has been used extensively in older children, there have been limited studies in neonates. Ketamine increases blood pressure and heart rate, increases the respiratory drive, and leads to bronchodilation.[182] Because ketamine does not affect cerebral blood flow significantly, it is a good choice for unstable, hypotensive neonates requiring procedures such as intubation or ECMO cannulation.[183] In the authors' laboratory, ketamine decreased neuronal cell death in the presence of repetitive pain in immature rodents, which would also make it attractive for preterm neonates,[184] although no significant differences occurred in human studies. The dose for effective management of the pain caused by endotracheal suctioning in ventilated neonates was 2 mg/kg in one Finnish study.[185] Despite these theoretic advantages, ketamine is a potent anesthetic with minimal study in neonates. Therefore, it should only be used for invasive procedures.

Dexmedetomidine Dexmedetomidine is a selective alpha-2 adrenergic receptor agonist that provides potent sedative and analgesic effects while causing minimal respiratory depression. Although dexmedetomidine is approved for sedation of patients undergoing surgical or other procedures, the clinical experience using this drug in neonates is limited. Ongoing research on its safety, dosing, and efficacy is being conducted in preterm and term infants, particularly following cardiac surgery.[186–192] Therefore, the routine use of this drug in ventilated neonates is not recommended until sufficient data demonstrating its safety and efficacy and its pharmacokinetics and pharmacodynamics have been published. Clinicians using this drug should note that the plasma levels producing sedation (0.4–0.8 mcg/L) are lower than those producing analgesia (0.6–1.25 µg/L), at least in older children,[193–196] and that it may cause seizures,[197] bradycardia,[198,199] and hypothermia[198] in neonates. However, it seems to be useful for radiological procedures[200–202] and supraventricular tachyarrhythmias[192,203] in infants and children.

Chloral hydrate Chloral hydrate is not available in the United States but is commonly used in European NICUs when sedation is required without analgesia. It is commonly used for radiological procedures, electroencephalography, echocardiography, and dental procedures in older patients. It is converted to trichloroethanol, which is also metabolically active.[204] A recent retrospective review found an increased incidence of apnea and desaturation in term neonates less than 1 month and in preterm neonates less than 60 weeks postconceptual age who were undergoing MRI.[205] One study evaluated the combination of chloral hydrate and acetaminophen in ophthalmologic surgery for retinopathy of prematurity, comparing it with IV opioid analgesia. Although there was a general reduction in pain scores, some of the infants in this study had very high pain scores with the chloral hydrate preparation, making this combination questionable at best.[206] In summary, this drug should be used for sedation without analgesia and with caution in preterm and young term neonates.

Acetaminophen (Paracetamol)

Acetaminophen inhibits the cyclooxygenase-2 (COX-2) enzymes in the brain; it has been well studied in newborns.[207] It is frequently used in conjunction with other types of pain relief to decrease opioid use, especially for postsurgical pain.[208] IV acetaminophen decreased the amount of opioids needed after surgery and is particularly useful for routine postsurgical care with opioid-sparing effects.[209] The main toxicity of this drug is liver damage; but when given in appropriate doses, it is safe and effective. One of the main concerns surrounding acetaminophen is drug overdosage, which can lead to significant liver toxicity.[210] Acetaminophen has also been used for procedural pain, such as immunizations or circumcision.[211]

In infants, oral, rectal, and IV formulations of acetaminophen have minimal adverse effects. In contrast to its use in older children or adults, acetaminophen rarely causes hepatic or renal toxicity in newborns.[211–215] In addition, IV acetaminophen does not induce hypothermia in neonates.[216] The prodrug is available as another IV formulation, marketed in European and other countries as propacetamol, although it causes more frequent side effects.[217–219]

In both preterm and term infants, the clearance of acetaminophen is slower than older children, so oral/rectal dosing is required less frequently.[218,220–226] Single *oral* doses of 10 to 15 mg/kg may be given every 6 to 8 hours, and 20 to 25 mg/kg can be given *rectally* at the same time intervals. These doses were primarily based on antipyretic dose-response studies and may not apply for pain control. Although limited data are available for *IV* acetaminophen in neonates, a pharmacokinetic analysis in 158 infants suggests a loading dose of 20 mg/kg and maintenance dosages of 10 mg/kg every 6 hours for infants at 32 to 44 weeks' postmenstrual age.[226] However, maintenance dosing for Extremely Low Gestational Age Neonates (ELGANs) is controversial and may be less than or equal to 7.5 mg/kg every 6 to 8 hours for neonates between 23 and 32 weeks' postmenstrual age.[209,226] The recommended total daily doses based on postmenstrual age are

- 24 to 30 weeks' gestation: 20 to 30 mg/kg/d
- 31 to 36 weeks' gestation: 35 to 50 mg/kg/d
- 37 to 42 weeks' gestation: 50 to 60 mg/kg/d
- 1 to 3 months' postnatal: 60 to 75 mg/kg/d

Wider use of acetaminophen as an analgesic will allow clearer definition of the adverse effects and safety profile of this useful drug in the neonatal population.[34]

Nonsteroidal antiinflammatory drugs

Nonsteroidal antiinflammatory drugs (NSAIDs) are used extensively for pain relief in children and adults, but drugs like indomethacin[227,228] and ibuprofen[229–231] are mainly used for patent ductus arteriosus closure in neonates. They act by inhibiting the cyclooxygenase enzymes (COX-1 and COX-2) responsible for converting arachidonic acid into prostaglandins, thus producing their analgesic, antipyretic, and antiinflammatory effects.[232] There are little data on the analgesic effects of NSAIDs in neonates. Concern over the side effects of renal dysfunction, platelet adhesiveness, and pulmonary hypertension have limited their study to this indication.[233] However, ibuprofen has demonstrated beneficial effects on cerebral circulation in human studies as well as beneficial effects on the development of chronic lung disease in baboon experiments,[234] making it potentially useful as an analgesic in preterm neonates.

IMPLEMENTING PAIN MANAGEMENT IN THE NEONATAL INTENSIVE CARE UNIT: A QUALITY IMPROVEMENT APPROACH

Pain in modern-day NICUs is inadequately treated, despite the overwhelming evidence depicting the adverse consequences of unrelieved pain/stress. Carbajal and colleagues[22] found that preterm neonates experienced 10 to 14 painful procedures daily, most of which (80%) were not preceded by specific analgesia. Numerous other NICUs have noted similar findings.[235–237] Even more concerning is the potential that chronic pain may be ignored, especially in mechanically ventilated neonates.[238] Barriers include inadequate ability to assess prolonged neonatal pain, lack of knowledge of therapeutic effectiveness, and exaggerated concerns over analgesic side effects.

Further, the inherent difficulties in conducting human pain research in neonates require an ethical approach that will leave most studies seriously flawed.

Developing Neonatal Intensive Care Unit: Specific Guidelines

A suggested approach to evidence-based recommendations for the treatment of neonatal pain includes the following[239]:

1. Recognition of neonatal pain as a valid concern
2. Recognition of acute procedural and chronic neonatal pain in need of treatment
3. Regular use of a validated assessment tool for neonatal pain
4. Educational resources for care givers and parents in the NICU
5. Protocolized stepwise treatment plan for the procedures and conditions encountered in the NICU using nonpharmacologic and pharmacologic approaches to treatment
6. Continued auditing to ascertain appropriate treatment of neonatal pain
7. Well-planned program of coordination, facilitation, and using local champions and project teams

Stevens and colleagues[240] identified 3 overarching themes that captured influences on optimal pain practices in the NICU:

1. A culture of collaboration and support among all health care providers *and patients' families*
2. Threats to autonomous decision making, such as autocratic leadership and hierarchical relationships
3. Complexities in care delivery, related to the complexities of the patients as well as the system of care

The authors recommend a quality-improvement approach, involving all members of the health care team and families to discuss the causes, prevention, and evidence-based treatment of pain. Education must be provided with continual assessment, which should be documented consistently according to the Joint Commission's requirements. By using this approach, the authors were able to decrease the number of painful procedures to less than 2 per day in neonates between 27 and 32 weeks' postconceptual age.[68]

Analgesia for Invasive Procedures

Analgesic approaches for specific procedures are listed in **Table 3**.

Postoperative Analgesia

Opiates remain the mainstay of postoperative pain relief. However, because of the concerns surrounding prolonged opiate therapy, many centers are using IV acetaminophen to augment opiate therapy. Its use has decreased the amount of opiates received by postoperative patients.[209]

Analgesia for Mechanical Ventilation

Mechanical ventilation is one of the most common sources of chronic pain in modern NICUs. Newer, more effective surfactants, the use of prenatal steroids, and improved nutrition has brought about a new generation of survivors, many of whom require several months of assisted ventilation. Despite several well-conducted studies in ventilated preterm neonates, the ideal method of analgesia for assisted ventilation in preterm neonates is still unknown.[112,115,161] Thus, analgesia for mechanical ventilation is controversial for a variety of reasons.[145]

Table 3
Summary of procedures and recommendations for pain relief

Skin-Breaking Procedures[a,b]	Proposed Interventions	Comments
Heel stick	Use nonpharmacologic measures + mechanical lance, squeezing the heel is the most painful phase	Venipuncture is more efficient, less painful; local anesthetics, acetaminophen, heel warming do not reduce heel stick pain
Venipuncture	Nonpharmacologic measures, use topical local anesthetics	Requires less time & less resampling than heel stick
Arterial puncture	Nonpharmacologic measures, use topical and subcutaneous local anesthetics	More painful than venipuncture
IV cannulation	Nonpharmacologic measures, use topical local anesthetics	—
Central line placement	Nonpharmacologic measures, use topical local anesthetics, consider low-dose opioids or deep sedation based on clinical factors	Some centers prefer using general anesthesia
Finger stick	Nonpharmacologic measures and use mechanical device	Venipuncture is more efficient, less painful; local anesthetics, acetaminophen, or warming may not reduce finger stick pain
Subcutaneous injection	Avoid if possible, use nonpharmacologic measures and topical local anesthetics if procedure cannot be avoided	—
Intramuscular injection	Avoid if possible, use nonpharmacologic measures and topical local anesthetics if procedure cannot be avoided	—
Lumbar puncture	Nonpharmacologic measures and topical local anesthetic, lidocaine infiltration, careful positioning	Use IV analgesia/sedation, if patients are intubated and ventilated
Peripheral arterial line	Nonpharmacologic measures and topical local anesthetic, lidocaine infiltration, consider IV opioids	—
Circumcision	Nonpharmacologic measures and topical local anesthetic, lidocaine infiltration, IV/PO acetaminophen before and after procedure	Lidocaine infiltration for distal, ring, or dorsal penile nerve blocks (DPNB); liposomal lidocaine is more effective than DPNB
Suprapubic bladder aspiration	Nonpharmacologic measures and topical local anesthetic, lidocaine infiltration, consider IV fentanyl (0.5–1.0 mcg/kg)	—

(continued on next page)

Table 3
(continued)

Skin-Breaking Procedures[a,b]	Proposed Interventions	Comments
Arterial or venous cutdown	Nonpharmacologic measures and topical local anesthetic, lidocaine infiltration, IV fentanyl (1–2 mcg/kg), consider deep sedation	Most arterial or venous cutdowns can be avoided, consider referral to interventional radiology
Peripherally inserted central catheter (PICC)	Nonpharmacologic measures and topical local anesthetic, lidocaine infiltration, consider IV fentanyl (1 mcg/kg) or IV ketamine (1 mg/kg)	Some centers prefer using deep sedation or general anesthesia
ECMO Cannulation	Propofol 2–4 mg/kg, ketamine 1–2 mg/kg, fentanyl 1–3 mcg/kg, muscle relaxant as needed	—
Tracheal intubation (eg, for mechanical ventilation)	Give fentanyl (1 mcg/kg) or morphine (10–30 mcg/kg), with midazolam (50–100 mcg/kg), ketamine (1 mg/kg), use muscle relaxant only if experienced clinician, consider atropine	Superiority of one drug regimen over another has not been investigated
Gastric tube insertion	Nonpharmacologic measures, consider local anesthetic gel	Perform rapidly, use lubricant, avoid injury
Chest physiotherapy	Gentle positioning, fentanyl (1 mcg/kg) if a chest tube is present	Avoid areas of injured or inflamed skin, areas with indwelling drains or catheters
Removal of IV catheter	Solvent swab, consider nonpharmacologic measures	—
Wound treatment	Nonpharmacologic measures, use topical local anesthetics, consider low-dose opioids, or deep sedation based on extent of injury	See also "Dressing change"
Umbilical catheterization	Nonpharmacologic measures, IV acetaminophen (10 mg/kg), avoid sutures to the skin	Cord tissue is not innervated, but avoid injury to skin
Bladder compression	Consider nonpharmacologic measures or IV acetaminophen (10 mg/kg) if severe or prolonged	—
Tracheal extubation	Use solvent swab for tape, consider nonpharmacologic measures	
Dressing change	Nonpharmacologic measures and topical local anesthetic, consider deep sedation if extensive	—

[a] Nonpharmacologic measures include pacifier, oral sucrose, swaddling, skin-to-skin contact with mother.
[b] The frequency of procedures can be reduced without sacrificing the quality of neonatal intensive care.

Mechanical ventilation leads to changes in neuroendocrine parameters, pain scores, and physiologic responses.[134,241] Assisted ventilation in neonates is presumed to be associated with chronic repetitive pain, which in turn is associated with adverse long-term sequelae.[242] Ventilated neonates treated with opiates have demonstrated improved ventilator synchrony[243]; improved pulmonary function; and decreased neuroendocrine responses, including cortisol, beta-endorphin, and catecholamines.[145] Reasons not to treat include the well-known adverse side effects of analgesics, especially the opiates, including hypotension from morphine[113]; chest wall rigidity from fentanyl and alfentanil[105]; and tolerance, dependence, and withdrawal from both opiates and benzodiazepines. Additionally, adverse effects, such as death and IVH, are not improved with preemptive treatment and may lead to adverse short-term effects.[112]

Chronic pain assessment is poorly validated and difficult to assess in this patient population, since most studies have only evaluated acute pain scores.[238] If patients are treated, opiates are the most common class of drugs, with morphine being the most well studied. Fentanyl may be advantageous in hypotensive and/or younger neonates because it has fewer cardiovascular effects. One recent study demonstrated improved acute pain scores with fentanyl, but time on the ventilator was prolonged compared with placebo.[146] Remifentanil, especially when short-term intubation is needed,[107] and dexmedetomidine are promising agents; but neonatal data are limited.[244,245] The benzodiazepines, midazolam and lorazepam, have been used in ventilated neonates; but midazolam has been associated with adverse effects in one small study.[161] Significant gaps in our knowledge exist, especially in regard to long-term effects of treatment, or lack thereof, and in chronic pain assessment associated with assisted ventilation. Recent data from the NEOPAIN trial suggest improved long-term outcomes at school age from the morphine-treated group, with fewer children requiring special education (Hall RW, personal communication, 2013).

In conclusion

- If neonatal patients exhibit irritability on assisted ventilation, first optimize oxygenation and ventilation.
- Treat acute pain and stress episodically as needed.
- Do not treat ventilated patients preemptively.
- There is no clear-cut advantage for any opioid in the management of ventilated preterm neonates.
- Key questions remain regarding chronic pain assessment, long-term outcomes, and safety.

SUMMARY

Pain management in neonates has made great strides over the last several years. Because of the serious short- and long-term adverse effects of pain and because of humanitarian reasons, all NICU patients deserve a focus on pain prevention, routine pain assessments, and evidence-based strategies for pain management, using both nonpharmacologic and pharmacologic approaches. Because pain strategies continue to fall short, future research should address systems-based practice and knowledge-transfer approaches on how to improve pain management in NICUs; how best to assess pain, especially prolonged or chronic pain; and how to incorporate the many variables affecting pain found in modern-day neonatology, such as light, sound, touch, parental separation, thermal stress, and extrauterine malnutrition. Continued emphasis on neonatal pain management research may help to decrease some of the adverse neurodevelopmental outcomes commonly found in our NICU graduates.

REFERENCES

1. Unruh AM. Voices from the past: ancient views of pain in childhood. Clin J Pain 1992;8:247–54.
2. Wesson SC. Ligation of the ductus arteriosus: anesthesia management of the tiny premature infant. AANA J 1982;50:579–82.
3. Anand KJ, Hickey PR. Pain and its effects in the human neonate and fetus. N Engl J Med 1987;317:1321–9.
4. Rodkey EN, Pillai Riddell R. The infancy of infant pain research: the experimental origins of infant pain denial. J Pain 2013;14:338–50.
5. Watson JB. Psychology as the behaviorist views it. Psychol Rev 1913;20: 158–77.
6. McGraw M. Neural maturation as exemplified in the changing reactions of the infant to pin prick. Child Dev 1941;12:31–42.
7. Dobbing J. Undernutrition and the developing brain. The relevance of animal models to the human problem. Am J Dis Child 1970;120:411–5.
8. Raiha N, Hjelt L. The correlation between the development of the hypophysial portal system and the onset of neurosecretory activity in the human fetus and infant. Acta Paediatr 1957;46:610–6.
9. Anand KJ, Brown MJ, Causon RC, et al. Can the human neonate mount an endocrine and metabolic response to surgery? J Pediatr Surg 1985;20:41–8.
10. Anand KJ, Hansen DD, Hickey PR. Hormonal-metabolic stress responses in neonates undergoing cardiac surgery. Anesthesiology 1990;73:661–70.
11. Anand KJ, Sippell WG, Aynsley-Green A. Randomised trial of fentanyl anaesthesia in preterm babies undergoing surgery: effects on the stress response. Lancet 1987;1:243–8.
12. Anand KJ, Sippell WG, Schofield NM, et al. Does halothane anaesthesia decrease the metabolic and endocrine stress responses of newborn infants undergoing operation? Br Med J (Clin Res Ed) 1988;296:668–72.
13. Anand KJ, Hickey PR. Halothane-morphine compared with high-dose sufentanil for anesthesia and postoperative analgesia in neonatal cardiac surgery. N Engl J Med 1992;326:1–9.
14. Franck LS. A national survey of the assessment and treatment of pain and agitation in the neonatal intensive care unit. J Obstet Gynecol Neonatal Nurs 1987;16: 387–93.
15. Krechel SW, Bildner J. CRIES: a new neonatal postoperative pain measurement score. Initial testing of validity and reliability. Paediatr Anaesth 1995;5:53–61.
16. Batton DG, Barrington KJ, Wallman C. Prevention and management of pain in the neonate: an update. Pediatrics 2006;118:2231–41.
17. Ferguson SA, Ward WL, Paule MG, et al. A pilot study of preemptive morphine analgesia in preterm neonates: effects on head circumference, social behavior, and response latencies in early childhood. Neurotoxicol Teratol 2012;34:47–55.
18. de Graaf J, van Lingen RA, Simons SH, et al. Long-term effects of routine morphine infusion in mechanically ventilated neonates on children's functioning: five-year follow-up of a randomized controlled trial. Pain 2011;152:1391–7.
19. Grunau R, Tu MT. Long-term consequences of pain in human neonates. In: Anand KJ, Stevens B, McGrath P, editors. Pain in neonates and infants. 3rd edition. Philadelphia: Elsevier Science B.V.; 2007. p. 45–55.
20. Anand KJ, Palmer FB, Papanicolaou AC. Repetitive neonatal pain and neurocognitive abilities in ex-preterm children. Pain 2013;154:1899–901.

21. Doesburg SM, Chau CM, Cheung TP, et al. Neonatal pain-related stress, functional cortical activity and visual-perceptual abilities in school-age children born at extremely low gestational age. Pain 2013;154:1946–52.
22. Carbajal R, Rousset A, Danan C, et al. Epidemiology and treatment of painful procedures in neonates in intensive care units. JAMA 2008;300:60–70.
23. Johnston C, Barrington KJ, Taddio A, et al. Pain in Canadian NICUs: have we improved over the past 12 years? Clin J Pain 2011;27:225–32.
24. Taylor BJ, Robbins JM, Gold JI, et al. Assessing postoperative pain in neonates: a multicenter observational study. Pediatrics 2006;118:e992–1000.
25. Anand KJ, Aranda JV, Berde CB, et al. Summary proceedings from the neonatal pain-control group. Pediatrics 2006;117:S9–22.
26. Simons SH, van Dijk M, Anand KJ, et al. Do we still hurt newborn babies? A prospective study of procedural pain and analgesia in neonates. Arch Pediatr Adolesc Med 2003;157:1058–64.
27. Ranger M, Johnston CC, Anand KJ. Current controversies regarding pain assessment in neonates. Semin Perinatol 2007;31:283–8.
28. Sharek PJ, Powers R, Koehn A, et al. Evaluation and development of potentially better practices to improve pain management of neonates. Pediatrics 2006; 118(Suppl 2):S78–86.
29. Walden M, Carrier C. The ten commandments of pain assessment and management in preterm neonates. Crit Care Nurs Clin North Am 2009;21:235–52.
30. Stapelkamp C, Carter B, Gordon J, et al. Assessment of acute pain in children: development of evidence-based guidelines. Int J Evid Based Healthc 2011;9: 39–50.
31. Duhn LJ, Medves JM. A systematic integrative review of infant pain assessment tools. Adv Neonatal Care 2004;4:126–40.
32. Anand KJ. Pain assessment in preterm neonates. Pediatrics 2007;119:605–7.
33. Guedj R, Danan C, Daoud P, et al. Neonatal pain management is not the same during days and nights in intensive care units: analysis from the EPIPPAIN Study. BMJ Open 2014;4(2):e004086.
34. Anand KJ. Pain panacea for opiophobia in infants? JAMA 2013;309:183–4.
35. Anand KJ, Clark AE, Willson DF, et al. Opioid analgesia in mechanically ventilated children: results from the multicenter Measuring Opioid Tolerance Induced by Fentanyl study. Pediatr Crit Care Med 2013;14:27–36.
36. Anand KJ, Willson DF, Berger J, et al. Tolerance and withdrawal from prolonged opioid use in critically ill children. Pediatrics 2010;125:e1208–25.
37. Hummel P, van Dijk M. Pain assessment: current status and challenges. Semin Fetal Neonatal Med 2006;11:237–45.
38. Johnston CC, Stevens B. Pain assessment in newborns. J Perinat Neonatal Nurs 1990;4:41–52.
39. Stevens B, Johnston C, Petryshen P, et al. Premature infant pain profile: development and initial validation. Clin J Pain 1996;12:13–22.
40. Gibbins S, Stevens B, McGrath PJ, et al. Comparison of pain responses in infants of different gestational ages. Neonatology 2008;93:10–8.
41. Grunau RE, Oberlander T, Holsti L, et al. Bedside application of the Neonatal Facial Coding System in pain assessment of premature neonates. Pain 1998; 76:277–86.
42. Holsti L, Grunau RE. Initial validation of the behavioral indicators of infant pain (BIIP). Pain 2007;132(3):264–72.
43. Ballantyne M, Stevens B, McAllister M, et al. Validation of the premature infant pain profile in the clinical setting. Clin J Pain 1999;15:297–303.

44. McNair C, Ballantyne M, Dionne K, et al. Postoperative pain assessment in the neonatal intensive care unit. Arch Dis Child Fetal Neonatal Ed 2004;89:F537–41.

45. Hummel P, Puchalski M, Creech SD, et al. Clinical reliability and validity of the N-PASS: neonatal pain, agitation and sedation scale with prolonged pain. J Perinatol 2008;28:55–60.

46. Hummel P, Lawlor-Klean P, Weiss MG. Validity and reliability of the N-PASS assessment tool with acute pain. J Perinatol 2010;30:474–8.

47. Lawrence J, Alcock D, McGrath P, et al. The development of a tool to assess neonatal pain. Neonatal Netw 1993;12:59–66.

48. Porter FL, Wolf CM, Miller JP. Procedural pain in newborn infants: the influence of intensity and development. Pediatrics 1999;104:e13.

49. Johnston CC, Stevens BJ, Franck LS, et al. Factors explaining lack of response to heel stick in preterm newborns. J Obstet Gynecol Neonatal Nurs 1999;28:587–94.

50. Johnston CC, Stevens BJ, Yang F, et al. Differential response to pain by very premature neonates. Pain 1995;61:471–9.

51. Ganzewinkel CJ, Anand KJ, Kramer BW, et al. Chronic pain in the newborn: toward a definition. Clin J Pain 2013. [Epub ahead of print].

52. van Dijk M, Koot HM, Saad HH, et al. Observational visual analog scale in pediatric pain assessment: useful tool or good riddance? Clin J Pain 2002;18:310–6.

53. Stevens BJ, Pillai Riddell R. Looking beyond acute pain in infancy. Pain 2006;124:11–2.

54. Pillai Riddell R, Racine N. Assessing pain in infancy: the caregiver context. Pain Res Manag 2009;14:27–32.

55. Holsti L, Grunau RE, Shany E. Assessing pain in preterm infants in the neonatal intensive care unit: moving to a 'brain-oriented' approach. Pain Manag 2011;1:171–9.

56. Ismail AQ, Gandhi A. Non-pharmacological analgesia: effective but underused. Arch Dis Child 2011;96:784–5.

57. Ernst E. Chiropractic manipulation for non-spinal pain–a systematic review. N Z Med J 2003;116:U539.

58. Eisenberg DM, Davis RB, Ettner SL, et al. Trends in alternative medicine use in the United States, 1990-1997: results of a follow-up national survey. JAMA 1998;280:1569–75.

59. Bewley S, Ross N, Braillon A, et al. Clothing naked quackery and legitimising pseudoscience. BMJ 2011;343:d5960.

60. Hall RW. Anesthesia and analgesia in the NICU. Clin Perinatol 2012;39:239–54.

61. Holsti L, Grunau RE, Oberlander TF, et al. Prior pain induces heightened motor responses during clustered care in preterm infants in the NICU. Early Hum Dev 2005;81:293–302.

62. Holsti L, Grunau RE, Whifield MF, et al. Behavioral responses to pain are heightened after clustered care in preterm infants born between 30 and 32 weeks gestational age. Clin J Pain 2006;22:757–64.

63. Karlsson V, Heinemann AB, Sjors G, et al. Early skin-to-skin care in extremely preterm infants: thermal balance and care environment. J Pediatr 2012;161:422–6.

64. Cong X, Cusson RM, Walsh S, et al. Effects of skin-to-skin contact on autonomic pain responses in preterm infants. J Pain 2012;13:636–45.

65. Johnston C, Campbell-Yeo M, Fernandes A, et al. Skin-to-skin care for procedural pain in neonates. Cochrane Database Syst Rev 2014;(1):CD008435.

66. Morelius E, Theodorsson E, Nelson N. Salivary cortisol and mood and pain profiles during skin-to-skin care for an unselected group of mothers and infants in neonatal intensive care. Pediatrics 2005;116:1105–13.

67. McCain GC, Ludington-Hoe SM, Swinth JY, et al. Heart rate variability responses of a preterm infant to kangaroo care. J Obstet Gynecol Neonatal Nurs 2005;34: 689–94.

68. Mitchell AJ, Yates CC, Williams DK, et al. Does daily kangaroo care provide sustained pain and stress relief in preterm infants? J Neonatal Perinatal Med 2013;6:45–52.

69. Mitchell AJ, Yates C, Williams K, et al. Effects of daily kangaroo care on cardiorespiratory parameters in preterm infants. J Neonatal Perinatal Med 2013;6:243–9.

70. Axelin A, Salantera S, Lehtonen L. 'Facilitated tucking by parents' in pain management of preterm infants-a randomized crossover trial. Early Hum Dev 2006; 82:241–7.

71. Cignacco EL, Sellam G, Stoffel L, et al. Oral sucrose and "facilitated tucking" for repeated pain relief in preterms: a randomized controlled trial. Pediatrics 2012; 129:299–308.

72. de Freitas RL, Kubler JM, Elias-Filho DH, et al. Antinociception induced by acute oral administration of sweet substance in young and adult rodents: the role of endogenous opioid peptides chemical mediators and mu(1)-opioid receptors. Pharmacol Biochem Behav 2012;101:265–70.

73. Liaw JJ, Zeng WP, Yang L, et al. Nonnutritive sucking and oral sucrose relieve neonatal pain during intramuscular injection of hepatitis vaccine. J Pain Symptom Manage 2011;42:918–30.

74. Corbo MG, Mansi G, Stagni A, et al. Nonnutritive sucking during heelstick procedures decreases behavioral distress in the newborn infant. Biol Neonate 2000;77:162–7.

75. Mitchell A, Waltman PA. Oral sucrose and pain relief for preterm infants. Pain Manag Nurs 2003;4:62–9.

76. Bueno M, Yamada J, Harrison D, et al. A systematic review and meta-analyses of nonsucrose sweet solutions for pain relief in neonates. Pain Res Manag 2013; 18:153–61.

77. O'Sullivan A, O'Connor M, Brosnahan D, et al. Sweeten, soother and swaddle for retinopathy of prematurity screening: a randomised placebo controlled trial. Arch Dis Child Fetal Neonatal Ed 2010;95:F419–22.

78. Kristoffersen L, Skogvoll E, Hafstrom M. Pain reduction on insertion of a feeding tube in preterm infants: a randomized controlled trial. Pediatrics 2011;127:e1449–54.

79. Holsti L, Grunau RE. Considerations for using sucrose to reduce procedural pain in preterm infants. Pediatrics 2010;125:1042–7.

80. Stevens B, Yamada J, Ohlsson A. Sucrose for analgesia in newborn infants undergoing painful procedures. Cochrane Database Syst Rev 2010;(1):CD001069.

81. Marin Gabriel MA, del Rey Hurtado de Mendoza B, Jimenez Figueroa L, et al. Analgesia with breastfeeding in addition to skin-to-skin contact during heel prick. Arch Dis Child Fetal Neonatal Ed 2013;98:F499–503.

82. Field T, Diego M, Hernandez-Reif M. Preterm infant massage therapy research: a review. Infant Behav Dev 2010;33:115–24.

83. Jain S, Kumar P, McMillan DD. Prior leg massage decreases pain responses to heel stick in preterm babies. J Paediatr Child Health 2006;42:505–8.

84. Diego MA, Field T, Hernandez-Reif M, et al. Preterm infant massage elicits consistent increases in vagal activity and gastric motility that are associated with greater weight gain. Acta Paediatr 2007;96:1588–91.

85. Procianoy RS, Mendes EW, Silveira RC. Massage therapy improves neurodevelopment outcome at two years corrected age for very low birth weight infants. Early Hum Dev 2010;86:7–11.

86. Woo YM, Lee MS, Nam Y, et al. Effects of contralateral electroacupuncture on brain function: a double-blind, randomized, pilot clinical trial. J Altern Complement Med 2006;12:813–5.

87. Taddio A, Katz J, Ilersich AL, et al. Effect of neonatal circumcision on pain response during subsequent routine vaccination. Lancet 1997;349:599–603.

88. Lander J, Brady-Fryer B, Metcalfe JB, et al. Comparison of ring block, dorsal penile nerve block, and topical anesthesia for neonatal circumcision: a randomized controlled trial [see comment]. JAMA 1997;278:2157–62.

89. Garcia OC, Reichberg S, Brion LP, et al. Topical anesthesia for line insertion in very low birth weight infants. J Perinatol 1997;17:477–80.

90. Kaur G, Gupta P, Kumar A. A randomized trial of eutectic mixture of local anesthetics during lumbar puncture in newborns. Arch Pediatr Adolesc Med 2003; 157:1065–70.

91. Gradin M, Eriksson M, Holmqvist G, et al. Pain reduction at venipuncture in newborns: oral glucose compared with local anesthetic cream. Pediatrics 2002;110: 1053–7.

92. Biran V, Gourrier E, Cimerman P, et al. Analgesic effects of EMLA cream and oral sucrose during venipuncture in preterm infants. Pediatrics 2011;128:e63–70.

93. Baxter AL, Ewing PH, Young GB, et al. EMLA application exceeding two hours improves pediatric emergency department venipuncture success. Adv Emerg Nurs J 2013;35:67–75.

94. Hui-Chen F, Hsiu-Lin C, Shun-Line C, et al. The effect of EMLA cream on minimizing pain during venipuncture in premature infants. J Trop Pediatr 2013;59: 72–3.

95. Lemyre B, Hogan DL, Gaboury I, et al. How effective is tetracaine 4% gel, before a venipuncture, in reducing procedural pain in infants: a randomized double-blind placebo controlled trial. BMC Pediatr 2007;7:7.

96. O'Brien L, Taddio A, Lyszkiewicz DA, et al. A critical review of the topical local anesthetic amethocaine (Ametop) for pediatric pain. Paediatr Drugs 2005;7:41–54.

97. Taddio A, Lee CM, Parvez B, et al. Contact dermatitis and bradycardia in a preterm infant given tetracaine 4% gel. Ther Drug Monit 2006;28:291–4.

98. Frey B, Kehrer B. Toxic methaemoglobin concentrations in premature infants after application of a prilocaine-containing cream and peridural prilocaine. Eur J Pediatr 1999;158:785–8.

99. Brisman M, Ljung BM, Otterbom I, et al. Methaemoglobin formation after the use of EMLA cream in term neonates. Acta Paediatr 1998;87:1191–4.

100. Taddio A, Ohlsson A, Einarson TR, et al. A systematic review of lidocaine-prilocaine cream (EMLA) in the treatment of acute pain in neonates. Pediatrics 1998;101:E1.

101. Essink-Tebbes CM, Wuis EW, Liem KD, et al. Safety of lidocaine-prilocaine cream application four times a day in premature neonates: a pilot study. Eur J Pediatr 1999;158:421–3.

102. Larsson BA, Norman M, Bjerring P, et al. Regional variations in skin perfusion and skin thickness may contribute to varying efficacy of topical, local anaesthetics in neonates. Paediatr Anaesth 1996;6:107–10.

103. Fitzgerald M, Millard C, McIntosh N. Cutaneous hypersensitivity following peripheral tissue damage in newborn infants and its reversal with topical anaesthesia. Pain 1989;39:31–6.

104. Schmidt B, Adelmann C, Stutzer H, et al. Comparison of sufentanil versus fentanyl in ventilated term neonates. Klin Padiatr 2010;222:62–6.
105. Saarenmaa E, Huttunen P, Leppaluoto J, et al. Alfentanil as procedural pain relief in newborn infants. Arch Dis Child Fetal Neonatal Ed 1996;75:F103–7.
106. Pokela ML, Koivisto M. Physiological changes, plasma beta-endorphin and cortisol responses to tracheal intubation in neonates. Acta Paediatr 1994;83:151–6.
107. e Silva YP, Gomez RS, Marcatto Jde O, et al. Early awakening and extubation with remifentanil in ventilated premature neonates. Paediatr Anaesth 2008;18:176–83.
108. Stoppa F, Perrotta D, Tomasello C, et al. Low dose remifentanyl infusion for analgesia and sedation in ventilated newborns. Minerva Anestesiol 2004;70:753–61.
109. Alencar AJ, Sanudo A, Sampaio VM, et al. Efficacy of tramadol versus fentanyl for postoperative analgesia in neonates. Arch Dis Child Fetal Neonatal Ed 2012;97:F24–9.
110. Quinn MW, Vokes A. Effect of morphine on respiratory drive in trigger ventilated pre-term infants. Early Hum Dev 2000;59:27–35.
111. Dyke MP, Kohan R, Evans S. Morphine increases synchronous ventilation in preterm infants. J Paediatr Child Health 1995;31:176–9.
112. Anand KJ, Hall RW, Desai N, et al. Effects of morphine analgesia in ventilated preterm neonates: primary outcomes from the NEOPAIN randomised trial [see comment]. Lancet 2004;363:1673–82.
113. Hall RW, Kronsberg SS, Barton BA, et al. Morphine, hypotension, and adverse outcomes among preterm neonates: who's to blame? Secondary results from the NEOPAIN trial. Pediatrics 2005;115:1351–9.
114. Menon G, Boyle EM, Bergqvist LL, et al. Morphine analgesia and gastrointestinal morbidity in preterm infants: secondary results from the NEOPAIN trial. Arch Dis Child Fetal Neonatal Ed 2008;93:F362–7.
115. Simons SH, van Dijk M, van Lingen RA, et al. Routine morphine infusion in preterm newborns who received ventilatory support: a randomized controlled trial. JAMA 2003;290:2419–27.
116. Bellu R, de Waal K, Zanini R. Opioids for neonates receiving mechanical ventilation: a systematic review and meta-analysis. Arch Dis Child Fetal Neonatal Ed 2010;95:F241–51.
117. MacGregor R, Evans D, Sugden D, et al. Outcome at 5-6 years of prematurely born children who received morphine as neonates. Arch Dis Child Fetal Neonatal Ed 1998;79:F40–3.
118. Ranger M, Synnes AR, Vinall J, et al. Internalizing behaviours in school-age children born very preterm are predicted by neonatal pain and morphine exposure. Eur J Pain 2014;18:844–52.
119. de Graaf J, van Lingen RA, Valkenburg AJ, et al. Does neonatal morphine use affect neuropsychological outcomes at 8 to 9 years of age? Pain 2013;154:449–58.
120. Angeles DM, Wycliffe N, Michelson D, et al. Use of opioids in asphyxiated term neonates: effects on neuroimaging and clinical outcome. Pediatr Res 2005;57:873–8.
121. El Sayed MF, Taddio A, Fallah S, et al. Safety profile of morphine following surgery in neonates. J Perinatol 2007;27:444–7.
122. Bouwmeester NJ, Hop WC, van Dijk M, et al. Postoperative pain in the neonate: age-related differences in morphine requirements and metabolism. Intensive Care Med 2003;29:2009–15.

123. Bouwmeester NJ, van den Anker JN, Hop WC, et al. Age- and therapy-related effects on morphine requirements and plasma concentrations of morphine and its metabolites in postoperative infants. Br J Anaesth 2003; 90:642–52.
124. van Dijk M, Bouwmeester NJ, Duivenvoorden HJ, et al. Efficacy of continuous versus intermittent morphine administration after major surgery in 0-3-year-old infants; a double-blind randomized controlled trial. Pain 2002; 98:305–13.
125. Rouss K, Gerber A, Albisetti M, et al. Long-term subcutaneous morphine administration after surgery in newborns. J Perinat Med 2007;35:79–81.
126. Lynn AM, Nespeca MK, Bratton SL, et al. Ventilatory effects of morphine infusions in cyanotic versus acyanotic infants after thoracotomy. Paediatr Anaesth 2003;13:12–7.
127. Lynn AM, Nespeca MK, Bratton SL, et al. Intravenous morphine in postoperative infants: intermittent bolus dosing versus targeted continuous infusions. Pain 2000;88:89–95.
128. Lynn AM, Nespeca MK, Opheim KE, et al. Respiratory effects of intravenous morphine infusions in neonates, infants, and children after cardiac surgery. Anesth Analg 1993;77:695–701.
129. Carbajal R, Lenclen R, Jugie M, et al. Morphine does not provide adequate analgesia for acute procedural pain among preterm neonates. Pediatrics 2005;115: 1494–500.
130. Taddio A, Lee C, Yip A, et al. Intravenous morphine and topical tetracaine for treatment of pain in neonates undergoing central line placement. JAMA 2006; 295:793–800.
131. Cignacco E, Hamers JP, van Lingen RA, et al. Pain relief in ventilated preterms during endotracheal suctioning: a randomized controlled trial. Swiss Med Wkly 2008;138:635–45.
132. Anand KJ, Anderson BJ, Holford NH, et al. Morphine pharmacokinetics and pharmacodynamics in preterm and term neonates: secondary results from the NEOPAIN trial. Br J Anaesth 2008;101:680–9.
133. Aguado-Lorenzo V, Weeks K, Tunstell P, et al. Accuracy of the concentration of morphine infusions prepared for patients in a neonatal intensive care unit. Arch Dis Child 2013;98:975–9.
134. Guinsburg R, Kopelman BI, Anand KJ, et al. Physiological, hormonal, and behavioral responses to a single fentanyl dose in intubated and ventilated preterm neonates. J Pediatr 1998;132:954–9.
135. Lago P, Benini F, Agosto C, et al. Randomised controlled trial of low dose fentanyl infusion in preterm infants with hyaline membrane disease. Arch Dis Child Fetal Neonatal Ed 1998;79:F194–7.
136. Orsini AJ, Leef KH, Costarino A, et al. Routine use of fentanyl infusions for pain and stress reduction in infants with respiratory distress syndrome. J Pediatr 1996;129:140–5.
137. Gitto E, Pellegrino S, Manfrida M, et al. Stress response and procedural pain in the preterm newborn: the role of pharmacological and non-pharmacological treatments. Eur J Pediatr 2012;171:927–33.
138. Lago P. Premedication for non-emergency intubation in the neonate. Minerva Pediatr 2010;62:61–3.
139. Lucas da Silva PS, Oliveira Iglesias SB, Leao FV, et al. Procedural sedation for insertion of central venous catheters in children: comparison of midazolam/fentanyl with midazolam/ketamine. Paediatr Anaesth 2007;17:358–63.

140. Roberts KD, Leone TA, Edwards WH, et al. Premedication for nonemergent neonatal intubations: a randomized, controlled trial comparing atropine and fentanyl to atropine, fentanyl, and mivacurium. Pediatrics 2006;118:1583–91.
141. VanLooy JW, Schumacher RE, Bhatt-Mehta V. Efficacy of a premedication algorithm for nonemergent intubation in a neonatal intensive care unit. Ann Pharmacother 2008;42:947–55.
142. Lago P, Tiozzo C, Boccuzzo G, et al. Remifentanil for percutaneous intravenous central catheter placement in preterm infant: a randomized controlled trial. Paediatr Anaesth 2008;18:736–44.
143. Pereira e Silva Y, Gomez RS, Marcatto Jde O, et al. Morphine versus remifentanil for intubating preterm neonates. Arch Dis Child Fetal Neonatal Ed 2007;92: F293–4.
144. Aranda JV, Carlo W, Hummel P, et al. Analgesia and sedation during mechanical ventilation in neonates. Clin Ther 2005;27:877–99.
145. Hall RW, Boyle E, Young T. Do ventilated neonates require pain management? Semin Perinatol 2007;31:289–97.
146. Ancora G, Lago P, Garetti E, et al. Efficacy and safety of continuous infusion of fentanyl for pain control in preterm newborns on mechanical ventilation. J Pediatr 2013;163:645–51.e1.
147. Franck LS, Vilardi J, Durand D, et al. Opioid withdrawal in neonates after continuous infusions of morphine or fentanyl during extracorporeal membrane oxygenation. Am J Crit Care 1998;7:364–9.
148. Ionides SP, Weiss MG, Angelopoulos M, et al. Plasma beta-endorphin concentrations and analgesia-muscle relaxation in the newborn infant supported by mechanical ventilation. J Pediatr 1994;125:113–6.
149. Saarenmaa E, Huttunen P, Leppaluoto J, et al. Advantages of fentanyl over morphine in analgesia for ventilated newborn infants after birth: a randomized trial. J Pediatr 1999;134:144–50.
150. Fahnenstich H, Steffan J, Kau N, et al. Fentanyl-induced chest wall rigidity and laryngospasm in preterm and term infants. Crit Care Med 2000;28: 836–9.
151. Hammer GB, Ramamoorthy C, Cao H, et al. Postoperative analgesia after spinal blockade in infants and children undergoing cardiac surgery. Anesth Analg 2005;100:1283–8.
152. Pirat A, Akpek E, Arslan G. Intrathecal versus IV fentanyl in pediatric cardiac anesthesia. Anesth Analg 2002;95:1207–14 [Table of contents].
153. Hickey PR, Hansen DD. Fentanyl- and sufentanil-oxygen-pancuronium anesthesia for cardiac surgery in infants. Anesth Analg 1984;63:117–24.
154. Hickey PR, Hansen DD, Wessel DL, et al. Blunting of stress responses in the pulmonary circulation of infants by fentanyl. Anesth Analg 1985;64:1137–42.
155. Welzing L, Roth B. Experience with remifentanil in neonates and infants. Drugs 2006;66:1339–50.
156. Marlow N, Weindling AM, Van Peer A, et al. Alfentanil pharmacokinetics in preterm infants. Arch Dis Child 1990;65:349–51.
157. Durrmeyer X, Vutskits L, Anand KJ, et al. Use of analgesic and sedative drugs in the NICU: integrating clinical trials and laboratory data. Pediatr Res 2010;67: 117–27.
158. Blumer JL. Clinical pharmacology of midazolam in infants and children. Clin Pharmacokinet 1998;35:37–47.
159. Benini F, Farina M, Capretta A, et al. Sedoanalgesia in paediatric intensive care: a survey of 19 Italian units. Acta Paediatr 2010;99:758–62.

160. Arya V, Ramji S. Midazolam sedation in mechanically ventilated newborns: a double blind randomized placebo controlled trial [see comment]. Indian Pediatr 2001;38:967–72.

161. Anand KJ, Barton BA, McIntosh N, et al. Analgesia and sedation in preterm neonates who require ventilatory support: results from the NOPAIN trial. Neonatal Outcome and Prolonged Analgesia in Neonates. Arch Pediatr Adolesc Med 1999;153:331–8 [Erratum appears in Arch Pediatr Adolesc Med 1999;153(8):895].

162. Shehab N, Lewis CL, Streetman DD, et al. Exposure to the pharmaceutical excipients benzyl alcohol and propylene glycol among critically ill neonates. Pediatr Crit Care Med 2009;10:256–9.

163. Ng E, Taddio A, Ohlsson A. Intravenous midazolam infusion for sedation of infants in the neonatal intensive care unit. Cochrane Database Syst Rev 2012;(6):CD002052.

164. Mekitarian Filho E, de Carvalho WB, Gilio AE, et al. Aerosolized intranasal midazolam for safe and effective sedation for quality computed tomography imaging in infants and children. J Pediatr 2013;163:1217–9.

165. Lane RD, Schunk JE. Atomized intranasal midazolam use for minor procedures in the pediatric emergency department. Pediatr Emerg Care 2008;24:300–3.

166. Ranger M, Celeste Johnston C, Rennick JE, et al. A multidimensional approach to pain assessment in critically ill infants during a painful procedure. Clin J Pain 2013;29:613–20.

167. Chess PR, D'Angio CT. Clonic movements following lorazepam administration in full-term infants. Arch Pediatr Adolesc Med 1998;152:98–9.

168. Treluyer JM, Zohar S, Rey E, et al. Minimum effective dose of midazolam for sedation of mechanically ventilated neonates. J Clin Pharm Ther 2005;30: 479–85.

169. de Wildt SN, de Hoog M, Vinks AA, et al. Pharmacodynamics of midazolam in pediatric intensive care patients. Ther Drug Monit 2005;27:98–102.

170. de Wildt SN, Kearns GL, Hop WC, et al. Pharmacokinetics and metabolism of oral midazolam in preterm infants. Br J Clin Pharmacol 2002;53:390–2.

171. Altintas O, Karabas VL, Demirci G, et al. Evaluation of intranasal midazolam in refraction and fundus examination of young children with strabismus. J Pediatr Ophthalmol Strabismus 2005;42:355–9.

172. Ince I, de Wildt SN, Wang C, et al. A novel maturation function for clearance of the cytochrome P450 3A substrate midazolam from preterm neonates to adults. Clin Pharmacokinet 2013;52:555–65 [Erratum appears in Clin Pharmacokinet 2013;52(7):611 Note: Wang, Chengueng [corrected to Wang, Chenguang]].

173. Bhatt-Meht V, Annich G. Sedative clearance during extracorporeal membrane oxygenation. Perfusion 2005;20:309–15.

174. McDermott CA, Kowalczyk AL, Schnitzler ER, et al. Pharmacokinetics of lorazepam in critically ill neonates with seizures. J Pediatr 1992;120:479–83.

175. Gonzalez-Darder JM, Ortega-Alvaro A, Ruz-Franzi I, et al. Antinociceptive effects of phenobarbital in "tail-flick" test and deafferentation pain. Anesth Analg 1992;75:81–6.

176. Ebner N, Rohrmeister K, Winklbaur B, et al. Management of neonatal abstinence syndrome in neonates born to opioid maintained women. Drug Alcohol Depend 2007;87:131–8.

177. Jenkins IA, Playfor SD, Bevan C, et al. Current United Kingdom sedation practice in pediatric intensive care. Paediatr Anaesth 2007;17:675–83.

178. Shah PS, Shah VS. Propofol for procedural sedation/anaesthesia in neonates. Cochrane Database Syst Rev 2011;(3):CD007248.

179. Ghanta S, Abdel-Latif ME, Lui K, et al. Propofol compared with the morphine, atropine, and suxamethonium regimen as induction agents for neonatal endotracheal intubation: a randomized, controlled trial [see comment]. Pediatrics 2007;119:e1248–55.
180. Allegaert K, Peeters MY, Verbesselt R, et al. Inter-individual variability in propofol pharmacokinetics in preterm and term neonates. Br J Anaesth 2007;99:864–70.
181. Welzing L, Kribs A, Eifinger F, et al. Propofol as an induction agent for endotracheal intubation can cause significant arterial hypotension in preterm neonates. Paediatr Anaesth 2010;20:605–11.
182. Chambliss CR, Anand KJ. Pain management in the pediatric intensive care unit. Curr Opin Pediatr 1997;9:246–53.
183. Betremieux P, Carre P, Pladys P, et al. Doppler ultrasound assessment of the effects of ketamine on neonatal cerebral circulation. Dev Pharmacol Ther 1993;20:9–13.
184. Anand KJ, Soriano SG. Anesthetic agents and the immature brain: are these toxic or therapeutic? [see comment]. Anesthesiology 2004;101:527–30.
185. Saarenmaa E, Neuvonen PJ, Huttunen P, et al. Ketamine for procedural pain relief in newborn infants. Arch Dis Child Fetal Neonatal Ed 2001;85:F53–6.
186. Barton KP, Munoz R, Morell VO, et al. Dexmedetomidine as the primary sedative during invasive procedures in infants and toddlers with congenital heart disease. Pediatr Crit Care Med 2008;9:612–5.
187. Carroll CL, Krieger D, Campbell M, et al. Use of dexmedetomidine for sedation of children hospitalized in the intensive care unit. J Hosp Med 2008;3:142–7.
188. Bejian S, Valasek C, Nigro JJ, et al. Prolonged use of dexmedetomidine in the paediatric cardiothoracic intensive care unit. Cardiol Young 2009;19:98–104.
189. Chrysostomou C, Sanchez De Toledo J, Avolio T, et al. Dexmedetomidine use in a pediatric cardiac intensive care unit: can we use it in infants after cardiac surgery? Pediatr Crit Care Med 2009;10:654–60.
190. Potts AL, Anderson BJ, Holford NH, et al. Dexmedetomidine hemodynamics in children after cardiac surgery. Paediatr Anaesth 2010;20:425–33.
191. Lam F, Bhutta AT, Tobias JD, et al. Hemodynamic effects of dexmedetomidine in critically ill neonates and infants with heart disease. Pediatr Cardiol 2012;33:1069–77.
192. Chrysostomou C, Morell VO, Wearden P, et al. Dexmedetomidine: therapeutic use for the termination of reentrant supraventricular tachycardia. Congenit Heart Dis 2013;8:48–56.
193. Diaz SM, Rodarte A, Foley J, et al. Pharmacokinetics of dexmedetomidine in postsurgical pediatric intensive care unit patients: preliminary study. Pediatr Crit Care Med 2007;8:419–24.
194. Potts AL, Anderson BJ, Warman GR, et al. Dexmedetomidine pharmacokinetics in pediatric intensive care–a pooled analysis. Paediatr Anaesth 2009;19:1119–29.
195. Su F, Nicolson SC, Gastonguay MR, et al. Population pharmacokinetics of dexmedetomidine in infants after open heart surgery. Anesth Analg 2010;110:1383–92.
196. Vilo S, Rautiainen P, Kaisti K, et al. Pharmacokinetics of intravenous dexmedetomidine in children under 11 yr of age. Br J Anaesth 2008;100:697–700.
197. Kubota T, Fukasawa T, Kitamura E, et al. Epileptic seizures induced by dexmedetomidine in a neonate. Brain Dev 2013;35:360–2.
198. Finkel JC, Quezado ZM. Hypothermia-induced bradycardia in a neonate receiving dexmedetomidine. J Clin Anesth 2007;19:290–2.

199. Berkenbosch JW, Tobias JD. Development of bradycardia during sedation with dexmedetomidine in an infant concurrently receiving digoxin. Pediatr Crit Care Med 2003;4:203–5.

200. Mason KP, Zgleszewski SE, Prescilla R, et al. Hemodynamic effects of dexmedetomidine sedation for CT imaging studies. Paediatr Anaesth 2008;18:393–402.

201. Mason KP. Sedation trends in the 21st century: the transition to dexmedetomidine for radiological imaging studies. Paediatr Anaesth 2010;20:265–72.

202. Mason KP, Zurakowski D, Zgleszewski S, et al. Incidence and predictors of hypertension during high-dose dexmedetomidine sedation for pediatric MRI. Paediatr Anaesth 2010;20:516–23.

203. Chrysostomou C, Beerman L, Shiderly D, et al. Dexmedetomidine: a novel drug for the treatment of atrial and junctional tachyarrhythmias during the perioperative period for congenital cardiac surgery: a preliminary study. Anesth Analg 2008;107:1514–22.

204. Mayers DJ, Hindmarsh KW, Gorecki DK, et al. Sedative/hypnotic effects of chloral hydrate in the neonate: trichloroethanol or parent drug? Dev Pharmacol Ther 1992;19:141–6.

205. Litman RS, Soin K, Salam A. Chloral hydrate sedation in term and preterm infants: an analysis of efficacy and complications. Anesth Analg 2010;110:739–46.

206. Novitskaya ES, Kostakis V, Broster SC, et al. Pain score assessment in babies undergoing laser treatment for retinopathy of prematurity under sub-tenon anaesthesia. Eye 2013;27:1405–10.

207. Menon G, Anand KJ, McIntosh N. Practical approach to analgesia and sedation in the neonatal intensive care unit. Semin Perinatol 1998;22:417–24.

208. Wong I, St John-Green C, Walker SM. Opioid-sparing effects of perioperative paracetamol and nonsteroidal anti-inflammatory drugs (NSAIDs) in children. Paediatr Anaesth 2013;23:475–95.

209. van den Anker JN, Tibboel D. Pain relief in neonates: when to use intravenous paracetamol. Arch Dis Child 2011;96:573–4.

210. Nevin DG, Shung J. Intravenous paracetamol overdose in a preterm infant during anesthesia. Paediatr Anaesth 2010;20:105–7.

211. Howard CR, Howard FM, Weitzman ML. Acetaminophen analgesia in neonatal circumcision: the effect on pain. Pediatrics 1994;93:641–6.

212. Allegaert K, Rayyan M, De Rijdt T, et al. Hepatic tolerance of repeated intravenous paracetamol administration in neonates. Paediatr Anaesth 2008;18:388–92.

213. Truog R, Anand KJ. Management of pain in the postoperative neonate. Clin Perinatol 1989;16:61–78.

214. Shah V, Taddio A, Ohlsson A. Randomised controlled trial of paracetamol for heel prick pain in neonates. Arch Dis Child Fetal Neonatal Ed 1998;79:F209–11.

215. Morris JL, Rosen DA, Rosen KR. Nonsteroidal anti-inflammatory agents in neonates. Paediatr Drugs 2003;5:385–405.

216. Hopchet L, Kulo A, Rayyan M, et al. Does intravenous paracetamol administration affect body temperature in neonates? Arch Dis Child 2011;96:301–4.

217. Rod B, Monrigal JP, Lepoittevin L, et al. Traitement de la douleur postoperatoire chez l'enfant en salle de reveil. Utilisation de la morphine et du propacetamol par voie intraveineuse. Cah Anesthesiol 1989;37:525–30.

218. Allegaert K, Anderson BJ, Naulaers G, et al. Intravenous paracetamol (propacetamol) pharmacokinetics in term and preterm neonates. Eur J Clin Pharmacol 2004;60:191–7.

219. Anderson BJ, Pons G, Autret-Leca E, et al. Pediatric intravenous paracetamol (propacetamol) pharmacokinetics: a population analysis. Paediatr Anaesth 2005;15:282–92.

220. Hopkins CS, Underhill S, Booker PD. Pharmacokinetics of paracetamol after cardiac surgery [see comments]. Arch Dis Child 1990;65:971–6.

221. Autret E, Dutertre JP, Breteau M, et al. Pharmacokinetics of paracetamol in the neonate and infant after administration of propacetamol chlorhydrate. Dev Pharmacol Ther 1993;20:129–34.

222. Lin YC, Sussman HH, Benitz WE. Plasma concentrations after rectal administration of acetaminophen in preterm neonates. Paediatr Anaesth 1997;7:457–9.

223. van Lingen RA, Deinum HT, Quak CM, et al. Multiple-dose pharmacokinetics of rectally administered acetaminophen in term infants. Clin Pharmacol Ther 1999; 66:509–15.

224. Anderson BJ, Woollard GA, Holford NH. A model for size and age changes in the pharmacokinetics of paracetamol in neonates, infants and children. Br J Clin Pharmacol 2000;50:125–34.

225. Anderson BJ, van Lingen RA, Hansen TG, et al. Acetaminophen developmental pharmacokinetics in premature neonates and infants: a pooled population analysis. Anesthesiology 2002;96:1336–45.

226. Allegaert K, Palmer GM, Anderson BJ. The pharmacokinetics of intravenous paracetamol in neonates: size matters most. Arch Dis Child 2011;96:575–80.

227. Fowlie PW. Prophylactic indomethacin: systematic review and meta-analysis. Arch Dis Child Fetal Neonatal Ed 1996;74:F81–7.

228. Sakhalkar VS, Merchant RH. Therapy of symptomatic patent ductus arteriosus in preterms using mefenemic acid and indomethacin. Indian Pediatr 1992;29:313–8.

229. Mosca F, Bray M, Lattanzio M, et al. Comparative evaluation of the effects of indomethacin and ibuprofen on cerebral perfusion and oxygenation in preterm infants with patent ductus arteriosus. J Pediatr 1997;131:549–54.

230. Van Overmeire B, Smets K, Lecoutere D, et al. A comparison of ibuprofen and indomethacin for closure of patent ductus arteriosus [see comment]. N Engl J Med 2000;343:674–81.

231. Varvarigou A, Bardin CL, Beharry K, et al. Early ibuprofen administration to prevent patent ductus arteriosus in premature newborn infants. JAMA 1996;275: 539–44.

232. Anand KJ, Hall RW. Pharmacological therapy for analgesia and sedation in the newborn. Arch Dis Child Fetal Neonatal Ed 2006;91:F448–53.

233. Allegaert K, Vanhole C, de Hoon J, et al. Nonselective cyclo-oxygenase inhibitors and glomerular filtration rate in preterm neonates. Pediatr Nephrol 2005;20: 1557–61.

234. Naulaers G, Delanghe G, Allegaert K, et al. Ibuprofen and cerebral oxygenation and circulation. Arch Dis Child Fetal Neonatal Ed 2005;90:F75–6.

235. Johnston CC, Fernandes AM, Campbell-Yeo M. Pain in neonates is different. Pain 2011;152:S65–73.

236. Byrd PJ, Gonzales I, Parsons V. Exploring barriers to pain management in newborn intensive care units: a pilot survey of NICU nurses. Adv Neonatal Care 2009;9:299–306.

237. Cong X, Delaney C, Vazquez V. Neonatal nurses' perceptions of pain assessment and management in NICUs: a national survey. Adv Neonatal Care 2013; 13:353–60.

238. Pillai Riddell RR, Stevens BJ, McKeever P, et al. Chronic pain in hospitalized infants: health professionals' perspectives. J Pain 2009;10:1217–25.

239. Spence K, Henderson-Smart D. Closing the evidence-practice gap for newborn pain using clinical networks. J Paediatr Child Health 2011;47:92–8.

240. Stevens B, Riahi S, Cardoso R, et al. The influence of context on pain practices in the NICU: perceptions of health care professionals. Qual Health Res 2011;21: 757–70.

241. Aretz S, Licht C, Roth B. Endogenous distress in ventilated full-term newborns with acute respiratory failure. Biol Neonate 2004;85:243–8.

242. Grunau RE, Whitfield MF, Petrie J. Children's judgments about pain at age 8-10 years: do extremely low birthweight (< or = 1000 g) children differ from full birth-weight peers? J Child Psychol Psychiatry 1998;39:587–94.

243. Boyle EM, Freer Y, Wong CM, et al. Assessment of persistent pain or distress and adequacy of analgesia in preterm ventilated infants. Pain 2006;124:87–91.

244. Giannantonio C, Sammartino M, Valente E, et al. Remifentanil analgosedation in preterm newborns during mechanical ventilation. Acta Paediatr 2009;98: 1111–5.

245. O'Mara K, Gal P, Ransommd JL, et al. Successful use of dexmedetomidine for sedation in a 24-week gestational age neonate. Ann Pharmacother 2009;43: 1707–13.

Vascular Endothelial Growth Factor Antagonist Therapy for Retinopathy of Prematurity

 CrossMark

M. Elizabeth Hartnett, MD

KEYWORDS

- Vascular endothelial growth factor • Physiologic retinal vascular development (PRVD)
- Intravitreal neovascularization (IVNV) • Bevacizumab • Angiogenesis
- Oxygen-induced retinopathy (OIR)

KEY POINTS

- Before considering anti-vascular endothelial growth factor (VEGF) agents in preterm infants, more studies are needed to determine long-term effects on safety, proper doses, or even the type of anti-VEGF agent or other drug.
- Retinopathy of prematurity phenotypes may vary throughout the world based on environmental factors and potential differences in genetic variants. These considerations are important when comparing outcomes from clinical reports after anti-VEGF therapy.
- Although there is promise with anti-VEGF treatment, there is clinical risk of poor outcome and safety concerns potentially from systemic reduction of VEGF. Other treatments are needed.

INTRODUCTION

Over the past several decades, vascular endothelial growth factor (VEGF) has become recognized as an important pathologic angiogenic factor in several eye diseases, including age-related macular degeneration (AMD),[1–3] diabetic retinopathy,[4,5] retinal vein occlusion,[4] and retinopathy of prematurity (ROP). Before US Food and Drug Administration (FDA) approval of anti-VEGF agents for AMD, a disease affecting elderly adults, preclinical studies tested VEGF inhibitors in animal models of angiogenesis, including models of oxygen-induced retinopathy (OIR) in which blood vessels grow into the vitreous cavity similar to what occurs in diabetic retinopathy and ROP.[6,7] After proven efficacy that anti-VEGF agents reduced intravitreal angiogenesis

Disclosure: NIH grants: NEI R01EY017011, NEI R01EY015130. March of Dimes grant: FY-13-75.
Department of Ophthalmology and Visual Sciences, John A. Moran Eye Center, University of Utah, 65 Mario Capecchi Drive, Salt Lake City, UT 84108, USA
E-mail address: me.hartnett@hsc.utah.edu

Clin Perinatol 41 (2014) 925–943
http://dx.doi.org/10.1016/j.clp.2014.08.011
perinatology.theclinics.com
0095-5108/14/$ – see front matter © 2014 Elsevier Inc. All rights reserved.

in preclinical testing in models of OIR and aberrant angiogenesis in clinical trials for neovascular AMD and adult eye diseases, a clinical trial was performed to test the effect of inhibiting the bioactivity of VEGF using the monoclonal antibody, bevacizumab, in severe ROP.[8] Success was reported in a subgroup of preterm infants with zone I, stage 3 ROP with plus disease. However, concerns remain.

No dosing studies were performed to determine an effective and safe dose or optimal agent for ROP. VEGF is an important angiogenic factor in development, a survival factor of newly formed capillaries, and also plays a role in the homeostasis of already developed vasculature.[9,10] In adults, repeated treatment with anti-VEGF agents, the standard of care for AMD, has been associated with geographic atrophy, another cause of vision loss in AMD.[11] VEGF is also a neuroprotective agent for retinal neurons.[12] Therefore, concerns of damaging effects from anti-VEGF were raised, particularly in the developing infant retina. In addition, anti-VEGF agents injected into the vitreous cavity reduced serum VEGF for several weeks,[13,14] raising additional concern of the effects of removing systemic VEGF on the development of organs, particularly kidney, brain, and lung in the preterm infant. Following the publication of the clinical trial, complications were reported after a single intravitreal injection of bevacizumab. These complications included persistent avascular retina, recurrent intravitreal angiogenesis, and stage 5 retinal detachment.[15,16] Therefore, before considering anti-VEGF agents in preterm infants, more studies are needed to determine long-term effects on safety, proper doses, or even the type of anti-VEGF agent or other drug.

In this article, the growing problem of ROP worldwide, the standard of care laser treatment in severe ROP, and the need for new treatments are discussed. Also discussed are the reasons to consider inhibiting the VEGF signaling pathway in ROP and the concerns about broad inhibition. Finally, the potential role of VEGF in ROP based on studies in OIR models, the effects of anti-VEGF based on basic research data, and the clinical relevance of these data are covered.

THE PROBLEM: RETINOPATHY OF PREMATURITY IS INCREASING WORLDWIDE AND HAS DIFFERENT PHENOTYPES

With increases in preterm births, ROP has become one of the leading causes of childhood blindness worldwide.[17] In the United States, ~14% of childhood blindness is attributed to ROP and in some developing nations estimates are greater than 20%.[18] In addition, some countries have developed the ability to save preterm infants but lack resources to regulate oxygen and are experiencing not only cases of ROP from extreme prematurity but also additional cases of ROP in larger and older infants from high oxygen-induced damage to newly formed retinal capillaries similar to what occurred in the 1940s and 1950s in the United States, United Kingdom, and Canada.[15,19,20] Compounding these increases in ROP cases throughout the world, the number of adequately trained ophthalmologists to diagnose and treat ROP is not increasing to meet the need.[19] There also appears to be a heritable component to ROP,[20] and genetic pools differ throughout the world. Thus, ROP phenotypes may vary throughout the world based on environmental factors and, potentially, differences in genetic variants. These considerations are important when comparing outcomes from clinical reports after anti-VEGF therapy.

CURRENT TREATMENT FOR RETINOPATHY OF PREMATURITY AND REASONS FOR BETTER THERAPIES

When ROP was first diagnosed as retrolental fibroplasia in the 1940s in the United States, studies in animal models were performed that revealed that high oxygen at birth was a cause.[21] Oxygen damaged newly formed retinal capillaries and led to broad areas of avascular retina.[21,22] When the infant was moved from high oxygen to a relatively hypoxic environment, cells within the avascular retina were stimulated by hypoxia and thought to increase the expression of angiogenic growth factors.[23] Now several mechanisms are proposed, including the stabilization and nuclear translocation of hypoxia-inducible factors that cause transcription of angiogenic factors, including VEGF.[24] However, rather than vascular growth into the avascular retina to relieve the hypoxic stimulus, vessels grow into the vitreous. Efforts were made to reduce oxygen, which drastically reduced cases of ROP but also increased infant morbidity and mortality. With advances in neonatal care and the ability to regulate oxygen, ROP re-emerged as smaller and younger preterm infants were surviving.

In the 1990s, the Supplemental Therapeutic Oxygen for Prethreshold ROP multicenter trial tested the hypothesis that increased supplemental oxygen treatment would reduce the hypoxic stimulus for vasoproliferation and thereby prevent severe ROP (**Table 1**). However, only in a post-hoc analysis was reduced progression to severe ROP noted in a subgroup with higher oxygen saturation (94%–99% Sao_2) compared with conventional oxygen saturation (89%–94% Sao_2).[25] Other smaller studies reported that supplemental oxygen later in the neonatal course in the nursery reduced severe ROP.[25,26] More recent studies tested the hypotheses that lower than conventional oxygen saturation targets would reduce severe ROP.[27–29] In 2 studies, the Surfactant, Positive Airway Pressure, Pulse Oximetry Randomized Trial[30] and Benefits of Oxygen Saturation Targeting,[30] low oxygen saturation targets were associated with lower incidence of ROP but higher mortality, whereas in the Canadian Oxygen Trial,[29] there was no effect on ROP or mortality.[30] However, the studies had important differences, including potentially regional differences in the phenotype of ROP of enrolled infants (see **Table 1**).[31] The conclusion from these studies is that even when oxygen is regulated, ROP can still occur in the smallest and youngest preterm infants.

Fluctuations in oxygenation have also been associated with severe ROP.[32] There is speculation that strict control of oxygen levels may lead to more fluctuations in oxygenation in preterm infants because of the difficulty in maintaining oxygen saturation levels within a tight range.[33] Repeated fluctuations in oxygen delivery in animal models leads to increased oxidative compounds,[34] overexpression of VEGF and VEGF receptor 2 (VEGFR2), and also overactivation of signaling cascades involving VEGFR2.[3,35] Besides fluctuations in oxygenation, risks for human ROP have included associations with poor infant growth[36] and increased oxidative stress.[37–39]

The current standard of care for ROP of all causes is treatment of the peripheral avascular retina with laser, preferably to cryotherapy, when a level of severity (type 1 ROP) develops (**Tables 2** and **3**).[40] There are several considerations for successful treatment. First, timing of treatment is critical. Early treatment of type 1 ROP before threshold ROP[40] occurs led to the prevention of blindness in more than 90% of enrolled infants whereas about a 75% success rate was reported in the multicenter study, Cryotherapy for ROP (see **Table 2**; **Table 4**).[41] Eyes that advance in severity of ROP beyond threshold do not respond well to laser, cryotherapy, or surgery.[42] Diagnosis and treatment with laser or cryotherapy require skill using an indirect ophthalmoscope and a scleral depressor.[43] Although wide-angle retinal imaging is being used as an aid in diagnosis,[44] treatment with laser or cryotherapy still requires ability with an indirect ophthalmoscope to target the appropriate areas in the retina. Subsequently, it is essential to have adequately trained ophthalmologists and staff who can diagnose[45] and treat severe ROP. Unfortunately, there is a shortage of suitably trained ophthalmologists who are willing to diagnose and treat preterm infants for ROP.[17,44] Adequate treatment and ability to determine when re-treatment is needed

Table 1
List of major oxygen trials

Trial	Dates	Enrolled	Exclusion	% Not Meeting Inclusion Criteria	Geography	Birth Weight (Mean or Range)	Intervention	Outcome	Mortality
STOP-ROP	1994–1999	30–48 wk GA with prethreshold ROP in one eye and median Sao_2 <94%	Median Sao_2>94% or congenital abnormality	34%	US	726 g	Infants randomized to Sao_2 ranges of 89%–94% or 96%–99%	No significant difference in threshold ROP. In subgroup, threshold ROP < infants without Plus disease in 96%–99% Sao_2 group	Not assessed formally, 7 infants in lower oxygen tension group vs 9 infants in the higher tension group died
SUPPORT	2005–2009	24–27 wk GA 6 d at birth who underwent full resuscitation	Infants with major congenital abnormalities	6.6%	US	825–836 g	1. Randomized to early CPAP or early surfactant 2. Randomized to Sao_2 of 85%–89% or 91%–95%	Decreased ROP in 85%–89% Sao_2 group	Increased mortality in 85%–89% Sao_2 group

Trial	Years	GA	Exclusion criteria	%	Countries	Weight	Randomization	ROP outcome	Mortality/disability outcome
BOOST II	2006–2011	<28 wk GA	1. Unlikely to survive 2. Major congenital abnormality 3. Unavailable for follow-up	9%	Australia, UK, New Zealand	826-837 g	Randomized to SaO_2 of 85%–89% or 91%–95%	Decreased ROP in 85%–89% SaO_2 group	Increased mortality when targeting SaO_2 <90%
COT	2006–2012	>23 wk–27 wk and 6 d GA	1. Not viable 2. Persistent pulmonary hypertension 3. Dysmorphic features or congenital malformations 4. Cyanotic heart disease 5. Unavailable for follow-up	16%	Canada, US, Argentina, Finland, Germany, Israel	827-845 g	Randomized to SaO_2 of 85%–89% or 91%–95%	No significant difference between SaO_2 targets on ROP at 18 mo	No significant difference between SaO_2 targets on death or disability at 18 mo

Abbreviations: BOOST, Benefits of Oxygen Saturation Targeting; COT, Canadian Oxygen Trial; GA, gestational age; SaO_2, oxygen saturation; STOP-ROP, Supplemental Therapeutic Oxygen for Prethreshold Retinopathy of Prematurity; SUPPORT, Surfactant, Positive Airway Pressure, Pulse Oximetry Randomized Trial.

Table 2 Prethreshold and threshold ROP	
Type 1 ROP, (high-risk) prethreshold ROP	
Zone I	Any stage with plus disease
Zone I, stage 3	Without plus disease
Zone II, stage 2 or 3	With plus disease
Type 2 ROP, (low risk) prethreshold ROP	
Zone I, stage 1 or 2	Without plus disease
Zone II, stage 3	Without plus disease

are important, and only a few studies have addressed the factors associated with progression of retinal detachment following laser treatment and the window of surgical opportunity.[46,47] Finally, laser treatment for severe ROP may take 2 or more hours to perform, whereas the time to perform an intravitreal injection is often less than 30 minutes. This shorter length of treatment time adds an incentive to find methods of treatment besides laser for ROP. However, adequate research and testing for safety and efficacy are needed.

TOWARD A TREATMENT SOLUTION

It is important to review new evidence regarding the pathophysiology of ROP that has been realized since early studies by Ashton and colleagues,[48] Patz,[21] and preclinical studies before the FDA approval of anti-VEGF agents in adult diseases. Because it is not possible to safely obtain tissue or vitreous samples from the preterm infant eye to study ROP without risks of bleeding, cataract, or inoperable retinal detachment,[42] animal models of OIR have been used. It is important to know strengths and limitations of different models when reviewing the evidence. First, all models use newborn, and not premature, animals, unlike the human infant with ROP. Second, most studies have used the mouse OIR model,[49] which exposes newborn mice to high oxygen levels. This model may reflect ROP in places that lack resources to regulate oxygen[50] or ROP that occurred in the United States and United Kingdom in the 1950s[51,52] but is not as representative of ROP in places where oxygen is regulated (**Table 5**). A benefit of the mouse OIR model is the ability to use transgenic mice to study mechanisms of angiogenesis, high oxygen, and relative hypoxia. In contrast, the rat 50/10 OIR model ("rat ROP model")[53,54] reflects the conditions associated with the pathogenesis of human ROP because it reproduces arterial oxygen levels of preterm infants with severe ROP.[32,55] It also causes extrauterine growth restriction.[56] It is the most representative model of ROP today.[52] Previously, mechanistic studies relied mainly on pharmacologic manipulations, but recently, methods have been developed using a gene therapy approach that permits knockdown of VEGF in specific cells in the retina that overexpress VEGF.[57,58] These new approaches have been valuable in understanding the mechanisms whereby overexpressed VEGF causes aberrant intravitreal angiogenesis as well as the effect of various methods to inhibit VEGF bioactivity on developing retinal vasculature and developing systemic organs.

THE BEVACIZUMAB ELIMINATES THE ANGIOGENIC THREAT OF RETINOPATHY OF PREMATURITY STUDY

Although several clinical series had been reported previously, the Bevacizumab Eliminates the Angiogenic Threat of Retinopathy of Prematurity (BEAT-ROP) was the first

Table 3 Current management of ROP	
Screening guidelines	
US	≤30 wk GA or ≤1500 g BW (and preterm infants with an unstable clinical course)[45]
UK	≤31 wk GA or ≤1500 g BW
Canada	≤30 6/7 wk GA or ≤1250 g
Timing of screening and examinations	
First examination at 4–6 wk chronologic age or 31 wk postgestational age	
Repeated examinations recommended by examining ophthalmologist based on retinal findings and suggested schedule	
Type of examination	
Dilated binocular indirect ophthalmoscopy	
Ongoing studies of validation and reliability of retinal imaging as a potential telemedicine alternative for screening	
Parameters of ROP determined in examinations	
Zone: Area of retinal vascularization	I: Retinal vasculature extends within a circle centered on the optic nerve, the radius of which is twice the optic nerve-to-macula distance II: Retinal vasculature extends beyond zone I within the limits of a circular area, the radius of which is the distance from the optic nerve to the nasal ora serrata III: The remaining area outside zones I or II
Stage: Disease severity **(Fig. 1)**	1: Line 2: Ridge (with volume) 3: IVNV 4: Partial retinal detachment 5: Total retinal detachment Plus disease, dilation and tortuosity of retinal vessels
Treatment	
Application of laser to peripheral avascular retina for type 1 ROP (high-risk prethreshold)	Zone I: stage 3 Zone I: any stage with plus disease Zone II: stage 2 or 3 with plus disease
In some cases, anti-VEGF for stage 3 and plus disease in zone I	Additional study needed to determine dose, safety, and type of anti-VEGF
Visual rehabilitation	Refractive correction very often needed for associated refractive errors (ametropia and anisometropia); protective eyewear and low vision aids

Abbreviations: BW, birth weight; GA, gestational age.

published clinical trial that tested intravitreal anti-VEGF antibody, bevacizumab (0.625 mg in 0.025 mL), compared with laser treatment in 150 infants.[59] Infants rather than eyes were enrolled to reduce confounding from crossover effects of the antibody. A benefit for infants with zone I/posterior zone II, stage 3+ ROP was reported in patients ($P = .003$). In many of these eyes, physiologic vascularization progressed to

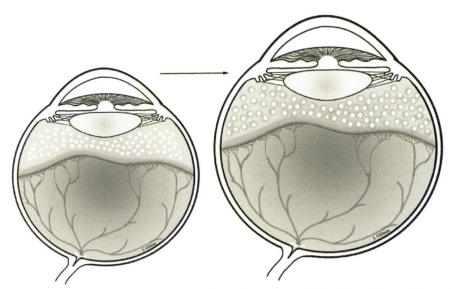

Fig. 1. As the eye grows, there is increased avascular retina peripherally and thus an increase in area between laser spots. Avascular retina leads to hypoxia, which can stimulate angiogenic signaling through hypoxia-inducible factors that translocate to the nucleus and bind to DNA promoter to cause transcription of multiple angiogenic factors, like VEGF, erythropoietin, angiopoietins, as examples.

zone II after intravitreal angiogenesis was inhibited. The study was too small to assess safety and effects on future development of brain and other tissues. The study also did not address dose or anti-VEGF agent. The study follow-up was continued through 54 weeks' postgestational age. However, later studies of infants treated with intravitreal bevacizumab and followed through 60 weeks' postgestational age reported associated complications, including persistent peripheral avascular retina, new intravitreal neovascularization (IVNV), retinal detachment, and macular dragging.[16,60] Other studies reported reduced serum VEGF in infants who received bevacizumab or ranibizumab even 2 weeks following the intravitreal injection.[13,14] Although there is some promise with anti-VEGF treatment, there is clinical risk of poor outcome and safety concerns potentially from systemic reduction of VEGF. Better treatments are needed.

CONSIDERATION OF ANTI-VASCULAR ENDOTHELIAL GROWTH FACTOR AGENTS IN SEVERE RETINOPATHY OF PREMATURITY: KNOWLEDGE FROM ANIMAL MODELS
Pro: Evidence That Inhibiting Vascular Endothelial Growth Factor Inhibits Intravitreal Angiogenesis in Severe Retinopathy of Prematurity

ROP has been characterized by 2 phases based on clinical observations and animal models.[48,61,62] Human ROP also has a third, fibrovascular phase, in which retinal detachment occurs. Few animal models reflect this. The first "epidemic" of ROP occurred in the United States and the United Kingdom in the 1950s. Using a model in kittens, Ashton described phase 1 as high oxygen-induced vaso-obliteration and phase 2 as later hypoxia-induced vasoproliferation.[48] Since then, with changes in neonatal practices and technologic improvements in oxygen regulation and monitoring, the 2-phase description has been refined.[52] In phase I ROP, mainly peripheral avascular retina occurs from a delay in physiologic retinal vascular development

Table 4
Major clinical trials in ROP

Trial (Enrollment)	Criteria	Number Enrolled	Endpoint (Follow-up)	Outcome Measures	Results
CRYO-ROP (1/1/86–1/22/88)	<1251 g BW; survived 28 d of life; no major systemic or ocular anomalies	4099 (291 with threshold ROP randomized to cryotherapy or observation, 254 analyzed at 15 y)	Reports at 3 mo, 1 through 15 y	Visual function; structural findings	At 15 y: 44.7% cryotherapy vs 64.3% observation had <20/200 and 30.0% vs 51.9% had unfavorable structural outcomes; P<.001
ETROP (10/9–10/02)	<1251 g BW; prethreshold ROP	828 infants (730 studied); 401 high-risk prethreshold (≥15% risk of unfavorable outcome = type 1 ROP), 329 low risk (<15% risk = type 2 ROP)	9 mo, 6 y early treatment (prethreshold) vs conventional (threshold) ROP	Vision at 9 mo (Teller Acuity Cards) and 6 y follow-up; secondary outcomes retinal structure, myopia, amblyopia, strabismus	Early treatment, reduced unfavorable visual outcome (19.8%–14.3%, P = .01) at 9 mo and for type 1 ROP at 6 y (16.4% early vs 25.2% conventional); significantly reduced unfavorable outcome (15.6% vs 9.0%; P<.001 at 9 mo and 15.2%–8.9% at 6 y)
BEAT-ROP (3/13/08–8/4/10)	≤ 1500 g BW, ≤30 wk, stage 3+ ROP in zone I or zone II	150 infants (67 with zone I, 83 with posterior zone II) enrolled, 143 survived; 75 randomized to conventional laser, 75 to intravitreal bevacizumab	54 wk PMA	Recurrence of ROP (primary outcome), interval from treatment to recurrence, need for surgery	Reduced recurrence of stage 3 ROP in zone I ROP after intravitreal bevacizumab (4%) compared with laser (22%); no effect for zone II disease

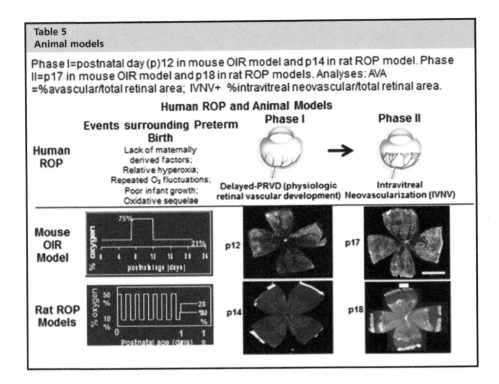

Table 5
Animal models

Phase I=postnatal day (p)12 in mouse OIR model and p14 in rat ROP model. Phase II=p17 in mouse OIR model and p18 in rat ROP models. Analyses: AVA =%avascular/total retinal area; IVNV+ %intravitreal neovascular/total retinal area.

Human ROP and Animal Models

(PRVD)[52] and, in places with insufficient resources to regulate oxygen, hyperoxia-induced vaso-attenuation.[50] With delayed PRVD but continued eye growth, the peripheral avascular retina can increase in area (eye growth can also expand avascular retina between laser spots and is hypothesized to create an additional hypoxic stimulus for the development of recurrent intravitreal angiogenesis after laser treatment in very small immature preterm infants; see **Fig. 1**).[63]

In phase II ROP, IVNV occurs from hypoxia or potentially oxidative stress or metabolic demands.[49,52,64,65] VEGF is an important angiogenic factor in both PRVD and in IVNV, and inhibition of its bioactivity would be predicted to inhibit both normal (PRVD) and pathologic (IVNV) angiogenesis. However, evidence from OIR models suggests that inhibition of VEGF signaling to a certain degree may not adversely inhibit PRVD and still reduce IVNV (**Table 6**). From the mouse OIR model, initial

Table 6
Pros and cons for inhibiting VEGF signaling in ROP

Pros	Cons
Orders developing retinal angiogenesis	Reduces serum VEGF in infants
Preclinical studies showing effects in models of OIR	Recurrent intravitreal NV in preterm infants occurs often much later than after laser
	Survival factor in adult homeostasis and in developing vascular and neural beds
	Animal models show reduced body weight gain, loss of retinal capillary support, cell death in photoreceptors, reduced serum VEGF, recurrent IVNV

observations suggested that the central vaso-obliterated retina induced by high oxygen was not increased after an anti-VEGF neutralizing antibody was delivered into the vitreous at a dose that was found to effectively inhibit IVNV.[66] Later, studies by Geisen and colleagues[67] and Budd and colleagues[68] used quantitative methods in the rat 50/10 OIR model and found that neither a neutralizing antibody to VEGF nor a VEGFR2 tyrosine kinase inhibitor increased the avascular retinal area at doses that significantly inhibited IVNV. Because a single allele knockout of VEGF or one of its splice variants or receptors is lethal in mice, studies done in an embryonic stem cell model were performed to understand the mechanisms whereby inhibition of an angiogenic factor would reduce intravitreal, but not systemic, intraretinal angiogenesis. Using a knockout of VEGFR1 (*flt1*) in the embryonic stem cell model permitted VEGF to trigger signaling mainly through VEGFR2 by overactivating the receptor. This model demonstrated that overactivation of VEGFR2 disordered angiogenesis and caused a pattern of growth similar in appearance to IVNV. The pattern of growth could be rescued and physiologic vascularization restored with the addition of a transgene of VEGFR1 containing a CD31 promoter to target endothelial cells.[69] This work demonstrated that not only overactivated VEGFR2 but also VEGFR2 specifically in endothelial cells was responsible for aberrant angiogenesis. Then, in the rat 50/10 OIR model, the relationship between the long axis of lectin-labeled retinal vessels and the anti-phospho-histone H3-labeled cleavage planes of dividing endothelial cells to a tortuosity index in lectin stained arteries and veins was determined following treatment with a neutralizing antibody to rat VEGF compared with a nonimmune immunoglobulin G (IgG) control. The neutralizing antibody was found to reduce dilation and tortuosity in the OIR model.[70] This study supported the development of the hypothesis that overactivation of VEGFR2 disordered dividing endothelial cells, allowing them to grow in a pattern similar to IVNV and that by down-regulating VEGFR2 signaling, intraretinal vascularization occurred. More recently, a lentivector gene therapy approach was developed in the rat 50/10 OIR model to reduce overexpressed VEGF in Müller cells, where the VEGF signal was found.[57] A short hairpin RNA to knockdown vascular endothelial growth factor A (VEGFA) in Müller cells only was introduced into the model and found to reduce VEGFR2 signaling in endothelial cells[57] and significantly inhibit IVNV, but not PRVD. Also, down-regulating overactivated VEGFR2 in endothelial cells ordered the cleavage planes of dividing endothelial cells into a physiologic pattern, promoting vessel elongation.[71] Thus, experimental evidence supports the premise that inhibiting the VEGF/VEGFR2 signaling cascade not only inhibits IVNV but also permits PRVD by restoring the normal orientation to dividing endothelial cells; this suggests that regulating VEGFR2 to physiologic signaling may be a promising approach to reduce IVNV without interfering with PRVD. However, VEGF is also important in physiologic development and homeostasis of retinal neurons and glial cells,[10,58] so efforts to target signaling effectors downstream of VEGF/VEGFR2 activation appear important.

Con: Evidence That Vascular Endothelial Growth Factor Inhibition Can Lead to Harm

Most studies regarding retinal vascular development have been done in animals. Evidence concerning vascular development exists up through 22 weeks' gestation in human preterm infant eyes. Based on careful immunohistochemical studies, retinal vascularization occurred through a process of vasculogenesis at about 12 weeks' gestation in the human embryonic retina and continued through at least 22 weeks' gestation, allowing for inner retinal plexus vascularization through zone I.[72] Vasculogenesis is the formation of blood vessels de novo from endothelial precursor cells or angioblasts.

After 22 weeks, it is less clear how the retinal vasculature extends to the ora serrata because of the difficulty in obtaining human eyes in adequate condition for study, but based on mice and other animals that vascularize their retinas after birth, vascularization is thought to occur through angiogenesis (ie, the budding of new vessels from existing blood vessels). Both processes appear to involve VEGF.[73] Besides its role in angiogenesis, VEGF is also a survival factor for other cells of the retina, including neurons, and is important in other organ development.[12] These issues are important when considering anti-VEGF agents in the developing preterm infant. However, many infants at risk of severe ROP also have delayed central nervous system development. Therefore, sorting out the effects of anti-VEGF treatment for ROP from prematurity and periventricular leukomalacia may be difficult.

Since the BEAT-ROP study, reports of reduced serum VEGF levels have been reported for at least 2 weeks following intravitreal anti-VEGF agents.[13,14] There have also been numerous reports on associations of intravitreal anti-VEGF agents[8] with prolonged, persistent avascular retina, recurrent IVNV, and even blindness from retinal detachment.[16,74] Early studies reported that the risk of ROP following laser or cryotherapy generally was removed after about 45 weeks' postgestational age.[75] However, recurrences after anti-VEGF were reported at 60 weeks' postgestational age.[60] The causes of the recurrences remain unclear. In one study using the rat 50/10 OIR model, investigators found recurrence after higher doses of anti-VEGF agents in association with other angiogenic factors, including erythropoietin.[76]

In another study, PRVD in retinal flat mounts was determined in retinal plexi by 2 methods.[71] The first method was the ratio of the areas of vascularized retina, determined by extent of coverage of lectin-stained retinal vessels, to total retina. In the second method, the number of pixels of fluorescence from lectin-stained vessels was determined and a ratio was created between pixels of lectin fluorescence to total retinal area. The latter measurement took into account both extent of retinal vascularization and capillary density. Two treatments were used: a broad intravitreal antibody to VEGF or a lentivector gene therapy approach to reduce overexpressed VEGF with an shRNA to VEGFA in Müller cells. Each treatment was compared with its respective control, either intravitreal IgG for the intravitreal anti-VEGF antibody or a control shRNA to the nonmammalian gene, luciferase, for the lentivector gene therapy strategy. Compared with respective controls, each treatment reduced IVNV 4-fold and did not adversely affect PRVD determined by extent of lectin-stained vascular coverage. However, the broad intravitreal anti-VEGF antibody reduced pixels of lectin fluorescence and, therefore, capillary density in retinal vascular plexi, whereas targeted VEGF knockdown did not.[71] In addition, intravitreal anti-VEGF antibody also reduced body weight gain[76] and serum VEGF levels, whereas targeted VEGF knockdown in Müller cells did not.[57] These results suggest that targeted VEGF knockdown in Müller cells may be safer than broad anti-VEGF inhibition. Also, VEGF appeared to be important for already developed retinal capillaries, and these studies suggested that reduced capillary density may be a possible mechanism for late recurrent IVNV reported after intravitreal anti-VEGF antibody.[76]

In an additional study, the question was posed whether knockdown of a VEGF splice variant might be safer that knockdown of the full VEGFA sequence. In the rat 50/10 OIR model, a gene therapy approach was used to knockdown VEGF or a splice variant in Müller cells using shRNAs to VEGFA, VEGF$_{164}$ splice variant, or luciferase as a control.[58] Initially, shRNAs to either VEGFA or VEGF$_{164}$ significantly reduced IVNV compared with control but only the VEGF$_{164}$ knockdown maintained IVNV inhibition at the later time point studied. Also, targeted Müller cell knockdown of VEGFA caused increased TUNEL+ cell death and retinal thinning of the outer nuclear layer, whereby the photoreceptor nuclei are located. From these studies, targeted knockdown of VEGFA in Müller cells following repeated fluctuations in oxygenation appears safer than broad intravitreal anti-VEGF antibody, but may still cause photoreceptor loss. (Photoreceptors, ie, rods and cones, are essential to visual development and to vision, generally.) Targeting Müller cell VEGF$_{164}$ may therefore be potentially safer. However, more studies are needed to determine the long-term effects of targeted knockdown of VEGF splice variants on visual and retinal function and structure. Also, it appears that measurements of body weight gain, vascular coverage or persistent avascular retina, and recurrence of IVNV are insufficient to determine safety in preterm infant retinas receiving anti-VEGF treatment because none of these was adversely affected by knockdown of either VEGFA or VEGF$_{164}$ in Müller cells.

As infants become older, examination of the peripheral retina without anesthesia becomes more difficult and less accurate. Several clinicians may perform laser treatment of the peripheral avascular retina after anti-VEGF agents with signs of recurrence or when the infant grows large enough that the ability to perform an adequate retinal examination without anesthesia is impaired. However, the question whether persistent avascular retina should be treated is difficult to address, because all OIR models have regression of IVNV and vascularization of the avascular retina. It is possible that some human preterm retinas may be incapable of supporting retinal vasculature, but in other eyes, vascularization might occur or avascular retina might persist without ever causing IVNV (see **Table 6**).

CONSIDERATIONS REGARDING ADULT/PRETERM INFANT SIZE AND DOSE CONSIDERATIONS

No anti-VEGF agent has been FDA-approved for treatment of ROP. Ranibizumab (Genentech) or aflibercept (Regeneron) are the FDA-approved agents for adult eye diseases. The BEAT-ROP clinical trial used bevacizumab, which has not been FDA-approved for any eye disease, but has been tested head-to-head with ranibizumab in a clinical trial for adult AMD and shown to be noninferior.[77] Bevacizumab is a humanized monoclonal antibody to VEGF that was tested as an anticancer agent but was not formally tested or formulated for use in the eye. Ranibizumab was tested for use in the eye and is the Fab fragment of a monoclonal anti-VEGF antibody. Treatment with bevacizumab is approximately 1/20th the cost of ranibizumab. The dose of either ranibizumab (0.5 mg) or bevacizumab (1.25 mg) is injected into the adult eye in a volume of 0.05 mL. Because no pharmacologic formulation is available for preterm infant eyes, the same dosing and volume have often been chosen because of the difficulty in drawing up smaller volumes accurately and the lack of knowledge as to appropriate dose in the preterm infant eye.

It is unknown what a normal VEGF level is in the blood or vitreous in a preterm infant who does not develop ROP. There also is no way to safely measure VEGF in the vitreous of a preterm infant, so the dose to neutralize VEGF cannot currently be determined for individual infants or eyes. Both ranibizumab and bevacizumab can reduce serum VEGF levels in preterm infants,[13,14] even though in adults, a study comparing bevacizumab, ranibizumab, and pegaptanib (an aptamer to VEGF splice variant, VEGF$_{165}$) found that only bevacizumab reduced serum VEGF.[78] The different concentrations of serum VEGF between adults and preterm infants may in part reflect the differences in eye/blood volumes. A preterm infant's vitreous volume is about 1 mL, whereas an adult's is approximately 4 mL. However, a preterm infant's blood volume is about 120 mL at a postgestational age of 35 to 39 weeks when severe ROP occurs, and an adult's blood volume is usually more than 5000 mLs. Therefore, even though the concentration of active VEGF is not known, there is less effect from dilution of the drug in the preterm infant's blood volume compared with the adult's blood volume. In addition, ROP develops often 2 or 3 months after birth. In the United States, an infant that develops severe ROP is often much smaller (and blood volume less) than an infant with severe ROP in other countries where ROP occurs in larger and older infants. Therefore, the safety profile from studies that test anti-VEGF in severe ROP from these countries may not be comparable to that of the United States. Anti-angiogenic treatment may need to be individualized based on the eye and infant. These potential considerations are rarely discussed when comparing anti-VEGF treatment outcomes or side effects in infants from developing nations or the United States.

GUIDELINES IF CONSIDERING ANTI-VASCULAR ENDOTHELIAL GROWTH FACTOR TREATMENT

Bevacizumab is not FDA-approved. However, there are more studies reported on bevacizumab than on ranibizumab, for which there is no clinical trial for ROP reported to date (**Table 7**). However, there have been opinions as to which anti-VEGF agent is optimal. Bevacizumab causes longer-term reduction in systemic VEGF levels in adults compared with ranibizumab and, therefore, may be more damaging to the preterm infant. However, in preterm infants, ranibizumab also reduced serum VEGF. Ranibizumab penetrates more deeply into the eye, and there is concern this might affect the choroidal circulation, which provides oxygen to the developing retina and is thought important in the pathophysiology of ROP.[79] The American Academy of Pediatrics

Table 7
Guidelines for use of anti-VEGF in ROP

Indications for Use	Informed Consent	Log	Follow-up
Clinical trial BEAT-ROP found effect in zone I, Stage 3+ disease	Agents not FDA approved	Age, date, eye treated, dose and agent used, volume	Monitor weekly after treatment until vascularization is complete to ora serrata
No clinical trial evidence of effect with less severe ROP	Questions remain regarding long-term safety, dose, timing, visual outcomes and long-term effects, including systemically	Communicate with neonatologist and ophthalmologist during transfer or discharge	Longer follow-up is needed because recurrences following bevacizumab occurred later than laser treatment
		Communication with parents is essential, including the need for follow-up examinations and risks, and documentation must be performed	Unknown what to do if avascular retina persists after 60 wk chronologic age when awake examinations are difficult; consider ablative treatment

Data from Fierson WM, American Academy of Pediatrics Section on Ophthalmology, American Academy of Ophthalmology, et al. Screening examination of premature infants for retinopathy of prematurity. Pediatrics 2013;131:189–95.

and the American Academy of Ophthalmology have developed guidelines for ROP and the consideration of anti-VEGF treatment.[45] Because no clinical trial has been performed for ranibizumab at the time of this writing, the recommendations are based on bevacizumab. If bevacizumab is contemplated in cases in which corneal, lenticular, or vitreous opacities preclude treatment with laser, it should only be used for stage 3+ ROP in zone I and not for zone II ROP. Also, a detailed informed consent outlining the potential risks is required. If bevacizumab is used, infants must be examined weekly until full vascularization of the retina occurs. Follow-up must be performed for a longer period of time than after conventional laser treatment, because recurrent stage 3 ROP has been reported at later time points than after conventional laser (16 ± 4.6 weeks vs 6.2 ± 5.7 weeks). Also, a log of infants treated and dates of treatment is recommended. Good and clear communication between the treating ophthalmologist and neonatologist is essential on transfer or discharge.

FUTURE

Studies are ongoing to determine pharmacologic approaches that target signaling downstream of VEGF receptors to safely and effectively inhibit pathologic angiogenesis without interfering with ongoing retinal vascular development. More clinical studies are needed to determine potential safe doses of anti-VEGF agents, and dose escalation studies are being considered. In addition, studies to promote normal retinal vascular development may be considered through the use of nutrients, such as peptides,[80] omega-3 fatty acids,[81] and growth factors, including insulin-like growth factor 1.[82] Clinical studies are also being performed testing early use of erythropoietin on later cognitive function. There is some evidence that erythropoietin can be angiogenic in preterm infants.[83] A recent clinical study in preterm infants testing darbepoietin, a form of erythropoietin, reported no increased, but also no reduced risk of severe ROP; however, numbers were small.[84] Further studies are warranted. Because heritability may be associated with ROP,[20] studies on the association of severe ROP and genetic variants are needed. Potentially, phenotype/genotype studies may identify infants at great risk of severe ROP and also help in understanding the pathophysiology of disease so as to develop new treatments.

REFERENCES

1. Churchill AJ, Carter JG, Lovell HC, et al. VEGF polymorphisms are associated with neovascular age-related macular degeneration. Hum Mol Genet 2006;15:2955–61.
2. Bird AC. Therapeutic targets in age-related macular disease. J Clin Invest 2010;120:3033–41.
3. Yang Z, Wang H, Jiang Y, et al. VEGFA activates erythropoietin receptor and enhances VEGFR2-mediated pathological angiogenesis. Am J Pathol 2014;184:1230–9.
4. Aiello LP, Avery RL, Arrigg PG, et al. Vascular endothelial growth factor in ocular fluid of patients with diabetic retinopathy and other retinal disorders. N Engl J Med 1994;331:1480–7.
5. Nicholson B, Schachat A. A review of clinical trials of anti-VEGF agents for diabetic retinopathy. Graefes Arch Clin Exp Ophthalmol 2010;248:915–30.
6. Cooke RW, Drury JA, Mountford R, et al. Genetic polymorphisms and retinopathy of prematurity. Invest Ophthalmol Vis Sci 2004;45:1712–5.
7. Mititelu M, Chaudhary KM, Lieberman RM. An evidence-based meta-analysis of vascular endothelial growth factor inhibition in pediatric retinal diseases: part 1. Retinopathy of prematurity. J Pediatr Ophthalmol Strabismus 2012;49:332–40.

8. Mintz-Hittner HA, Kennedy KA, Chuang AZ. Efficacy of intravitreal bevacizumab for stage 3+ retinopathy of prematurity. N Engl J Med 2011;364:603–15.

9. Saint-Geniez M, Kurihara T, Sekiyama E, et al. An essential role for RPE-derived soluble VEGF in the maintenance of the choriocapillaris. Proc Natl Acad Sci U S A 2009;106:18751–6.

10. Saint-Geniez M, Maharaj AS, Walshe TE, et al. Endogenous VEGF is required for visual function: evidence for a survival role on muller cells and photoreceptors. PLoS One 2008;3:e3554.

11. Rofagha S, Bhisitkul RB, Boyer DS, et al. Seven-year outcomes in ranibizumab-treated patients in ANCHOR, MARINA, and HORIZON: a Multicenter Cohort Study (SEVEN-UP). Ophthalmology 2013;120:2292–9.

12. Nishijima K, Ng YS, Zhong L, et al. Vascular endothelial growth factor-A is a survival factor for retinal neurons and a critical neuroprotectant during the adaptive response to ischemic injury. Am J Pathol 2007;171:53–67.

13. Sato T, Wada K, Arahori H, et al. Serum concentrations of bevacizumab (Avastin) and vascular endothelial growth factor in infants with retinopathy of prematurity. Am J Ophthalmol 2012;153:327–33.

14. Hoerster R, Muether P, Dahlke C, et al. Serum concentrations of vascular endothelial growth factor in an infant treated with ranibizumab for retinopathy of prematurity. Acta Ophthalmol 2013;91:e74–5.

15. Hu J. Reactivation of retinopathy of prematurity after bevacizumab injection. Arch Ophthalmol 2012;130:1000–6.

16. Patel RD, Blair MP, Shapiro MJ, et al. Significant treatment failure with intravitreous bevacizumab for retinopathy of prematurity. Arch Ophthalmol 2012;130:801–2.

17. Gilbert C. Retinopathy of prematurity: a global perspective of the epidemics, population of babies at risk and implications for control. Early Hum Dev 2008; 84:77–82.

18. Kong L, Fry M, Al-Samarraie M, et al. An update on progress and the changing epidemiology of causes of childhood blindness worldwide. J AAPOS 2012;16:501–7.

19. Kemper AR, Freedman SF, Wallace DK. Retinopathy of prematurity care: patterns of care and workforce analysis. J AAPOS 2008;12:344–8.

20. Bizzarro MJ, Hussain N, Jonsson B, et al. Genetic susceptibility to retinopathy of prematurity. Pediatrics 2006;118:1858–63.

21. Patz A. Studies on retinal neovascularization. Friedenwald Lecture. Invest Ophthalmol Vis Sci 1980;19:1133–8.

22. Ashton N, Cook C. Direct observation of the effect of oxygen on developing vessels: preliminary report. Br J Ophthalmol 1954;38:433–40.

23. Ashton N. Editorial: retrolental fibroplasia now retinopathy of prematurity. Br J Ophthalmol 1984;68:689.

24. Shweiki D, Itin A, Soffer D, et al. Vascular endothelial growth factor induced by hypoxia may mediate hypoxia-initiated angiogenesis. Nature 1992;359:843–5.

25. Group TS-RMS. Supplemental therapeutic oxygen for prethreshold retinopathy of prematurity (STOP-ROP), a randomized, controlled trial. I: primary outcomes. Pediatrics 2000;105:295–310.

26. Gaynon MW. Rethinking stop-ROP: is it worthwhile trying to modulate excessive VEGF levels in prethreshold ROP eyes by systemic intervention? A review of the role of oxygen, light adaptation state, and anemia in prethreshold ROP. Retina 2006;26:S18–23.

27. SUPPORT Study Group of the Eunice Kennedy Shriver NICHD Neonatal Research Network, Finer NN, Carlo WA, et al. Early CPAP versus surfactant in extremely preterm infants. N Engl J Med 2010;362:1970–9.

28. Stenson BJ, Tarnow-Mordi WO, Darlow BA, et al. Oxygen saturation and outcomes in preterm infants. N Engl J Med 2013;368:2094–104.
29. Schmidt B, Whyte RK, Asztalos EV, et al. Effects of targeting higher vs lower arterial oxygen saturations on death or disability in extremely preterm infants: a randomized clinical trial. JAMA 2013;309:2111–20.
30. Hartnett ME, Lane RH. Effects of oxygen on the development and severity of retinopathy of prematurity. J AAPOS 2013;17:229–34.
31. Owen L, Hartnett ME. Current concepts of oxygen management and ROP. J Ophthalmic Vis Res 2014;9:94–100.
32. York JR, Landers S, Kirby RS, et al. Arterial oxygen fluctuation and retinopathy of prematurity in very-low-birth-weight infants. J Perinatol 2004;24:82–7.
33. Hauspurg AK, Allred EN, Vanderveen DK, et al. Blood gases and retinopathy of prematurity: the ELGAN Study. Neonatology 2011;99:104–11.
34. Saito Y, Geisen P, Uppal A, et al. Inhibition of NAD(P)H oxidase reduces apoptosis and avascular retina in an animal model of retinopathy of prematurity. Mol Vis 2007;13:840–53.
35. Budd SJ, Thompson H, Hartnett ME. Association of retinal vascular endothelial growth factor with avascular retina in a rat model of retinopathy of prematurity. Arch Ophthalmol 2010;128:1014–21.
36. Hellstrom A, Hard AL, Engstrom E, et al. Early weight gain predicts retinopathy in preterm infants: new, simple, efficient approach to screening. Pediatrics 2009; 123:e638–45.
37. Penn JS. Oxygen-induced retinopathy in the rat: possible contribution of peroxidation reactions. Doc Ophthalmol 1990;74:179–86.
38. Phelps DL. Vitamin E and retinopathy of prematurity: the clinical investigator's perspective on antioxidant therapy: side effects and balancing risks and benefits. Birth Defects Orig Artic Ser 1988;24:209–18.
39. Raju TN, Langenberg P, Bhutani V, et al. Vitamin E prophylaxis to reduce retinopathy of prematurity: a reappraisal of published trials. J Pediatr 1997;131:844–50.
40. Early Treatment for Retinopathy of Prematurity Cooperative Group. Revised indications for the treatment of retinopathy of prematurity: results of the early treatment for retinopathy of prematurity randomized trial. Arch Ophthalmol 2003;121: 1684–94.
41. Cryotherapy for Retinopathy of Prematurity Cooperative Group. Multicenter trial of cryotherapy for retinopathy of prematurity. Snellen visual acuity and structural outcome at 51/2 years after randomization. Arch Ophthalmol 1996;114: 417–24.
42. Hartnett ME. Features associated with surgical outcome in patients with stages 4 and 5 retinopathy of prematurity. Retina 2003;23:322–9.
43. Wong RK, Ventura CV, Espiritu MJ, et al. Training fellows for retinopathy of prematurity care: a web-based survey. J AAPOS 2012;16:177–81.
44. Ells AL, Holmes JM, Astle WF, et al. Telemedicine approach to screening for severe retinopathy of prematurity: a pilot study. Ophthalmology 2003;110:2113–7.
45. Fierson WM, American Academy of Pediatrics Section on Ophthalmology, American Academy of Ophthalmology, et al. Screening examination of premature infants for retinopathy of prematurity. Pediatrics 2013;131:189–95.
46. Coats DK. Retinopathy of prematurity: involution, factors predisposing to retinal detachment, and expected utility of preemptive surgical reintervention. Trans Am Ophthalmol Soc 2005;103:281–312.
47. Hartnett ME, McColm JR. Retinal features predictive of progressive stage 4 retinopathy of prematurity. Retina 2004;24:237–41.

48. Ashton N, Ward B, Serpell G. Effect of oxygen on developing retinal vessels with particular reference to the problem of retrolental fibroplasia. Br J Ophthalmol 1954;38:397–430.
49. Smith LE, Wesolowski E, McLellan A, et al. Oxygen-induced retinopathy in the mouse. Invest Ophthalmol Vis Sci 1994;35:101–11.
50. Shah PK, Narendran V, Kalpana N. Aggressive posterior retinopathy of prematurity in large preterm babies in South India. Arch Dis Child Fetal Neonatal Ed 2012;97:F371–5.
51. Patz A. Oxygen studies in retrolental fibroplasia. Am J Ophthalmol 1954;38:291–308.
52. Hartnett ME, Penn JS. Mechanisms and management of retinopathy of prematurity. N Engl J Med 2012;367:2515–26.
53. Penn JS, Henry MM, Tolman BL. Exposure to alternating hypoxia and hyperoxia causes severe proliferative retinopathy in the newborn rat. Pediatr Res 1994;36: 724–31.
54. Berkowitz BA, Zhang W. Significant reduction of the panretinal oxygenation response after 28% supplemental oxygen recovery in experimental ROP. Invest Ophthalmol Vis Sci 2000;41:1925–31.
55. Cunningham S, Fleck BW, Elton RA, et al. Transcutaneous oxygen levels in retinopathy of prematurity. Lancet 1995;346:1464–5.
56. Holmes JM, Duffner LA. The effect of postnatal growth retardation on abnormal neovascularization in the oxygen exposed neonatal rat. Curr Eye Res 1996;15:403–9.
57. Wang H, Smith GW, Yang Z, et al. Short hairpin RNA-mediated knockdown of VEGFA in muller cells reduces intravitreal neovascularization in a rat model of retinopathy of prematurity. Am J Pathol 2013;183:964–74.
58. Jiang Y, Wang H, Culp D, et al. Targeting Müller cell-derived VEGF164 to reduce intravitreal neovascularization in the rat model of retinopathy of prematurity. Invest Ophthalmol Vis Sci 2014;55:824–31.
59. Mintz-Hittner HA. Treatment of retinopathy of prematurity with vascular endothelial growth factor inhibitors. Early Hum Dev 2012;88:937–41.
60. Hu J, Blair MP, Shapiro MJ, et al. Reactivation of retinopathy of prematurity after bevacizumab injection. Arch Ophthalmol 2012;130:1000–6.
61. Smith LE. Through the eyes of a child: understanding retinopathy through ROP the Friedenwald lecture. Invest Ophthalmol Vis Sci 2008;49:5177–82.
62. An International Committee for the Classification of Retinopathy of Prematurity. The international classification of retinopathy of prematurity revisited. Arch Ophthalmol 2005;123:991–9.
63. Hartnett ME. Retinopathy of prematurity: a template for studying retinal vascular disease. In: Werner JS, Chalupa LM, editors. The New Visual Neurosciences. Cambridge (MA): MIT Press; 2014. p. 1483–501.
64. Byfield G, Budd S, Hartnett ME. The role of supplemental oxygen and JAK/STAT signaling in intravitreous neovascularization in a ROP rat model. Invest Ophthalmol Vis Sci 2009;50:3360–5.
65. Saito Y, Uppal A, Byfield G, et al. Activated NAD(P)H oxidase from supplemental oxygen induces neovascularization independent of VEGF in retinopathy of prematurity model. Invest Ophthalmol Vis Sci 2008;49:1591–8.
66. Sone H, Kawakami Y, Kumagai AK, et al. Effects of intraocular or systemic administration of neutralizing antibody against vascular endothelial growth factor on the murine experimental model of retinopathy. Life Sci 1999;65:2573–80.
67. Geisen P, Peterson L, Martiniuk D, et al. Neutralizing antibody to VEGF reduces intravitreous neovascularization and does not interfere with vascularization of avascular retina in an ROP model. Mol Vis 2008;14:345–57.

68. Budd S, Byfield G, Martiniuk D, et al. Reduction in endothelial tip cell filopodia corresponds to reduced intravitreous but not intraretinal vascularization in a model of ROP. Exp Eye Res 2009;89:718–27.
69. Zeng G, Taylor SM, McColm JR, et al. Orientation of endothelial cell division is regulated by VEGF signaling during blood vessel formation. Blood 2007;109: 1345–52.
70. Hartnett ME, Martiniuk D, Byfield G, et al. Neutralizing VEGF decreases tortuosity and alters endothelial cell division orientation in arterioles and veins in a rat model of ROP: relevance to plus disease. Invest Ophthalmol Vis Sci 2008;49:3107–14.
71. Wang H, Yang Z, Jiang Y, et al. Quantitative analyses of retinal vascular area and density after different methods to reduce VEGF in a rat model of retinopathy of prematurity. Invest Ophthalmol Vis Sci 2014;55:737–44.
72. Hasegawa T, McLeod DS, Prow T, et al. Vascular precursors in developing human retina. Invest Ophthalmol Vis Sci 2008;49:2178–92.
73. Chan-Ling T, Gock B, Stone J. The effect of oxygen on vasoformative cell division: evidence that 'physiological hypoxia' is the stimulus for normal retinal vasculogenesis. Invest Ophthalmol Vis Sci 1995;36:1201–14.
74. Jalali S, Balakrishnan D, Zeynalova Z, et al. Serious adverse events and visual outcomes of rescue therapy using adjunct bevacizumab to laser and surgery for retinopathy of prematurity. The Indian Twin Cities Retinopathy of Prematurity Screening database Report number 5. Arch Dis Child Fetal Neonatal Ed 2013;98:F327–33.
75. Reynolds JD, Dobson V, Quinn GE, et al. Evidence-based screening criteria for retinopathy of prematurity: natural history data from the CRYO-ROP and LIGHT-ROP studies. Arch Ophthalmol 2002;120:1470–6.
76. McCloskey M, Wang H, Jiang Y, et al. Anti-VEGF antibody leads to later atypical intravitreous neovascularization and activation of angiogenic pathways in a rat model of retinopathy of prematurity. Invest Ophthalmol Vis Sci 2013;54:2020–6.
77. Martin DF, Maguire MG, Ying GS, et al. Ranibizumab and bevacizumab for neovascular age-related macular degeneration. N Engl J Med 2011;364:1897–908.
78. Zehetner C, Kirchmair R, Huber S, et al. Plasma levels of vascular endothelial growth factor before and after intravitreal injection of bevacizumab, ranibizumab and pegaptanib in patients with age-related macular degeneration, and in patients with diabetic macular oedema. Br J Ophthalmol 2013;97:454–9.
79. Chemtob S, Hardy P, Abran D, et al. Peroxide-cyclooxygenase interactions in postasphyxial changes in retinal and choroidal hemodynamics. J Appl Physiol (1985) 1995;78:2039–46.
80. Neu J, Afzal A, Pan H, et al. The Dipeptide Arg-Gln inhibits retinal neovascularization in the mouse model of oxygen-induced retinopathy. Invest Ophthalmol Vis Sci 2006;47:3151–5.
81. Connor KM, SanGiovanni JP, Lofqvist C, et al. Increased dietary intake of omega-3-polyunsaturated fatty acids reduces pathological retinal angiogenesis. Nat Med 2007;13:868–73.
82. Hellström A, Smith LE, Dammann O. Retinopathy of prematurity. Lancet 2013; 382:1445–57.
83. Brown MS, Baron AE, France EK, et al. Association between higher cumulative doses of recombinant erythropoietin and risk for retinopathy of prematurity. J AAPOS 2006;10:143–9.
84. Ohls RK, Christensen RD, Kamath-Rayne BD, et al. A randomized, masked, placebo-controlled study of darbepoetin alfa in preterm infants. Pediatrics 2013;132:e119–27.

Preventing Herpes Simplex Virus in the Newborn

Swetha G. Pinninti, MD[a], David W. Kimberlin, MD[b],*

KEYWORDS

- HSV • Genital herpes • Acyclovir • PCR • Antiviral therapy

KEY POINTS

- Herpes simplex virus (HSV) infection in the newborn is an uncommon disease with devastating consequences.
- Early diagnosis and parenteral antiviral therapy followed by long-term oral suppressive therapy have improved the prognosis of newborns with HSV infection.
- Vaccine development and interventions to decrease neonatal transmission remain a challenge.

VIRAL STRUCTURE

Herpes simplex viruses (HSV-1 and HSV-2) are large, enveloped virions with a double-stranded DNA core. There is considerable cross-reactivity between most HSV-1 and HSV-2 glycoproteins, which mediate attachment to and penetration into cells and evoke host immune responses. However, antibody responses to glycoprotein G allow for serologic distinction between HSV-1 and HSV-2.

MATERNAL GENITAL INFECTIONS DURING PREGNANCY

Terminology pertaining to herpes infections is outlined in **Box 1**. Genital herpes infections are caused by either HSV-1 or HSV-2, and most infections are asymptomatic.

Funding Sources: None (Dr S.G. Pinninti); National Institutes of Health, Cellex, GSK (All monies go directly to the University) (Dr D.W. Kimberlin).
Conflict of Interest: None.
This work was supported under contract with the Division of Microbiology and Infectious Diseases of the National Institute of Allergy and Infectious Diseases (NIAID) (N01-AI-30025, N01-AI-65306, N01-AI-15113, N01-AI-62554).
[a] Division of Pediatric Infectious Diseases, The University of Alabama at Birmingham, 1600 Seventh Avenue South, CHB 308, Birmingham, AL 35233, USA; [b] Division of Pediatric Infectious Diseases, The University of Alabama at Birmingham, 1600 Seventh Avenue South, CHB 303, Birmingham, AL 35233, USA
* Corresponding author.
E-mail address: dkimberlin@peds.uab.edu

Box 1
Terminology pertaining to herpes simplex virus infections

- Acquisition of HSV-1 or HSV-2 without prior exposure to either virus and hence no preformed antibodies is referred to as a *first-episode primary infection*.
- Acquisition of HSV-2 in an individual with prior HSV-1 antibodies and vice versa is referred to as a *first-episode nonprimary infection*.
- *Reactivation* refers to isolation of HSV-1 in a person who already has HSV-1 antibodies, or the isolation of HSV-2 in a person who already has HSV-2 antibodies.
- Presence of lesions characteristic of genital herpes with detectable HSV-1 or HSV-2 from the lesions by culture or PCR is referred to as *symptomatic shedding*.
- Detection of HSV-1 or HSV-2 from genital mucosa by culture or PCR in the absence of genital lesions is referred to as *subclinical shedding*.

HSV-2 seroprevalence among pregnant women is estimated to be 20% to 30%, with approximately 10% of HSV-2 seronegative women living with a seropositive partner and hence at risk for acquisition of genital herpes during pregnancy.[1,2] Among discordant couples, women seronegative for both HSV-1 and HSV-2 have an estimated 3.7% chance for seroconversion, while the risk for women already seropositive for HSV-1 to seroconvert to HSV-2 is estimated to be 1.7%.[3] Similar to nonpregnant women, two-thirds of women who acquire genital HSV infection during pregnancy are either asymptomatic or have nonspecific symptoms. Among women with a history of genital herpes acquired before pregnancy, 75% will have at least one recurrence during pregnancy, and 14% will have prodromal symptoms or lesions at the time of delivery.[4,5] For peripartum neonatal transmission, women must be shedding the virus symptomatically or asymptomatically around the time of delivery. It has been shown that 0.2% to 0.39%[6] of all pregnant women shed HSV in the genital tract around the time of delivery irrespective of prior history of HSV, and this incidence of shedding increases to 0.77% to 1.4% among women with prior history of recurrent genital herpes.[7,8]

The risk of transmission of HSV to the neonate remains significantly higher with primary maternal infections acquired closer to the time of delivery compared with recurrent infections (50%–60% with primary infections vs <3% for recurrent infections), most likely due to lack of transplacentally acquired antibodies in the neonate of women with primary infection as well as exposure in the birth canal of those women to larger quantities of virus for longer durations of time.[9]

HERPES SIMPLEX VIRUS IN THE NEWBORN

HSV infection of the neonate is uncommon, with an estimated rate of 1 in 3200 deliveries.[10] Approximately 1500 cases of neonatal HSV disease occur annually in the United States.[11]

Risk Factors for Transmission of Herpes Simplex Virus to the Newborn

The risk of neonatal acquisition of HSV is significantly higher with first episode primary and first episode nonprimary maternal infections when compared with recurrent genital infections (**Box 2**).[10] The risk of neonatal transmission in a large study was identified as 57% with first-episode primary infection, compared with 25% with first-episode nonprimary infection and 2% with recurrent genital HSV infections.[10] Other

---

Box 2
Risk factors for acquisition of herpes simplex virus in the newborn

- Primary maternal genital herpes during pregnancy > recurrent infection
- Vaginal delivery > cesarean section
- Prolonged rupture of membranes
- Use of fetal scalp electrodes
- Genital herpes with HSV-1 > HSV-2

---

statistically significant risk factors in this large study for transmission of HSV to neonate were isolation of HSV-1 from genital lesions when compared with HSV-2.

Cesarean delivery has been proven to be effective in preventing the transmission of HSV to the neonate,[12] although neonatal HSV cases have occurred despite cesarean delivery before rupture of membranes.[2,13] Evidence also exists for prolonged rupture of membranes[14] and disruption of mucocutaneous barrier by the use of fetal scalp electrodes and other instrumentation to affect the acquisition of neonatal HSV disease.[10,15] Although it has been shown that the chances of acquisition of HSV-1 are decreased in women who are seropositive for HSV-2, transmission of HSV-1 to the neonate has been documented to be high irrespective of primary or recurrent infection when compared with HSV-2 transmission patterns.[10]

Times of Herpes Simplex Virus Acquisition by the Newborn

Neonatal HSV is acquired during 1 of 3 time periods as outlined below:

1. In utero (5%)
2. Peripartum (85%)
3. Postnatal (10%)

Disease Classification and Clinical Presentations

HSV infection acquired in the peripartum or postnatal period is classified by extent of disease, with disease classification being predictive of both mortality and morbidity[16–20]:

1. Disseminated disease
2. Central nervous system (CNS) disease
3. Skin, eye, and/or mouth (SEM) disease

Disseminated Disease

- Accounts for ~25% of all neonatal herpes infections[10]
- Usually presents around day 10 to 12 of life
- Involves multiple organs, including the CNS, lungs, liver, adrenal, skin, eyes, and/or mouth
- Presents with viral sepsis, respiratory failure, hepatic failure, and disseminated intravascular coagulation
- Two-thirds of infants with disseminated disease also have concurrent encephalitis, and 40% never develop a vesicular rash during the entire illness.[2,20,21]

Central Nervous System Disease

- Accounts for one-third of cases of neonatal herpes disease
- Infants present around 16 to 19 days of life[20]

- Clinical manifestations include focal/generalized seizures, lethargy, irritability, poor feeding, temperature instability, and bulging fontanelle
- 60% to 70% of infants with CNS disease have skin lesions at some point during the course of the illness[20]

Skin, Eye, and/or Mouth Disease

- Infection confined to the skin, eye, and/or mouth of newborns; by definition, does not involve visceral organs or the CNS
- Since the introduction of antiviral therapy, ~45% of infants with neonatal HSV disease present with SEM disease[2]
- Infants present around day 10 to 12 of life
- 80% of infants with SEM disease present with a vesicular rash.

Diagnostic Modalities for Identifying Infants with Herpes Simplex Virus

Viral culture

- The definitive method for identifying newborns with HSV
- Swabs from conjunctivae, nasopharynx, mouth, and anus (surface cultures) are inoculated into cell culture systems and monitored for cytopathic effect[21]
- Other sites for HSV isolation include vesicular lesions, cerebrospinal fluid (CSF), and blood

Polymerase chain reaction

- The application of polymerase chain reaction (PCR) to CSF samples has revolutionized the diagnosis of CNS neonatal herpes disease[22–25]
- Sensitivity of CSF PCR in neonatal HSV disease ranges from 75% to 100%, and specificity ranges from 71% to 100%.[23,24] A positive CSF PCR for HSV DNA defines that patient as having CNS involvement (categorized as either CNS disease or disseminated disease with CNS involvement)
- Blood PCR in neonatal HSV has been evaluated to a lesser extent in the diagnosis of neonatal HSV infections.[24–26] A positive blood PCR for HSV DNA confirms infection but does not define disease classification, because all clinical disease categories (SEM, CNS, and disseminated) can have viremia and DNAemia[22,24]
- Blood PCR can be positive for weeks, with the clinical significance of this (if any) unknown. As such, no data exist to support use of serial blood PCR assay to monitor response to therapy.

Specimens to Obtain from Newborn Before Initiating Antiviral Therapy

Before initiation of empiric parenteral antiviral therapy, the following specimens should be collected to aid in the diagnosis of neonatal HSV disease or to determine if antiviral therapy may be discontinued if HSV has been excluded[21]:

1. CSF for indices, bacterial culture, and HSV DNA PCR
2. Swab for viral culture from the base of vesicles, suspicious areas, and mucous membrane lesions for viral culture; PCR may be performed in addition to cultures
3. Swab from mouth, conjunctiva, nasopharynx, and rectum (surface cultures) for viral culture; PCR may be performed in addition to cultures
4. Whole blood for HSV DNA PCR
5. Blood to determine alanine aminotransferase.

Recommendations for Treatment of Herpes Simplex Virus in the Newborn

- Treat with parenteral acyclovir given at 60 mg/kg/d divided every 8 hours[19,21]
- Treat newborns with SEM disease for 14 days, and neonates with CNS and disseminated disease for 21 days[21]
- In newborns with CNS involvement, repeat CSF PCR at the end of therapy to document a negative CSF PCR result
- In neonates with positive CSF PCR near the end of 21 days of parenteral therapy, intravenous acyclovir should be continued until PCR negativity is achieved[20,21,23]
- The significance of blood DNA PCR positivity remains unknown, and therefore, serial measurement of blood DNA PCR for assessing response to therapy is not recommended at this time[21]

Prognosis of Herpes Simplex Virus in the Newborn

With the utilization of the higher dose of acyclovir (60 mg/kg/d divided in 3 doses for 21 days), 1-year mortality has been reduced to 29% for disseminated disease and 4% for CNS disease.[19] With high-dose acyclovir, 83% of neonates with disseminated disease and 31% with CNS disease develop normally at 12 months of age.[16,19] Morbidity following SEM disease has dramatically improved after initiation of antiviral therapy, likely due to preemption of SEM disease progressing to disseminated disease and improved diagnostic classification of CNS disease with the availability of CSF PCR testing. None of the infants with SEM disease in the high-dose acyclovir study developed developmental disabilities at 12 months of age.[19]

Long-Term Antiviral Suppressive Therapy

A phase III, placebo-controlled trial performed by The National Institute of Allergy and Infectious Diseases Collaborative Antiviral Study Group supports the use of acyclovir suppressive therapy for 6 months after completion of intravenous therapy for neonatal HSV disease. Infants with CNS disease randomized to receive oral acyclovir had better neurodevelopmental outcomes compared with placebo group, with 69% and 30% developing normally, respectively. Infants with SEM disease had less frequent recurrence of skin lesions while receiving suppressive therapy.[27] Although almost half of the infants enrolled in an earlier small phase I/II trial had significant neutropenia,[28] the phase III trial of acyclovir suppressive therapy found similar rates of neutropenia in the treatment and placebo arms of the study[27] (although the P value approached statistical significance). Babies with neonatal HSV infection of any disease classification should receive oral acyclovir at 300 mg/m^2 per dose, 3 times a day for 6 months. Absolute neutrophil counts should be monitored at 2 and 4 weeks and monthly thereafter after initiation of suppressive therapy.[21]

Approach to an Infant Exposed to Active Maternal Primary or Recurrent Genital Herpes Simplex Virus

Recommendations for the management of infants exposed to HSV in the intrapartum period, until recently, were based on expert opinion and did not take into consideration the change in epidemiology of genital HSV (primary vs recurrent infections and HSV-1 vs HSV-2 infections in women). The most recent Clinical Report endorsed by the American Academy of Pediatrics provides evidence-based guidance on the management of neonates born to women with active genital herpetic lesions.[29]

The recommendations are applicable to institutions that have access to PCR and serologic test results in a rapid fashion. They require clinicians to work very closely across pediatric and obstetric lines. Moreover, the guidelines are only applicable to the care of infants exposed to HSV from maternal genital lesions present at the time of delivery and not to situations of asymptomatic shedding.

Testing of women in labor

- Viral culture and PCR from genital lesions suggestive of HSV
- Characterize virus type as HSV-1 or HSV-2
- Obtain maternal serologic status for HSV-1 and HSV-2
- Use these data to determine status of maternal infection (primary vs recurrent)

The information obtained from viral culture/PCR of genital lesions and maternal serologic status obtained at delivery allow the clinician to determine the type of maternal infection and the risk of transmission to the neonate and guide the approach to management of the neonate. Management of newborns born to women with genital lesions suggestive of HSV at delivery is outlined in **Figs. 1** and **2**.

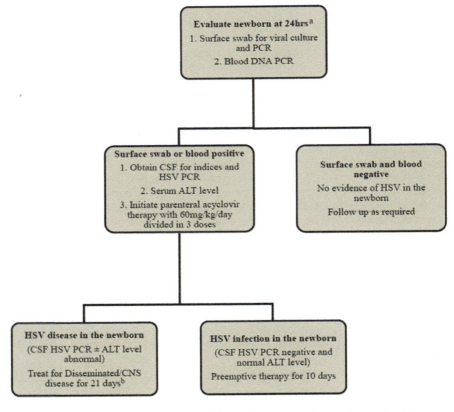

a Waiting for 24hrs after delivery is recommended to differentiate contamination of neonatal skin by maternal secretions versus true HSV infection of the baby.

b After completion of parenteral therapy, treat with oral acyclovir suppressive therapy for 6 months (300mg/m^2/dose three times per day)

Fig. 1. Algorithm for management of newborns born to women with HSV genital lesions at delivery and a prior history of genital herpes.

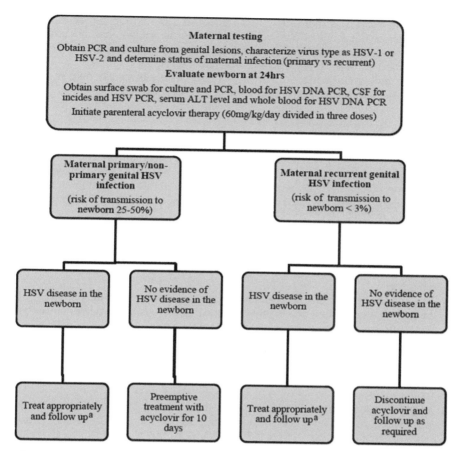

Fig. 2. Management of newborns born to women with lesions at delivery and no history of genital herpes before pregnancy.

Strategies for Prevention of Herpes Simplex Virus in the Newborn

Cesarean delivery

- Delivery by cesarean section decreases but does not entirely prevent transmission of HSV to the neonate. Transmission of HSV has been documented in circumstances where cesarean section was performed before rupture of membranes[2,13]
- This mode of delivery of the infant in women with active genital lesions can reduce the infant's risk of acquiring HSV[10,14] and is recommended when genital lesions or prodromal symptoms are present at the time of delivery[12]

- Cesarean delivery is more likely to be effective if performed before rupture of membranes, but in situations where rupture of membranes has occurred and genital lesions are observed on physical examination, cesarean delivery is recommended to minimize exposure of the neonate to HSV[12]
- It is not recommended for women with a prior history of genital herpes and no active lesions/prodromal symptoms at the time of delivery[12,30]

Antiviral suppressive therapy

- In women with active recurrent genital herpes, antiviral suppressive therapy with acyclovir/valacyclovir initiated at 36 weeks of gestation is associated with decreased likelihood of genital lesions at the time of delivery and decreased viral detection by culture/PCR, with associated reduced need for cesarean section, and currently is recommended by American College of Obstetricians and Gynecologists (ACOG).[12]
- Subclinical viral shedding is not entirely suppressed and the utility of such a practice in preventing neonatal HSV disease is not defined. A recent multicenter case series reported 8 cases of infants with neonatal HSV disease acquired from mothers despite receiving antiviral suppressive therapies beyond 36 weeks of gestation.[31]
- Although maternal antiviral suppressive therapy decreases the incidence of genital recurrences at labor, the extent to which these drugs prevent neonatal acquisition remains unknown and requires further research.

Herpes simplex virus vaccine

- Currently, no vaccine has proven to be effective for preventing acquisition of HSV-1 or HSV-2
- An HSV-2 glycoprotein D (gD) subunit vaccine, adjuvanted with alum, initially was found to be effective in preventing HSV-1 or HSV-2 genital herpes (~75% vaccine efficacy) and HSV-2 infection, but the efficacy was limited only to women who were HSV-1 and HSV-2 seronegative before vaccination with no reported efficacy in men or women who were HSV-1 seropositive before vaccination[32]
- In a subsequent randomized, double-blind trial evaluating the efficacy of the same HSV-2 gD subunit vaccine in women seronegative for HVS-1 and HSV-2, the vaccine was found to have an efficacy of 58% for preventing HSV-1 genital herpes but lacked efficacy for preventing HSV-2 genital herpes.[33]

Prevention of maternal herpes simplex virus acquisition during pregnancy

Various strategies have been recommended to prevent maternal acquisition during pregnancy but none have been tested in large scale trials.[34,35]

- The first approach is to screen all women with an immunoglobulin G-based assay at 24 to 28 weeks of gestation. Women identified to be seropositive but unaware of a prior infection would benefit from education regarding the significance of this finding and identification of recurrent lesions and prodromal symptoms, particularly at the time of labor. Women should be counseled regarding avoiding oro-genital contact. This strategy does not take into account the serostatus or exposure risk to the sexual partner.
- The second approach recommends screening all couples for HSV serology at 14 to 18 weeks, with appropriate counseling based on serology results for both

partners. This approach might not be applicable in situations where there are multiple partners or the partner changes during the course of pregnancy.
- The third approach is to advise all pregnant women to abstain from all forms of sexual contact during the third trimester of pregnancy. The final approach might particularly be applicable in situations where serologic testing is either unavailable or economically not feasible.

ACOG currently does not recommend routine screening of asymptomatic women for HSV during pregnancy.[12]

Prevention of postnatal acquisition

- Approximately 10% of cases are acquired in the postpartum period by exposure to the virus from open lesions of caretakers, or following Jewish ritual circumcision involving oro-genital contact[36]
- Infected household contacts and family members are recommended to avoid contact with a newborn
- Infected health care personnel with active herpetic whitlow lesions should not provide direct care for neonates[21]

SUMMARY

Although genital herpes infections remain common worldwide, HSV infection in the newborn fortunately is rare but when present contributes to significant long-term morbidity. Significant advances have been made for diagnosing and effectively treating neonatal HSV disease. Efforts in vaccine development to prevent maternal acquisition and subsequent transmission to the neonate have been unsuccessful so far.

REFERENCES

1. Kulhanjian JA, Soroush V, Au DS, et al. Identification of women at unsuspected risk of primary infection with herpes simplex virus type 2 during pregnancy. N Engl J Med 1992;326(14):916–20.
2. Whitley RJ, Corey L, Arvin A, et al. Changing presentation of herpes simplex virus infection in neonates. J Infect Dis 1988;158(1):109–16.
3. Brown ZA, Selke S, Zeh J, et al. The acquisition of herpes simplex virus during pregnancy. N Engl J Med 1997;337(8):509–15.
4. Sheffield JS, Hill JB, Hollier LM, et al. Valacyclovir prophylaxis to prevent recurrent herpes at delivery: a randomized clinical trial. Obstet Gynecol 2006; 108(1):141–7.
5. Watts DH, Brown ZA, Money D, et al. A double-blind, randomized, placebo-controlled trial of acyclovir in late pregnancy for the reduction of herpes simplex virus shedding and cesarean delivery. Am J Obstet Gynecol 2003;188(3): 836–43.
6. Brown ZA, Benedetti J, Ashley R, et al. Neonatal herpes simplex virus infection in relation to asymptomatic maternal infection at the time of labor. N Engl J Med 1991;324(18):1247–52.
7. Arvin AM, Hensleigh PA, Prober CG, et al. Failure of antepartum maternal cultures to predict the infant's risk of exposure to herpes simplex virus at delivery. N Engl J Med 1986;315(13):796–800.
8. Vontver LA, Hickok DE, Brown Z, et al. Recurrent genital herpes simplex virus infection in pregnancy: infant outcome and frequency of asymptomatic recurrences. Am J Obstet Gynecol 1982;143(1):75–84.

9. Sullender WM, Yasukawa LL, Schwartz M, et al. Type-specific antibodies to herpes simplex virus type 2 (HSV-2) glycoprotein G in pregnant women, infants exposed to maternal HSV-2 infection at delivery, and infants with neonatal herpes. J Infect Dis 1988;157(1):164–71.
10. Brown ZA, Wald A, Morrow RA, et al. Effect of serologic status and cesarean delivery on transmission rates of herpes simplex virus from mother to infant. JAMA 2003;289(2):203–9.
11. Kimberlin DW. Neonatal herpes simplex infection. Clin Microbiol Rev 2004;17(1):1–13.
12. ACOG Committee on Practice Bulletins. ACOG Practice Bulletin. Clinical management guidelines for obstetrician-gynecologists. No. 82 June 2007. Management of herpes in pregnancy. Obstet Gynecol 2007;109(6):1489–98.
13. Peng J, Krause PJ, Kresch M. Neonatal herpes simplex virus infection after cesarean section with intact amniotic membranes. J Perinatol 1996;16(5):397–9.
14. Nahmias AJ, Josey WE, Naib ZM, et al. Perinatal risk associated with maternal genital herpes simplex virus infection. Am J Obstet Gynecol 1971;110(6):825–37.
15. Kaye EM, Dooling EC. Neonatal herpes simplex meningoencephalitis associated with fetal monitor scalp electrodes. Neurology 1981;31(8):1045–7.
16. Whitley RJ, Nahmias AJ, Soong SJ, et al. Vidarabine therapy of neonatal herpes simplex virus infection. Pediatrics 1980;66(4):495–501.
17. Whitley R, Arvin A, Prober C, et al. A controlled trial comparing vidarabine with acyclovir in neonatal herpes simplex virus infection. Infectious Diseases Collaborative Antiviral Study Group. N Engl J Med 1991;324(7):444–9.
18. Whitley R, Arvin A, Prober C, et al. Predictors of morbidity and mortality in neonates with herpes simplex virus infections. The National Institute of Allergy and Infectious Diseases Collaborative Antiviral Study Group. N Engl J Med 1991;324(7):450–4.
19. Kimberlin DW, Lin CY, Jacobs RF, et al. Safety and efficacy of high-dose intravenous acyclovir in the management of neonatal herpes simplex virus infections. Pediatrics 2001;108(2):230–8.
20. Kimberlin DW, Lin CY, Jacobs RF, et al. Natural history of neonatal herpes simplex virus infections in the acyclovir era. Pediatrics 2001;108(2):223–9.
21. American Academy of Pediatrics. Herpes simplex. In: Pickering L, Baker C, Kimberlin D, et al, editors. Red book: 2012 report of the Committee on Infectious Diseases. 29th edition. Elk Grove Village (IL): American Academy of Pediatrics; 2012. p. 398–408.
22. Diamond C, Mohan K, Hobson A, et al. Viremia in neonatal herpes simplex virus infections. Pediatr Infect Dis J 1999;18(6):487–9.
23. Kimberlin DW, Lakeman FD, Arvin AM, et al. Application of the polymerase chain reaction to the diagnosis and management of neonatal herpes simplex virus disease. National Institute of Allergy and Infectious Diseases Collaborative Antiviral Study Group. J Infect Dis 1996;174(6):1162–7.
24. Kimura H, Futamura M, Kito H, et al. Detection of viral DNA in neonatal herpes simplex virus infections: frequent and prolonged presence in serum and cerebrospinal fluid. J Infect Dis 1991;164(2):289–93.
25. Malm G, Forsgren M. Neonatal herpes simplex virus infections: HSV DNA in cerebrospinal fluid and serum. Arch Dis Child Fetal Neonatal Ed 1999;81(1):F24–29.
26. Lewensohn-Fuchs I, Osterwall P, Forsgren M, et al. Detection of herpes simplex virus DNA in dried blood spots making a retrospective diagnosis possible. J Clin Virol 2003;26(1):39–48.

27. Kimberlin DW, Whitley RJ, Wan W, et al. Oral acyclovir suppression and neurodevelopment after neonatal herpes. N Engl J Med 2011;365(14):1284–92.
28. Kimberlin D, Powell D, Gruber W, et al. Administration of oral acyclovir suppressive therapy after neonatal herpes simplex virus disease limited to the skin, eyes and mouth: results of a phase I/II trial. Pediatr Infect Dis J 1996;15(3):247–54.
29. Kimberlin DW, Baley J, Committee on Infectious Diseases, Committee on Fetus and Newborn. Guidance on management of asymptomatic neonates born to women with active genital herpes lesions. Pediatrics 2013;131(2):383–6.
30. Roberts SW, Cox SM, Dax J, et al. Genital herpes during pregnancy: no lesions, no cesarean. Obstet Gynecol 1995;85(2):261–4.
31. Pinninti SG, Angara R, Feja KN, et al. Neonatal herpes disease following maternal antenatal antiviral suppressive therapy: a multicenter case series. J Pediatr 2012; 161(1):134–8.e1–3.
32. Stanberry LR, Spruance SL, Cunningham AL, et al. Glycoprotein-D-adjuvant vaccine to prevent genital herpes. N Engl J Med 2002;347(21):1652–61.
33. Belshe RB, Leone PA, Bernstein DI, et al. Efficacy results of a trial of a herpes simplex vaccine. N Engl J Med 2012;366(1):34–43.
34. Brown ZA, Gardella C, Wald A, et al. Genital herpes complicating pregnancy. Obstet Gynecol 2005;106(4):845–56.
35. Corey L, Wald A. Maternal and neonatal herpes simplex virus infections. N Engl J Med 2009;361(14):1376–85.
36. Centers for Disease Control and Prevention (CDC). Neonatal herpes simplex virus infection following Jewish ritual circumcisions that included direct orogenital suction - New York City, 2000-2011. MMWR Morb Mortal Wkly Rep 2012;61: 405–9.

Use of Cell-Free Fetal DNA in Maternal Plasma for Noninvasive Prenatal Screening

CrossMark

Amy J. Wagner, MD[a], Michael E. Mitchell, MD[b],
Aoy Tomita-Mitchell, PhD[b],*

KEYWORDS

- Noninvasive prenatal testing • Screening • Cell-free DNA • Aneuploidy

KEY POINTS

- Noninvasive prenatal testing (NIPT) using cell-free fetal (cfDNA) offers potential as a screening tool for fetal anomalies; it is more accurate than maternal serum markers and nuchal translucency tests.
- The accuracy of NIPT using cfDNA, with a lower false-positive rate than previous standard aneuploidy testing, decreases the overall number of invasive tests needed for a definitive diagnosis, subjecting fewer pregnancies to the risk of the invasive procedures.
- Women who undergo NIPT need informed consent before testing and accurate, sensitive counseling after results are available.

INTRODUCTION

Prenatal screening for aneuploidy has been available to pregnant women for more than three decades. Accurate prenatal screening is important for several reasons. It can provide reassurance early in pregnancy in some cases. For those receiving less encouraging news, it allows the opportunity to consider options, have ample time to make difficult decisions, and manage expectations. It also may help to predict the postnatal course and make appropriate delivery plans when needed. An ideal prenatal test is one that is accurate, can be completed early in gestation, and poses minimal or

Disclosures: M.E. Mitchell and A. Tomita-Mitchell are co-founders of Ariosa Diagnostics, a company that offers a noninvasive prenatal screening test in which they have a significant financial interest. Any financial conflicts of interest that may be related to the work presented here have been disclosed to The Medical College of Wisconsin as required per Federal Regulation(s) 42 CFR Part 50, Subpart F and 45 CFR Part 94. A.J. Wagner has no disclosures.
[a] Division of Pediatric Surgery, Department of Surgery, Medical College of Wisconsin, 999 North 92nd Street, Suite C320, Milwaukee, WI 53226, USA; [b] Division of Cardiothoracic Surgery, Department of Surgery, Medical College of Wisconsin, 8701 Watertown Plank Road, Milwaukee, WI 53226, USA
* Corresponding author.
E-mail address: amitchell@mcw.edu

Clin Perinatol 41 (2014) 957–966
http://dx.doi.org/10.1016/j.clp.2014.08.013
0095-5108/14/$ – see front matter © 2014 Elsevier Inc. All rights reserved.
perinatology.theclinics.com

no risk to the fetus and the mother. Over the past several years, the discovery of cell-free fetal DNA (cfDNA) in the maternal circulation has revolutionized prenatal screening and changed the standard of care.

Noninvasive maternal blood testing began in the early 1980s with the maternal serum test for α-fetoprotein (AFP). Since that time, many serum factors have been studied as screening tests for fetal anomalies. Maternal serum markers tested in the second trimester utilized the double (maternal serum beta-human chorionic gonadotropin [hCG] and AFP), triple (maternal serum beta-hCG, AFP, unconjugated estriol), and eventually quadruple (maternal serum beta-hCG, AFP, unconjugated estriol, and inhibin A) screens. The quadruple screen is associated with a false-positive rate of 7% and a sensitivity of less than 80%.[1] In 2007, the American College of Obstetricians and Gynecologists released guidelines that included nuchal translucency (a measurement of the thickness of the back of the fetal neck), serum pregnancy-associated plasma protein A (PAPP-A), and serum beta-hCG in the first trimester in addition to the quadruple screen in the second trimester. The nuchal translucency test has an overall sensitivity of 77% for trisomy 21 and a false-positive rate of 6%.[2] Combining the nuchal translucency and quad screens improves sensitivity, but there continues to be a 3% to 5% false-positive rate.[3]

The maternal serum markers AFP, beta-hCG, unconjugated estriol, and inhibin A (the quad screen) are now routinely utilized in screening pregnancies for trisomy 21. AFP is a major fetal plasma protein and has a structure similar to albumin that is found in postnatal life. AFP is made initially by the yolk sac, gastrointestinal tract, and liver. Fetal plasma levels peak at approximately 10 to 13 weeks gestation and then decline progressively until term, whereas maternal levels peak in the third trimester. Maternal and amniotic fluid levels of AFP are increased in pregnancies in which the fetus has a neural tube defect (ie, anencephaly and open spina bifida) or certain other fetal malformations, such as abdominal wall defects. Screening of maternal blood samples usually is done between weeks 16 and 18 of gestation.[4,5] Although neural tube defects have been associated with elevated levels of AFP, decreased levels have been associated with Down syndrome.

A complex glycoprotein, beta-hCG is produced exclusively by the outer layer of the trophoblast shortly after implantation in the uterine wall. It increases rapidly in the first 8 weeks of gestation, declines steadily until 20 weeks, and then plateaus. Unconjugated estriol is produced by the placenta from precursors provided by the fetal adrenal glands and liver. It increases steadily throughout pregnancy to a higher level than that normally produced by the liver. Unconjugated estriol levels are decreased in Down syndrome and trisomy 18. The last maternal serum marker that makes up the quadruple screen is inhibin-A. Inhibin A, which is secreted by the corpus luteum and fetoplacental unit, is also a maternal serum marker for fetal Down syndrome when levels are reduced.[6]

Another first trimester serum screening test for trisomy 21, or Down syndrome, is PAPP-A. PAPP-A, which is secreted by the placenta, has been shown to play an important role in promoting cell differentiation and proliferation in various body systems. The PAPP-A concentration increases with gestational age until term. Decreased PAPP-A levels in the first trimester (between 10 and 13 weeks) have been shown to be associated with Down syndrome. When used along with free β-hCG and ultrasound measurement of nuchal translucency, serum PAPP-A levels can reportedly detect 82% to 87% of affected pregnancies with a false-positive rate of approximately 5%.[7]

The limitations of these standard prenatal screening tools include high false-positive and false-negative rates. Additionally, the quadruple screen is drawn in the second trimester, which gives the patient less time to make challenging decisions regarding the pregnancy. Last, these screening tests need to be confirmed by an invasive test to obtain a sample of fetal tissue and a definitive diagnosis, either through chorionic villus sampling (CVS) or an amniocentesis. Both tests have a known risk of fetal loss to be approximately 1 in 200 to 1 in 300 procedures.[8,9]

As a positive screening test requires a confirmatory invasive CVS or amniocentesis, the high false-positive rate of these tests results in unnecessary procedures that put the fetus at risk (**Table 1**). Because of these limitations, other approaches with better diagnostic accuracy and without the invasive risk have been investigated.

FETAL CELL-FREE DNA

A major breakthrough in the approach to accurate, noninvasive prenatal screening occurred after the discovery of fetal cfDNA in the maternal serum in 1997.[10] Circulating cfDNA fragments are short fragments of DNA found in the blood. During pregnancy, there are cfDNA fragments from both the mother and fetus in the maternal circulation. Fetal cfDNA can be detected as early as 4 weeks gestation.[11] The total amount of fetal cfDNA in the maternal serum is known as the fetal fraction.

The fetal fraction varies between pregnancies and is affected by multiple factors including maternal weight, ethnicity, smoking status, gestational age, singleton versus

Table 1
Down syndrome screening tests and detection rates

Screening Test	Detection Rate (%)
First trimester	
NT measurement	64–70
NT measurement, PAPP-A, free or total beta-hCG	82–87
Second trimester	
Triple screen (maternal serum alpha-fetoprotein, hCG, unconjugated estriol)	69
Quadruple screen (maternal serum alpha-fetoprotein, hCG, unconjugated estriol, inhibin A)	81
First and second trimesters	
Integrated (NT, PAPP-A, quadruple screen)	94–96
Serum integrated (PAPP-A, quadruple screen)	85–88

Stepwise sequential
First-trimester test result
  Positive: Diagnostic test offered
  Negative: Second-trimester test offered
  Final: Risk assessment incorporates first- and second-trimester results
	95

Contingent sequential
First-trimester test result
  Positive: Diagnostic test offered
  Negative: No further testing
  Intermediate: Second-trimester test offered
  Final: Risk assessment incorporates first- and second-trimester results
	88–94

Note: Detection rates are based on a 5% positive screen rate.
Abbreviations: hCG, human chorionic gonadotropin; NT, nuchal translucency; PAPP-A, pregnancy-associated plasma protein A.
Adapted from ACOG Committee on Practice Bulletins. Screening for fetal chromosomal abnormalities. Obstet Gynecol 2007;109:218; with permission.

multiples, and fetal chromosomal abnormalities. The fetal fraction is about 10% of total circulating cfDNA on average and can range from 7% to 19%.[12] Levels of cfDNA have been shown to increase moderately during a normal pregnancy,[13] as well as during pathologic conditions of pregnancy such as preeclampsia.[14] The majority of cfDNA in plasma is thought to originate from the natural turnover of hematopoietic cells via apoptosis.[15,16]

cfDNA has a rapid turnover, with the mean half-life estimated to be 16.3 minutes (range, 4–30). Therefore, to maintain a constant fetal fraction despite a relatively short half-life, fetal DNA must be released into the maternal circulation at a rate of 2.24×10^4 copies per minute.[17] Because the half-life is so short, the fetal fragments are no longer detectable in the maternal circulation soon after birth.[18,19] Therefore, the cfDNA test should also be accurate in multigravid women with the results reflecting the current pregnancy, because cfDNA from previous pregnancies would have cleared.[20]

Initially, cfDNA was able to be detected in the maternal plasma using paternally inherited loci or loci on the Y chromosome.[21,22] This allowed maternal DNA to be differentiated from the male fetal DNA. However, the utility of the test was thus limited because it would be applicable only to male fetuses, loci on the Y chromosome, and heterozygous paternally inherited polymorphisms.[23]

In 2007, an advance in technology occurred that allowed aneuploidy detection from the maternal plasma regardless of fetal gender and theoretically to all chromosomes. This technology involved parallel shotgun DNA sequencing, also known as next-generation sequencing, followed by counting statistics.[24–26] A variety of other methods have demonstrated proof of concept for detecting fetal DNA including placentally expressed mRNA and others.

The first four companies to offer noninvasive cfDNA tests employ next-generation sequencing. Two of the tests use whole-genome shotgun sequencing[27,28] and two use a targeted approach.[29,30] Advantages of a targeted approach include reduced cost as well as shorter bioinformatics analysis.[31] Although, theoretically, whole-genome shotgun sequencing would be more comprehensive, there is uncertainty about clinically reportable findings which could result in a greater burden for clinicians and their patients.[32]

Before the commercial availability of these products, proof of concept studies were completed, which proved that noninvasive prenatal testing (NIPT) is feasible using cfDNA in the maternal plasma. These studies were completed in both aneuploid and euploid pregnancies.[20,24,33–35] The methods used included shotgun DNA sequencing in trisomies 13, 18,[35,36] and 21.[24,35,37] Tandem single nucleotide polymorphism analysis (short haplotype analysis) was also shown to be an effective and accurate means of diagnosing trisomy 21.[34] Additionally, an alternate method called digital analysis of selected regions was developed to detect fetal trisomies 21 and 18 in the maternal plasma. Digital analysis of selected regions has the benefits of increasing mapping efficiency and selective analysis of specific chromosomes, while decreasing cost and improving throughput.[33] Finally, an approach that assesses placentally expressed mRNA present in maternal plasma has shown moderate success for detecting trisomy 21.[38] Using single nucleotide polymorphisms on the *PLAC4* gene, 9 out of 10 trisomy 21 patients were identified (90% sensitivity).[38] However, there are inherent issues of RNA-based approaches. Limitations include the instability of RNA, currently only one gene seems to be reliably suitable for such analysis on chromosome 21, the number of potentially informative single nucleotide polymorphisms on the *PLAC4* gene is limited, and false positives are likely with certain maternal illnesses. Furthermore, because the approach is not DNA-based and requires more than a thousand-fold differential between placental RNA expression and maternal hematopoietic cells, the ability to expand toward other chromosomal regions and assays for trisomies 13 and 18 is limited.

After publication of these proof-of-concept trials, several clinical trials were published in women who were deemed high risk for trisomy 21, another aneuploidy, or any disorder.[28,29,39–43] Patients were defined as high risk if they had a positive screening test, advanced maternal age, ultrasound findings, or positive family history. The studies included results on trisomies 13, 18, and 21. A systematic review was published regarding the diagnostic accuracy of noninvasive detection of fetal trisomy 21 in high-risk patients.[44] This included a total of 681 pregnancies with an overall sensitivity of 125 of 125 (100%; 95% CI, 97.5%–100%) and specificity of 552 of 556 (99.3%; 95% CI, 98.7%–99.3%). This revealed that there is a high diagnostic accuracy to detect trisomy 21 in high-risk patients using fetal nucleic acids in the maternal plasma.

More recently, there have been studies investigating the accuracy of NIPT using cfDNA in non–high-risk subjects. It was important to examine the utility in low-risk patients, because the results of studies completed on high-risk individuals could not necessarily be generalized to the rest of the obstetric population. These studies also found that NIPT is highly accurate in this population to detect fetal aneuploidy.[45–49] Bianchi and colleagues[49] reported results from 1914 women with singleton pregnancies who were undergoing standard aneuploidy testing using serum biochemical assays with or without nuchal translucency measurement. They used massively parallel sequencing of maternal cfDNA. The false-positive rates with cfDNA testing were lower than those that had standard screening for trisomies 21 and 18 (0.3% vs 3.6% for trisomy 21 [$P = .001$]; 0.2% vs 0.6% for trisomy 18 [$P = .03$]).[49] Therefore, cfDNA was shown to have lower false-positive rates and higher positive predictive values than standard screening in the general obstetric population. A meta-analysis was also recently published that reviewed cfDNA for aneuploidy screening. The results for pooled detection rates and false-positive rates were 99.0% (95% CI, 98.2–99.6) and 0.08% (95% CI, 0.03–0.14) respectively, for trisomy 21; 96.8% (95% CI, 94.5–98.4) and 0.15% (95% CI, 0.08–0.25) for trisomy 18; and 92.1% (95% CI, 85.9–96.7) and 0.2% (95% CI, 0.04–0.46) for trisomy 13.[50]

Although cfDNA screening studies are promising and demonstrate high sensitivity and specificity with low false-positive rates, there are limitations to NIPT. Specificity and sensitivity are not uniform for all chromosomes, in part owing to differing content of cytosine and guanine nucleotide pairs.[51] False-positive screening results occur. Furthermore, the sequences derived from NIPT are derived from the placenta and, like CVS, may not reflect the true fetal karyotype. Therefore, invasive testing is recommended for confirmation of a positive screening test and should remain an option for patients seeking a definitive diagnosis.[51]

Despite these known limitations and the requirement for invasive testing to confirm a definitive diagnosis, the American College of Obstetricians and Gynecologists, the Society for Maternal-Fetal Medicine, the National Society of Genetic Counselors, and the International Society for Prenatal Diagnosis state that cfDNA testing should be offered to pregnant women at high risk for fetal aneuploidy as a screening test.[52–54]

In addition to advances in prenatal screening for aneuploidy, recent developments in the clinical application of genomic technologies have impacted prenatal diagnosis. Chromosomal microarray analysis allows identification of microdeletions and microduplications of chromosomes that are too small to be identified by karyotyping.[55] Another advantage of chromosomal microarray analysis is the rapidity of results. Standard cytogenetic karyotype requires 5 to 7 days of tissue culture, whereas chromosomal microarray analysis is able to be completed on uncultured samples. This more rapid result time is important in prenatal testing and counseling.[55]

CONTROVERSIES

Prenatal testing and counseling are inherently emotionally complex endeavors. The development of NIPT and the ability to provide additional information about the fetus earlier in gestation has raised many ethical issues including informed consent, terminations, changes in perceptions of those with disabilities, and appropriate counseling.

Practitioners discussing invasive testing such as CVS or an amniocentesis have a clear need to obtain informed consent because there is an inherent risk to the procedure. However, when the same emotionally complex issues regarding aneuploidy results are garnered through a peripheral blood draw, the question arises of whether or not the patient was properly prepared for the information she will receive. The first issue is the need for a confirmatory invasive test; NIPT is simply screening and not meant as a definitive diagnostic test. After a woman receives results that are concerning for aneuploidy, she needs to make the decision of whether or not to pursue an invasive test (CVS or amniocentesis) for a definitive diagnosis. It is important that the patient understand this will be recommended, and not be surprised when that is the next recommended step.[31]

In addition to the concern regarding appropriate informed consent for women undergoing NIPT, the concern has been raised that it may lead to an increase in the number of terminations. More accurate and reliable prenatal testing will likely lead to a greater number of fetuses diagnosed with not only aneuploidy, but also the possibility of diagnosing other genetic conditions early in the pregnancy. This will likely result in more pregnancy terminations. There is rarely an issue more passionately debated or contentious than that of reproductive rights. The concern is that NIPT will make abortion more common because the diagnoses will be available to a woman earlier in her pregnancy.[56] Fears of eugenics and termination over qualities such as gender, trait selection, or even the concern of creation of "savior siblings" have also been raised.[57] Additionally, implications have been raised that there may be a negative effect on the status and worth of those people currently living with disabilities as more people decide to terminate pregnancies with similar diagnoses. There have also been concerns raised about funding, research, treatment, awareness, and support of those with disabilities or aneuploidy.[57]

Women who are pregnant with a fetus with a prenatal diagnosis of aneuploidy or any disability require careful, thorough, and understandable prenatal counseling in a nondirective fashion. The question arises of how best to provide appropriate pretest genetic counseling before the decision to pursue NIPT is made. Currently, in California approximately two thirds of pregnant women undergo noninvasive screening for trisomy 21 and neural tube defects. If the same proportions of women in the United States choose to have NIPT, the number of genetic tests will go from 100,000 per year to more than 3 million.[57] If more women undergo NIPT, it is important to ensure that there are a sufficient number of genetic counselors to provide appropriate information regarding interpretation of results and expectations.

As more patients opt for NIPT, the responsibility of delivering the information will increasingly fall to the obstetricians because the information will exceed the number of genetic counselors available. Genetic counselors traditionally receive formal training on how to deliver a prenatal diagnosis to a pregnant mother.[58] In a 2004 survey of American College of Obstetricians and Gynecologists fellows, 45% rated their training regarding prenatal diagnosis and counseling as "barely adequate or nonexistent."[59] Unfortunately, as more of the NIPT responsibility falls to obstetricians who have not had the benefit of formal training, the mothers' experience when receiving the news has been reported to be less than positive. Mothers with a prenatal diagnosis of trisomy 21 state that the diagnosis was delivered to them in an "incomplete" or "inaccurate" fashion by their obstetrician.[60]

Ideally, obstetricians and pediatricians should coordinate their counseling to deliver news as parents preferred to receive the diagnosis together in a joint meeting with both providers.[61] When this is not possible, the obstetrician and the pediatrician should communicate to ensure that a consistent message is being conveyed.[61]

SUMMARY

NIPT using cfDNA offers tremendous potential as a screening tool owing to its increased accuracy over maternal serum markers and nuchal translucency tests. The American College of Obstetricians and Gynecologists recommends that all pregnant women, regardless of age, be offered prenatal screening and diagnostic testing by their obstetrician.[7] The recent and rapid adoption of NIPT in high-risk pregnancies in the United States suggests that NIPT may change the standard of care for genetic screening. This allows the advantages of an accurate test with results available early in the pregnancy. The accuracy of NIPT using cfDNA, with a lower false-positive rate than previous standard aneuploidy testing, decreases the overall number of invasive tests needed for a definitive diagnosis, subjecting fewer pregnancies to the risk of the invasive procedures. Women who undergo NIPT need informed consent before testing and accurate, sensitive counseling after results are available.

REFERENCES

1. Wald NJ, Huttly WJ, Hackshaw AK. Antenatal screening for Down's syndrome with the quadruple test. Lancet 2003;361(9360):835–6.
2. Malone FD, D'Alton ME, Society for Maternal-Fetal Medicine. First-trimester sonographic screening for Down syndrome. Obstet Gynecol 2003;102(5 Pt 1): 1066–79.
3. Malone FD, Canick JA, Ball RH, et al. First-trimester or second-trimester screening, or both, for Down's syndrome. N Engl J Med 2005;353(19):2001–11.
4. Nassbaum RL, McInnes RR, Willard HF, editors. Thompson & Thompson genetics in medicine. 7th edition. Philadelphia: Saunders Elsevier; 2007.
5. Graves JC, Miller KE, Sellers AD. Maternal serum triple analyte screening in pregnancy. Am Fam Physician 2002;65(5):915–20.
6. Lambert-Messerlian GM, Canick JA. Clinical application of inhibin a measurement: prenatal serum screening for Down syndrome. Semin Reprod Med 2004;22(3):235–42.
7. ACOG Committee on Practice Bulletins. ACOG practice bulletin no. 77: screening for fetal chromosomal abnormalities. Obstet Gynecol 2007;109(1): 217–27.
8. Antsaklis A, Papantoniou N, Xygakis A, et al. Genetic amniocentesis in women 20-34 years old: associated risks. Prenat Diagn 2000;20(3):247–50.
9. Evans MI, Andriole S. Chorionic villus sampling and amniocentesis in 2008. Curr Opin Obstet Gynecol 2008;20(2):164–8.
10. Lo YM, Corbetta N, Chamberlain PF, et al. Presence of fetal DNA in maternal plasma and serum. Lancet 1997;350(9076):485–7.
11. Illanes S, Denbow M, Kailasam C, et al. Early detection of cell-free fetal DNA in maternal plasma. Early Hum Dev 2007;83(9):563–6.

12. Ashoor G, Poon L, Syngelaki A, et al. Fetal fraction in maternal plasma cell-free DNA at 11-13 weeks' gestation: effect of maternal and fetal factors. Fetal Diagn Ther 2012;31(4):237–43.

13. Lo YM, Tein MS, Lau TK, et al. Quantitative analysis of fetal DNA in maternal plasma and serum: implications for noninvasive prenatal diagnosis. Am J Hum Genet 1998;62(4):768–75.

14. Zhong XY, Laivuori H, Livingston JC, et al. Elevation of both maternal and fetal extracellular circulating deoxyribonucleic acid concentrations in the plasma of pregnant women with preeclampsia. Am J Obstet Gynecol 2001;184(3):414–9.

15. Suzuki N, Kamataki A, Yamaki J, et al. Characterization of circulating DNA in healthy human plasma. Clin Chim Acta 2008;387(1–2):55–8.

16. Lui YY, Chik KW, Chiu RW, et al. Predominant hematopoietic origin of cell-free DNA in plasma and serum after sex-mismatched bone marrow transplantation. Clin Chem 2002;48(3):421–7.

17. Lo YM, Zhang J, Leung TN, et al. Rapid clearance of fetal DNA from maternal plasma. Am J Hum Genet 1999;64(1):218–24.

18. Hui L, Vaughan JI, Nelson M. Effect of labor on postpartum clearance of cell-free fetal DNA from the maternal circulation. Prenat Diagn 2008;28(4):304–8.

19. Smid M, Galbiati S, Vassallo A, et al. No evidence of fetal DNA persistence in maternal plasma after pregnancy. Hum Genet 2003;112(5–6):617–8.

20. Benn P, Cuckle H, Pergament E. Non-invasive prenatal testing for aneuploidy: current status and future prospects. Ultrasound Obstet Gynecol 2013;42(1): 15–33.

21. Dhallan R, Guo X, Emche S, et al. A non-invasive test for prenatal diagnosis based on fetal DNA present in maternal blood: a preliminary study. Lancet 2007;369(9560):474–81.

22. Lo YM. Noninvasive prenatal detection of fetal chromosomal aneuploidies by maternal plasma nucleic acid analysis: a review of the current state of the art. BJOG 2009;116(2):152–7.

23. Sifakis S, Papantoniou N, Kappou D, et al. Noninvasive prenatal diagnosis of Down syndrome: current knowledge and novel insights. J Perinat Med 2012; 40(4):319–27.

24. Fan HC, Quake SR. Detection of aneuploidy with digital polymerase chain reaction. Anal Chem 2007;79(19):7576–9.

25. Lo YM, Lun FM, Chan KC, et al. Digital PCR for the molecular detection of fetal chromosomal aneuploidy. Proc Natl Acad Sci U S A 2007;104(32):13116–21.

26. Bianchi DW, Wilkins-Haug L. Integration of noninvasive DNA testing for aneuploidy into prenatal care: what has happened since the rubber met the road? Clin Chem 2014;60(1):78–87.

27. Canick JA, Kloza EM, Lambert-Messerlian GM, et al. DNA sequencing of maternal plasma to identify Down syndrome and other trisomies in multiple gestations. Prenat Diagn 2012;32(8):730–4.

28. Bianchi DW, Platt LD, Goldberg JD, et al. Genome-wide fetal aneuploidy detection by maternal plasma DNA sequencing. Obstet Gynecol 2012;119(5): 890–901.

29. Norton ME, Brar H, Weiss J, et al. Non-invasive chromosomal evaluation (NICE) study: results of a multicenter prospective cohort study for detection of fetal trisomy 21 and trisomy 18. Am J Obstet Gynecol 2012;207(2):137.e1–8.

30. Zimmermann B, Hill M, Gemelos G, et al. Noninvasive prenatal aneuploidy testing of chromosomes 13, 18, 21, X, and Y, using targeted sequencing of polymorphic loci. Prenat Diagn 2012;32(13):1233–41.

31. Morain S, Greene MF, Mello MM. A new era in noninvasive prenatal testing. N Engl J Med 2013;369(6):499–501.
32. Dewey FE, Grove ME, Pan C, et al. Clinical interpretation and implications of whole-genome sequencing. JAMA 2014;311(10):1035–45.
33. Sparks AB, Wang ET, Struble CA, et al. Selective analysis of cell-free DNA in maternal blood for evaluation of fetal trisomy. Prenat Diagn 2012;32(1):3–9.
34. Ghanta S, Mitchell ME, Ames M, et al. Non-invasive prenatal detection of trisomy 21 using tandem single nucleotide polymorphisms. PLoS One 2010;5(10): e13184.
35. Sehnert AJ, Rhees B, Comstock D, et al. Optimal detection of fetal chromosomal abnormalities by massively parallel DNA sequencing of cell-free fetal DNA from maternal blood. Clin Chem 2011;57(7):1042–9.
36. Chen EZ, Chiu RW, Sun H, et al. Noninvasive prenatal diagnosis of fetal trisomy 18 and trisomy 13 by maternal plasma DNA sequencing. PLoS One 2011;6(7): e21791.
37. Chiu RW, Chan KC, Gao Y, et al. Noninvasive prenatal diagnosis of fetal chromo-somal aneuploidy by massively parallel genomic sequencing of DNA in maternal plasma. Proc Natl Acad Sci U S A 2008;105(51):20458–63.
38. Lo YM, Tsui NB, Chiu RW, et al. Plasma placental RNA allelic ratio permits nonin-vasive prenatal chromosomal aneuploidy detection. Nat Med 2007;13(2):218–23.
39. Chiu RW, Akolekar R, Zheng YW, et al. Non-invasive prenatal assessment of tri-somy 21 by multiplexed maternal plasma DNA sequencing: large scale validity study. BMJ 2011;342:c7401.
40. Ehrich M, Deciu C, Zwiefelhofer T, et al. Noninvasive detection of fetal trisomy 21 by sequencing of DNA in maternal blood: a study in a clinical setting. Am J Ob-stet Gynecol 2011;204(3):205.e1–11.
41. Palomaki GE, Kloza EM, Lambert-Messerlian GM, et al. DNA sequencing of maternal plasma to detect Down syndrome: an international clinical validation study. Genet Med 2011;13(11):913–20.
42. Ashoor G, Syngelaki A, Wagner M, et al. Chromosome-selective sequencing of maternal plasma cell-free DNA for first-trimester detection of trisomy 21 and tri-somy 18. Am J Obstet Gynecol 2012;206(4):322.e1–5.
43. Sparks AB, Struble CA, Wang ET, et al. Noninvasive prenatal detection and se-lective analysis of cell-free DNA obtained from maternal blood: evaluation for tri-somy 21 and trisomy 18. Am J Obstet Gynecol 2012;206(4):319.e1–9.
44. Verweij EJ, van den Oever JM, de Boer MA, et al. Diagnostic accuracy of nonin-vasive detection of fetal trisomy 21 in maternal blood: a systematic review. Fetal Diagn Ther 2012;31(2):81–6.
45. Lau TK, Chan MK, Lo PS, et al. Clinical utility of noninvasive fetal trisomy (NIFTY) test–early experience. J Matern Fetal Neonatal Med 2012;25(10):1856–9.
46. Nicolaides KH, Syngelaki A, Ashoor G, et al. Noninvasive prenatal testing for fetal trisomies in a routinely screened first-trimester population. Am J Obstet Gy-necol 2012;207(5):374.e1–6.
47. Dan S, Wang W, Ren J, et al. Clinical application of massively parallel sequencing-based prenatal noninvasive fetal trisomy test for trisomies 21 and 18 in 11,105 pregnancies with mixed risk factors. Prenat Diagn 2012;32(13):1225–32.
48. Gil MM, Quezada MS, Bregant B, et al. Implementation of maternal blood cell-free DNA testing in early screening for aneuploidies. Ultrasound Obstet Gy-necol 2013;42(1):34–40.
49. Bianchi DW, Parker RL, Wentworth J, et al. DNA sequencing versus standard prenatal aneuploidy screening. N Engl J Med 2014;370(9):799–808.

50. Gil MM, Akolekar R, Quezada MS, et al. Analysis of cell-free DNA in maternal blood in screening for aneuploidies: meta-analysis. Fetal Diagn Ther 2014; 35(3):156–73.
51. Gregg AR, Gross SJ, Best RG, et al. ACMG statement on noninvasive prenatal screening for fetal aneuploidy. Genet Med 2013;15(5):395–8.
52. Benn P, Borell A, Chiu R, et al. Position statement from the aneuploidy screening committee on behalf of the board of the international society for prenatal diagnosis. Prenat Diagn 2013;33(7):622–9.
53. Devers PL, Cronister A, Ormond KE, et al. Noninvasive prenatal testing/noninvasive prenatal diagnosis: the position of the national society of genetic counselors. J Genet Couns 2013;22(3):291–5.
54. American College of Obstetricians and Gynecologists Committee on Genetics. Committee opinion no. 545: noninvasive prenatal testing for fetal aneuploidy. Obstet Gynecol 2012;120(6):1532–4.
55. Wapner RJ, Levy B. The impact of new genomic technologies in reproductive medicine. Discov Med 2014;17(96):313–8.
56. Benn PA, Chapman AR. Ethical challenges in providing noninvasive prenatal diagnosis. Curr Opin Obstet Gynecol 2010;22(2):128–34.
57. Greely HT. Get ready for the flood of fetal gene screening. Nature 2011; 469(7330):289–91.
58. Skotko BG, Kishnani PS, Capone GT, Down Syndrome Diagnosis Study Group. Prenatal diagnosis of Down syndrome: how best to deliver the news. Am J Med Genet A 2009;149A(11):2361–7.
59. Cleary-Goldman J, Morgan MA, Malone FD, et al. Screening for Down syndrome: practice patterns and knowledge of obstetricians and gynecologists. Obstet Gynecol 2006;107(1):11–7.
60. Skotko BG. Prenatally diagnosed Down syndrome: mothers who continued their pregnancies evaluate their health care providers. Am J Obstet Gynecol 2005; 192(3):670–7.
61. Skotko BG, Capone GT, Kishnani PS, Down Syndrome Diagnosis Study Group. Postnatal diagnosis of Down syndrome: synthesis of the evidence on how best to deliver the news. Pediatrics 2009;124(4):e751–8.

Probiotics and Necrotizing Enterocolitis

Josef Neu, MD

KEYWORDS

- Probiotics • Necrotizing enterocolitis • Pathophysiology • Dysbiosis

KEY POINTS

- It is clear that routine use of probiotics for prevention of necrotizing enterocolitis (NEC) remains controversial.
- There are currently neonatologists who insist on using probiotics without additional safety and efficacy studies.
- Basic research on the developing microbiome and its interaction with the host will add to understanding of how it might be safely manipulated to prevent diseases such as NEC in the neonate.

INTRODUCTION

One of the most controversial areas in neonatology over the past few years is whether probiotics should be provided routinely to preterm infants for the prevention of necrotizing enterocolitis (NEC). The goals of this review are to (1) provide the reader with a brief overview of NEC and current concepts of its pathophysiology, including the role of intestinal microbes, (2) discuss the microbial ecology of the intestine in preterm infants and factors that may lead to an unhealthy microbial intestinal environment (a "dysbiosis"), (3) summarize studies of probiotics in preterm infants, (4) elaborate on the need for regulation in this area, and (5) discuss alternatives to probiotics and what is the future for the prevention of NEC.

NECROTIZING ENTEROCOLITIS: MORE THAN ONE DISEASE

In this section, several aspects of developmental gastroenterology will be described as they relate to increased susceptibility to intestinal injury such as that seen in NEC. I provide a brief description of NEC, the most fulminant gastrointestinal disease seen in neonatal intensive care. A more comprehensive review of NEC can be found in elsewhere.[1–3] Although NEC can present in several ways, a common characteristic is a

Disclosure: None.
University of Florida, Department of Pediatrics, Division of Neonatology, 1600 Southwest Archer Road, Human Development Building, HD 112, Gainesville, FL 32610, USA
E-mail address: neuj@peds.ufl.edu

Clin Perinatol 41 (2014) 967–978
http://dx.doi.org/10.1016/j.clp.2014.08.014
0095-5108/14/$ – see front matter © 2014 Elsevier Inc. All rights reserved.

perinatology.theclinics.com

subtle onset presenting as a slightly distended abdomen, nonspecific instability such as apneas or bradycardias, and changes in appearance and activity of the infant. These highly nonspecific signs and symptoms may subside, but occasionally will fulminate to severe intestinal necrosis with systemic inflammation and shock. Mortality ranges between 20% and 30%, with a greater association in the least mature infants; however, a diagnosis of NEC confers a much greater relative risk of mortality to the larger infants because their baseline mortality is lower.[4] Significant morbidities include severe neurodevelopmental delays, shortened intestine, and inflammatory processes that can affect other organs such as the liver with severe cholestasis.[5] It is thus a very expensive disease, not only in terms of its financial impact,[6] but also in terms of long-term physical disabilities and neurodevelopmental delays.

Progress in the treatment and prevention of NEC over the past several decades has been almost nil.[7] Attempts to decrease incidence have included prolonged periods of nulla per os (NPO), wherein preterm infants would not receive food by the enteral route for weeks after birth or extremely slow institution of enteral feedings,[8] but subsequent studies suggested that this was counterproductive.[9,10] Studies in animals show that lack of enteral nutrition may lead to mucosal atrophy, decreased motility, decreased trophic hormones, and increased inflammation.[11] Numerous studies have now shown that providing at least small amounts of enteral feeding, especially human milk from early on after birth, does not increase the incidence of NEC and may reduce the risk of other complications such as sepsis.[12,13]

Increased survival of very small infants who have a greater propensity to develop this disease than larger infants may be a partial reason for the lack of progress. Use of experimental animal models that do not directly reflect the highly multifactorial pathophysiology of this disease as seen in preterm infants is also a likely reason for lack of progress. For example, a recent study from Sweden showed an increase in NEC together with decreasing mortality between 1987 and 2009.[14] Likewise, what we have been recording in our databases as "NEC" consists of a variety of entities, some of which may not even involve a necrotic intestine or primary inflammatory process. Hence, aiming a "magic bullet" directed at a poorly delineated disease process is likely to miss the target.

For example, babies with congenital left-sided cardiac lesions, such as hypoplastic left ventricle, interrupted aortic arch, coarctation of the aorta, or even a severe left-to-right shunt owing to a persistently patent ductus arteriosus, are at increased risk to develop bowel ischemia, which does not involve a primary inflammatory process seen in typical NEC. Designing a preventative or therapeutic approach based on prevention of inflammation by altering the microbial environment in a disease that involves primarily a lack of intestinal blood flow does not represent a reasonable approach for these forms of ischemic intestinal necrosis. Another entity, spontaneous intestinal perforation (SIP), may present with signs and symptoms similar to NEC, but involves minimal inflammation or necrotic intestine.[15] It occurs early after birth often without the infant being enterally fed. However, the radiologic presentation may be similar to NEC (free intraperitoneal air) and the therapy often includes peritoneal drainage without direct surgical inspection of the bowel and definitive diagnosis of NEC or SIP not being differentiated. Thus, SIP, sometimes mistakenly called "NEC," is unlikely to be amenable to therapies or preventative measures that include manipulations of the inflammatory response, nutritional composition, or the intestinal microbial environment, and should not be clustered in a database with the diagnosis of "NEC," because it can be misleading.

Another often unappreciated fact is that NEC may be very difficult to diagnose. The Bells Staging criteria[16] are often unhelpful in this regard. "Stage 1 NEC" is highly nonspecific in that there are no criteria that provide for a definitive diagnosis. A distended abdomen, increased gastric residuals before the next feeding, and nonspecific signs such as increased apnea and bradycardia, all used in the diagnosis of "stage 1 NEC" do not signify that the bowel is necrotic. Hence, "stage 1 NEC," often used to name this set of signs and symptoms, is a poor term that when used for inclusion of subjects in studies of NEC can only be misleading. For "stage 2 NEC," the diagnosis relies on radiographic criteria such as pneumatosis intestinalis and portal venous gas. However, in many instances, this can also be misleading. Presented with the same radiograph, there is often disagreement among neonatologists, surgeons, and radiologists as to whether some of the "gas bubbles" seen in the intestinal radiographs represent intramural air or feces. Often babies with free intraperitoneal air on radiograph are treated with a peritoneal drain and thus differentiation between NEC and SIP cannot be made because the bowel is not directly visualized on laparotomy. These difficulties in diagnosis provide a major challenge to design of clinical trials of NEC.

A disposition to NEC relates to several immaturities of the gastrointestinal tract. These include poor barrier function leading to increased permeability[17] with an activation of the highly immunoreactive cells that underlie the epithelial surface. Other aspects include a highly immunoresponsive potential of the Toll-like receptor (TLR) pathways especially TLR4,[18] which can be found on several intestinal cell types, including the surface epithelium. Interaction of these receptors with microbial components is related to the intestinal inflammatory response, but the precise mechanism requires further elucidation.

Microbial dysbiosis (inappropriate colonization) has long been suspected to play a crucial role in the development of NEC.[19] Exploration of the microbial environment has recently undergone intensified scrutiny, largely because of newly developed technologies for microbial identification and funding engendered by the Human Microbiome Project. Several studies suggest that there is a progression of microbial taxonomy that differs in NEC patients versus controls before the onset of NEC.[20–22] This includes a high proportion of Proteobacteria compared with Firmicutes and Bacteroidetes at the phylum level. Other bacteria taxa such as *Klebsiella* have also been seen strongly associated with NEC using 16S sequencing techniques.[22] Current studies are focusing on a more specific delineation of the functional aspects of the microbial milieu (metabolomics, transcriptomics, microbe–host interactions) that may led to NEC.

There are several other aspects of development of the intestinal tract, which include the microvasculature and adaptive immune system, that may at least be partially responsible for the interesting finding that many of these babies do not develop the disease until several weeks after birth, with a propensity to develop the disease between 28 and 31 weeks postmenstrual age.[23]

Other developmental components of the gastrointestinal tract that may predispose to NEC that involve intestinal microbiota include a low basal output of gastrointestinal acid from the stomach.[24] This is of considerable interest because the studies show a correlation between the use of histamine receptor 2 antagonists and NEC or sepsis in preterm infants.[25,26] The mechanisms underlying this are poorly understood but studies suggest that Proteobacteria do not survive well in an acid environment and do better in a more basic milieu.[27] This fits well with the recent findings that Proteobacteria are present in high quantities relative to the Firmicutes phyla before the onset of NEC in preterm infants.[21,22] The Proteobacteria phylum contains many of the pathogenic microbes including *Escherichia coli* and *Klebsiella*. Such studies suggest that a targeted microbial bacteriotherapeutic approach that engineers the gut microbiota toward a "healthy" composition might be feasible.[28]

Currently, there is no treatment for NEC and there have been only minor changes in our treatment and preventative modalities in the past 40 years. It is clear that the best path toward eliminating this disease will be through interventions that interfere with the most proximal components of the pathophysiologic cascade. This would include dietary, microbial, and other environmental manipulations. The rapid progression of the disease likely precludes interventions such as anticytokine therapy that might be given once the disease is already suspected.

MICROBIAL ECOLOGY OF THE INTESTINE

Since the beginning of the Human Microbiome Project in 2007,[29] studies that previously relied on cultivation of microbes are being rapidly augmented with several non–culture-based techniques, including quantitative polymerase chain reaction, microarrays, 16SrRNA, and whole genome based studies. The conundrum termed the "great plate count anomaly"[30] (being able to see microbes in various settings without being able to culture them) is being explained by studies that rely on novel DNA-based sequencing technologies and bioinformatic techniques to identify and characterize the function of noncultivatable taxa. These taxa constitute the majority of microbes in the intestine. The promise that the new knowledge of the human microbiome holds has prompted some to use the term "our second genome"[31] for the genes comprising the microbiome in our bodies.

It is important to recognize that simply being able to name the taxa present in a certain niche before or during development of a disease process falls far short of being able to explain mechanisms of pathophysiology. Understanding how microbes interact with, what bioactive products they produce, and the interaction of these products with the host under various environmental (eg, nutrition, antibiotic) conditions is critical. For example, samples of intestinal contents can now be analyzed using nuclear magnetic resonance, mass spectrometry, or both for small molecules such as the short chain fatty acids acetate, propionate, and butyrate. Of these, butyrate is of special interest because of its strong relationship to the energy metabolism in the colon, its capability to induce proliferation, differentiation, formation of interepithelial tight junctions, and inhibition of histone deacetylase with resultant epigenetic potential.[32,33]

There are numerous factors that can affect the intestinal microbiota and lead to a dysbiosis. Of these factors, antibiotics are thought to play a major role and have been implicated to contribute to the development or exacerbation of various disease entities including NEC.[34,35] It can be argued that this association may not be causal because infants who are more ill initially may have both a higher incidence of NEC and the need for antibiotic use. However, several studies in animals are providing support for causality. Rakoff-Nahoum and colleagues[36] showed that obliteration of the microbial flora with broad-spectrum antibiotics resulted in a greater propensity to intestinal injury and lesser capability to induce repair. Interestingly, this impact on propensity to injury and capability to induce repair is similar to that seen in genetically modified animals lacking TLR4, TLR2, and the signaling molecule MyD88.[36] Several additional studies show the effects of antibiotics on alteration of transcriptional regulation mechanisms in the intestine of newborn animals, as well as their long-term effects on the microbiome and how these effects lead to increases susceptibility to injury either by chemical agents or other microbes including viral infections.[37–39]

Nutritional composition may also be of major importance. Human milk, especially that provided by the baby's own mother, seems to play a major protective role in the prevention of NEC.[40] Numerous factors in human milk have been implicated in this protective role, including bioactive molecules such as lactoferrin, oligosaccharides, long chain omega-3 fatty acids, and live immunocompetent cells.[41] More recently, the use of non–culture-based technologies have explored the microbial milieu of human milk and have found that this may be a source of microbes for the infant.[42] The hypothetical source of these microbes is reviewed elsewhere,[43] but an intriguing finding is that the microbes in the human milk from 1 mother seem to differ little over a period of several months, but the microbes in the milk from 1 mother differ significantly from the microbes of another mother, suggesting a mother-specific role for these microbes for each individual mothers' infant.[42]

Other factors are likely to also play major roles in the development of the microbial ecology of the preterm infants' gastrointestinal tracts. These include mode of delivery, postnatal bathing, the use of incubators versus radiant warmers, the frequency of checking gastric residuals, and caretaker hygiene (hand washing).

PROBIOTICS: THE CONTROVERSY

The definition of probiotics as defined by the World Health Organization is "live microorganisms which when administered in adequate amounts confer a health benefit on the host." Of interest, this definition implies a health claim and thus has triggered concern by safety authorities such as the European Food Safety Authority and the US Food and Drug Administration.[44] This concern becomes even more acute when considering claims for prevention of diseases such as NEC in a highly vulnerable population such as preterm infants.

The history of "probiotics" predates use of this term. Fermented food products have been used for centuries worldwide, but the relationship of microbes to these fermented foods was poorly described until the beginning of the 20th century, when Eli Metchnikoff, the Russian scientist and Nobel laureate, suggested that certain microbes may benefit the host by interfering with factors associated with the aging process. For the past several decades, the food industry has been a primary advocate for the widespread use of probiotics. Whether the paradigm of probiotics as a food to prevent NEC in preterm infants is appropriate needs to be questioned. This is addressed in greater detail elsewhere in this review.

One of the first probiotic studies in neonates evaluated the effects of adding *Lactobacillus* to formula on the growth of intestinal microorganisms, including pathogens.[45] The results showed there were no differences in the colonization patterns between the *Lactobacillus*-treated and the control infants. In the past 2 decades, several additional studies evaluated the effects of probiotics on neonatal outcomes including NEC.[46–49] Some of the initial studies relied on historical controls, but suggested benefit. Subsequent relatively small trials of probiotics for the prevention of NEC were done in preterm infants. Meta-analyses of these studies that have shown positive effects, which stimulated interest in this area.

The most controversial was published in 2010[50] along with a commentary that suggested it was no longer necessary to do further clinical trials on probiotics.[51] Questions were subsequently raised about the quality of the studies comprising the meta-analysis.[46,52–55] Further, and most important, is the fact that 10 different forms of probiotics were used in the individual studies rather than a single agent. This was subsequently followed by a Cochrane review that included 16 studies that yielded similar results.[56] Although not a direct analogy, this approach is not much different than performing a meta-analysis that draws from a series of studies that utilize 10 different antibiotics to treat pneumonia, and subsequently concludes that we should equally consider treating with ampicillin or chloramphenicol based on a few studies that demonstrated benefit. Of course, these are all antibiotics, but their spectrum of activity and safety is different. This raises several questions: Which probiotic might be the most beneficial? What dosage should be used and when should they be started? Should larger studies that actually have adequate sample size based on the a priori hypothesis of NEC prevention be done? If one does a sample size determination based on a 5% baseline NEC rate, a 30% decrease with the intervention, and corrects for possible dropout rate and uses strict criteria for NEC diagnosis, none of the studies reported in the meta-analyses had an adequate sample size (nearly 2000 needed in each arm of the study). Again, one of the strongest and most valid concerns raised pertains to the number of different agents in the studies that were meta-analyzed and the validity of combining agents with potentially different properties and mechanisms. In addition, safety concerns should also have been raised. In one of the largest studies, the smallest babies (<750 g) had higher sepsis in the probiotic group.[57]

IS THERE A NEED FOR REGULATION OF PROBIOTICS FOR USE IN NEONATES?

There remains heated debate on whether probiotics should be used routinely in preterm infants for the prevention of NEC. Although the prevalence is not known, many neonatologists have started prescribing probiotics in neonatal intensive care units for the prevention of NEC. Anecdotally, some of the agents being used are not even probiotics previously studied in preterm neonates. In the United States, there seem to be no probiotics that are "licensed" or for which there are well-developed access schemes detailing routine use in the prevention of NEC as suggested by 1 author for their use.[51] There are also no current standards for "quality control of a reconstituted product." Good manufacturing practices specifically for use of probiotics as drugs to prevent a specific disease such as NEC are not available. Regulatory agencies in the United States and Europe have strict criteria for studies and the use of certain agents for which specific health claims, such as prevention of NEC, are made. These include well-controlled, randomized studies that are adequately powered and studies of both safety and efficacy.

At this juncture, such studies have not been done in North America for probiotics. One of the largest (but still underpowered) studies to date was done in South America where 750 babies weighing 2000 g or less were evaluated with the probiotic Lactobacillus reuteri versus controls.[49] This study resulted in no difference in mortality, nosocomial infection, or NEC between the probiotic-treated and control infants. Another large, multicenter, randomized study performed in Australia used 3 different microbes in the probiotic preparation and employed late-onset sepsis (not NEC) as the primary outcome.[48] Approximately 1099 babies were evaluated, and their results showed that there was no difference in sepsis or the mortality rate between the 2 groups. These results, as in the study with L. reuteri,[49] did not support a decrease in mortality as seen in the meta-analysis.[47] However on secondary analysis in the Australian study, there was a decrease in the incidence of NEC in babies weighing more than 1000 g at birth, but not in smaller infants. The number needed to treat was 43 with a 95% CI of 23 to 333.[48] Thus, the question arises whether this actually incurs any true benefit if all preterm infants are treated routinely for the prevention of NEC.

From the perspective of the regulatory agencies, probiotics have not been treated as a drug but rather as a food, and thus are not being scrutinized with the same standards of a drug. This raises the question of quality and consistency of the product. It also needs to be remembered that probiotics are not a classic drug in that they are live agents that can proliferate and stay in the individual's gastrointestinal tract indefinitely, as seen in recent studies of the intestinal microbiome after Cesarean section versus vaginal delivery.[58,59] Furthermore, although authors of the meta-analyses suggest probiotics in preterm are safe, some studies on pancreatitis prophylaxis in adults,[60] studies in preterm piglets,[61] and the results in the extremely low birth weight infants (increased sepsis, intraventricular hemorrhage, periventricular leukomalacia)[57] provide evidence that we cannot ignore that support the need for caution. It is also clear that "probiotics safety should be considered on a strain by strain basis."[62] Stringent standards for detecting microbial infections using culture media specific for the probiotic bacteria or specific polymerase chain reaction techniques have not been done in these studies. As stated by several authors[53,54,63–66] as well as by the American Academy of Pedicatrics[67] and European Society for Paediatric Gastroenterology, Hepatology and Nutrition[68] committees on nutrition, despite showing promise, additional studies with adequate sample size and with an approved product as per US Food and Drug Administration (or equivalent for other countries) are advised.

DO WE HAVE ALTERNATIVES TO PROBIOTICS?

As described in previous sections, it is very possible that probiotics may play a role in the prevention of NEC in premature babies. However, if large, adequately done, randomized, controlled trials do not demonstrate safety and efficacy with certain probiotic preparations, it is unlikely that this will be repeated for several other single preparations. Thus, we need to begin to consider options for the use of probiotics in the prevention of NEC.

As previously mentioned, the use of the human milk is a known preventative measure. Of interest is the fact that recent studies have shown that there are microbes present in human milk,[42,43] and that these microbes may originate from the maternal gastrointestinal tract. In 1 study, microbes from each mother were stable over time but differed considerably when comparing 1 mother's milk to the other mothers' milk microbes.[42] This may suggest a specificity of the microbial composition of human milk for each mother's baby. Thus, we may already be providing "probiotics" for infants in their own mothers' (but not pasteurized donor) milk.

Several studies done in vitro and with animals suggest that certain components of microbes may stimulate the innate mechanisms of the gastrointestinal immune system and lead to a response that is actually protective in the gastrointestinal tract.[69] Thus, it is possible that heat-inactivated or ultraviolet radiation-inactivated microbes may benefit the host in terms of the prevention of an overtly active inflammatory response.[70] Certain molecules derived from the bacteria such as polysaccharide A, primarily derived from the Bacteroidetes phylum, may drive the conversion of naïve CD4 T cells to the production of regulatory T cells, which are active in the production of interleukin-10 and transforming growth factor-beta, which are important immunomodulatory molecules.[71]

The carbohydrate composition of milk that is provided to preterm babies may also be of importance in the regulation of microbial growth and NEC. Although not considered as a classic prebiotic, 1 agent that is present in human milk in large quantities is the disaccharide lactose. Even though it is thought that preterm infants may have difficulties in the hydrolysis of lactose because of immaturity and local activity of the brush border enzyme lactase,[72] it is known that microbial fermentation of lactose in the distal small intestine leads to the production of the short chain fatty acids such as acetate, propionate, and butyrate, the latter of which is critical in the energy metabolism of the colonic epithelial cells and is also important in proliferation, differentiation, and maintenance of junctional epithelial integrity.[73,74] Thus, if a formula that is devoid of lactose is given to preterm infants, this benefit may not be incurred.

Classically, prebiotics are nondigestible food ingredients, usually complex carbohydrates that cannot be digested by the human host, but can be utilized to stimulate the growth of beneficial intestinal bacteria. Several studies have shown that fructose oligosaccharides and glucose oligosaccharides (prebiotics) may actually soften stools and decrease crying in infants.[75,76] However, at this juncture there are no studies that show the prebiotics are effective in the prevention of NEC. Human milk has also been found to be a rich source of oligosaccharides.[77,78] Human milk oligosaccharides have been the focus of intensive investigation and studies in animal models suggests that human milk oligosaccharides may be beneficial in the prevention of intestinal injury.[79,80] Research is ongoing that may lead to their application in preterm infants.

Another area of major interest relates to fecal microbial therapeutics, 1 variant of which is the fecal transplant.[28] This has received considerable attention over the past decade largely because it has been effective in the treatment of the refractory *Clostridium difficile* infections.[81] There is emerging interest in using fecal transplants (or some variant) in ulcerative and Crohn's colitis, type I diabetes, and the prevention of NEC in preterm infants.[82–84] However, this is a very controversial area, and the logistics of this modality remains a challenge.

THE FUTURE

It is clear that routine use of probiotics for prevention of NEC remains a highly controversial topic. There are currently neonatologists who insist on using probiotics without additional safety and efficacy studies, nor do these neonatologists consider of choice of probiotic strain. The need to know which probiotic or strains to use is of the utmost importance because they are not all the same, just as not all antibiotics are the same. Meticulously designed studies that are adequately powered and controlled to test the safety and efficacy of individual probiotics are either underway or being planned with close collaboration of the regulatory agencies such as the US Food and Drug Administration. Once the studies are completed, it will be clearer that the product(s) being provided are truly safe and beneficial. In the meantime, basic research on the developing microbiome, and its interaction with the host will add to our understanding of how it might be safely manipulated to prevent diseases such as NEC in the neonate.

REFERENCES

1. Neu J, Walker WA. Necrotizing enterocolitis. N Engl J Med 2011;364:255–64.
2. Sharma R, Hudak ML. A clinical perspective of necrotizing enterocolitis: past, present, and future. Clin Perinatol 2013;40:27–51.
3. Lin PW, Stoll BJ. Necrotising enterocolitis. Lancet 2006;368:1271–83.
4. Fitzgibbons SC, Ching Y, Yu D, et al. Mortality of necrotizing enterocolitis expressed by birth weight categories. J Pediatr Surg 2009;44:1072–6.
5. Pike K, Brocklehorst P, Jones D, et al. Outcomes at 7 years for babies who developed neonatal necrotising enterocolitis: the ORACLE Children Study. Arch Dis Child Fetal Neonatal Ed 2012;97:F318–22.
6. Bisquera JA, Cooper TR, Berseth CL. Impact of necrotizing enterocolitis on length of stay and hospital charges in very low birth weight infants. Pediatrics 2002;109:423–8.
7. Obladen M. Necrotizing enterocolitis–150 years of fruitless search for the cause. Neonatology 2009;96:203–10.
8. Brown EG, Sweet AY. Preventing necrotizing enterocolitis in neonates. JAMA 1978;240:2452–4.

9. LaGamma EF, Ostertag SG, Birenbaum H. Failure of delayed oral feedings to prevent necrotizing enterocolitis. Results of study in very-low-birth-weight neonates. Am J Dis Child 1985;139:385–9.

10. Hay WW Jr. Aggressive nutrition of the preterm infant. Curr Pediatr Rep 2013;1.

11. Jacobi SK, Odle J. Nutritional factors influencing intestinal health of the neonate. Adv Nutr 2012;3:687–96.

12. Terrin G, Passariello A, Canani RB, et al. Minimal enteral feeding reduces the risk of sepsis in feed-intolerant very low birth weight newborns. Acta Paediatr 2009;98:31–5.

13. Taylor SN, Kiger J, Finch C, et al. Fluid, electrolytes, and nutrition: minutes matter. Adv Neonatal Care 2010;10:248–55.

14. Ahle M, Drott P, Andersson RE. Epidemiology and trends of necrotizing enterocolitis in Sweden: 1987-2009. Pediatrics 2013;132:e443–51.

15. Gordon PV, Attridge JT. Understanding clinical literature relevant to spontaneous intestinal perforations. Am J Perinatol 2009;26:309–16.

16. Bell MJ, Ternberg JL, Feigin RD, et al. Neonatal necrotizing enterocolitis: therapeutic decisions based upon clinical staging. Ann Surg 1978;187:1–6.

17. Anand RJ, Leaphart CL, Mollen KP, et al. The role of the intestinal barrier in the pathogenesis of necrotizing enterocolitis. Shock 2007;27:124–33.

18. Hackam DJ, Good M, Sodhi CP. Mechanisms of gut barrier failure in the pathogenesis of necrotizing enterocolitis: toll-like receptors throw the switch. Semin Pediatr Surg 2013;22:76–82.

19. Claud EC, Walker WA. Hypothesis: inappropriate colonization of the premature intestine can cause neonatal necrotizing enterocolitis. FASEB J 2001;15: 1398–403.

20. Wang Y, Hoenig JD, Qamar S, et al. 16S rRNA gene-based analysis of fecal microbiota from preterm infants with and without necrotizing enterocolitis. ISME J 2009;3:944–54.

21. Mai V, Young CM, Ukhanova M, et al. Fecal microbiota in premature infants prior to necrotizing enterocolitis. PLoS One 2011;6:e20647.

22. Torrazza RM, Ukhanova M, Wang X, et al. Intestinal microbial ecology and environmental factors affecting necrotizing enterocolitis. PLoS One 2013;8:e83304.

23. Neu J. Neonatal necrotizing enterocolitis: an update. Acta Paediatr Suppl 2005; 94:100–5.

24. Hyman PE, Clarke DD, Sonne B, et al. Gastric acid secretory function in preterm infants. J Pediatr 1985;106:467–71.

25. Guillet R, Stoll BJ, Cotton CM, et al. Association of H2-blocker therapy and higher incidence of necrotizing enterocolitis in very low birth weight infants. Pediatrics 2006;117:e137–42.

26. Terrin G, Passariello A, DeCurtis M, et al. Ranitidine is associated with infections, necrotizing enterocolitis, and fatal outcome in newborns. Pediatrics 2012;129: e40–5.

27. Duncan SH, Louis P, Thomson JM, et al. The role of pH in determining the species composition of the human colonic microbiota. Environ Microbiol 2009;11: 2112–22.

28. Petrof EO, Claud EC, Gloor GB, et al. Microbial ecosystems therapeutics: a new paradigm in medicine? Benef Microbes 2013;4:53–65.

29. Turnbaugh PJ, Ley RE, Hamady M, et al. The human microbiome project. Nature 2007;449:804–10.

30. Keller M, Zengler K. Tapping into microbial diversity. Nature reviews. Microbiology 2004;2:141–50.

31. Song S, Jarvie T, Hattori M. Our second genome-human metagenome: how next-generation sequencer changes our life through microbiology. Adv Microb Physiol 2013;62:119–44.

32. Leonel AJ, Alvarez-Leite JI. Butyrate: implications for intestinal function. Curr Opin Clin Nutr Metab Care 2012;15:474–9.

33. Chang PV, Hao L, Offermanns S, et al. The microbial metabolite butyrate regulates intestinal macrophage function via histone deacetylase inhibition. Proc Natl Acad Sci U S A 2014;111:2247–52.

34. Greenwood C, Morrow AL, Lagomarcino AJ, et al. Early empiric antibiotic use in preterm infants is associated with lower bacterial diversity and higher relative abundance of enterobacter. J Pediatr 2014;165:23–9.

35. Cotten CM, Taylor S, Stoll B, et al. Prolonged duration of initial empirical antibiotic treatment is associated with increased rates of necrotizing enterocolitis and death for extremely low birth weight infants. Pediatrics 2009;123:58–66.

36. Rakoff-Nahoum S, Paglino J, Eslami-Varzaneh F, et al. Recognition of commensal microflora by toll-like receptors is required for intestinal homeostasis. Cell 2004;118:229–41.

37. Russell SL, Gold MJK, Willing BP, et al. Perinatal antibiotic treatment affects murine microbiota, immune responses and allergic asthma. Gut Microbes 2013;4: 158–64.

38. Schumann A, Nutten S, Donnicola D, et al. Neonatal antibiotic treatment alters gastrointestinal tract developmental gene expression and intestinal barrier transcriptome. Physiol Genomics 2005;23:235–45.

39. Trasande L, Bluestein J, Liu M, et al. Infant antibiotic exposures and early-life body mass. Int J Obes (Lond) 2013;37:16–23.

40. Meinzen-Derr J, Poindexter B, Wrage L, et al. Role of human milk in extremely low birth weight infants' risk of necrotizing enterocolitis or death. J Perinatol 2009;29:57–62.

41. Neville MC, Anderson SM, McManaman JL, et al. Lactation and neonatal nutrition: defining and refining the critical questions. J Mammary Gland Biol Neoplasia 2012;17:167–88.

42. Hunt KM, Foster JA, Forney LJ, et al. Characterization of the diversity and temporal stability of bacterial communities in human milk. PLoS One 2011;6:e21313.

43. Jeurink PV, Bergenhenegouwan J, Jimenez E, et al. Human milk: a source of more life than we imagine. Benef Microbes 2013;4:17–30.

44. Rijkers GT, de Vos WM, Brummer RJ, et al. Health benefits and health claims of probiotics: bridging science and marketing. Br J Nutr 2011;106:1291–6.

45. Reuman PD, Duckworth DH, Smith KL, et al. Lack of effet of Lactobacillus on gastrointestinal bacterial colonization in premature infants. Pediatr Infect Dis 1986;5:663–8.

46. Mihatsch WA, Duckworth DH, Smith KL, et al. Critical systematic review of the level of evidence for routine use of probiotics for reduction of mortality and prevention of necrotizing enterocolitis and sepsis in preterm infants. Clin Nutr 2012; 31:6–15.

47. Deshpande G, Rao S, Patole S, et al. Updated meta-analysis of probiotics for preventing necrotizing enterocolitis in preterm neonates. Pediatrics 2010;125:921–30.

48. Jacobs SE, Tobin SE, Opie GF, et al. Probiotic effects on late-onset sepsis in very preterm infants: a randomized controlled trial. Pediatrics 2013;132: 1055–62.

49. Rojas MA, Lozano JM, Rojas MX, et al. Prophylactic probiotics to prevent death and nosocomial infection in preterm infants. Pediatrics 2012;130:e1113–20.

50. Deshpande G, Rao S, Patole S. Probiotics for prevention of necrotising entero-colitis in preterm neonates with very low birthweight: a systematic review of randomised controlled trials. Lancet 2007;369:1614–20.
51. Tarnow-Mordi WO, Wilkinson D, Trived IA, et al. Probiotics reduce all-cause mortality in necrotizing enterocolitis: it is time to change practice. Pediatrics 2010; 125(5):1068–70.
52. Soll RF. Probiotics: are we ready for routine use? Pediatrics 2010;125:1071–2.
53. Murguia-Peniche T, Mihatsch WA, Zegerra J, et al. Intestinal mucosal defense system, Part 2. Probiotics and prebiotics. J Pediatr 2013;162:S64–71.
54. Caplan M. Are probiotics ready for prime time? JPEN J Parenter Enteral Nutr 2012;36:6S.
55. Neu J, Mihatsch W. Recent developments in necrotizing enterocolitis. JPEN J Parenter Enteral Nutr 2012;36:30S–5S.
56. Alfaleh K, Anabrees J, Bassler D, et al. Probiotics for prevention of necrotizing enterocolitis in preterm infants. Cochrane Database Syst Rev 2011;(3):CD005496.
57. Lin HC, Hsu CH, Chen HL, et al. Oral probiotics prevent necrotizing enterocolitis in very low birth weight preterm infants: a multicenter, randomized, controlled trial. Pediatrics 2008;122:693–700.
58. Azad MB, Konya T, Maughan H, et al. Gut microbiota of healthy Canadian infants: profiles by mode of delivery and infant diet at 4 months. CMAJ 2013; 185:385–94.
59. Jakobsson HE, Abrahamsson TR, Jenmaier MC, et al. Decreased gut microbiota diversity, delayed Bacteroidetes colonisation and reduced Th1 responses in infants delivered by Caesarean section. Gut 2014;63:559–66.
60. McClave SA, Heyland DK, Wischmeyer PE. Comment on: probiotic prophylaxis in predicted severe acute pancreatitis: a randomized, double-blind, placebo-controlled trial. JPEN J Parenter Enteral Nutr 2009;33:444–6.
61. Cilieborg MS, Thymann T, Siggers R, et al. The incidence of necrotizing entero-colitis is increased following probiotic administration to preterm pigs. J Nutr 2011;141:223–30.
62. Shanahan F. A commentary on the safety of probiotics. Gastroenterol Clin North Am 2012;41:869–76.
63. Neu J. Routine probiotics for premature infants: let's be careful! J Pediatr 2011; 158:672–4.
64. Modi N. Probiotics and necrotising enterocolitis: the devil (as always) is in the detail. Commentary on N. Ofek Shlomai et al.: probiotics for preterm neonates: what will it take to change clinical practice? (Neonatology 2014;105:64-70). Neonatology 2014;105:71–3.
65. Claud EC. First do no harm. J Pediatr Pharmacol Ther 2012;17:298–301.
66. Martin CR. Probiotics for the prevention of necrotizing enterocolitis: not just which ones but also why? J Pediatr Gastroenterol Nutr 2013;57:3.
67. Thomas DW, Greer FR. Probiotics and prebiotics in pediatrics. Pediatrics 2010; 126:1217–31.
68. Braegger C, Chmielewska A, Decsi T, et al. Supplementation of infant formula with probiotics and/or prebiotics: a systematic review and comment by the ESPGHAN committee on nutrition. J Pediatr Gastroenterol Nutr 2011;52:238–50.
69. Kataria J, Li N, Wynn JL, et al. Probiotic microbes: do they need to be alive to be beneficial? Nutr Rev 2009;67:546–50.
70. Lopez M, Li N, Kataria J, et al. Live and ultraviolet-inactivated Lactobacillus rhamnosus GG decrease flagellin-induced interleukin-8 production in Caco-2 cells. J Nutr 2008;138:2264–8.

71. Mazmanian SK, Round JL, Kasper DL. A microbial symbiosis factor prevents intestinal inflammatory disease. Nature 2008;29:620–5.
72. Antonowicz I, Lebenthal E. Developmental pattern of small intestinal enterokinase and disaccharidase activities in the human fetus. Gastroenterology 1977;72:1299–303.
73. Kien CL, McClead RE, Cordero LJ. Effects of lactose intake on lactose digestion and colonic fermentation in preterm infants. J Pediatr 1998;133:401–5.
74. Kien CL, Chang JC, Cooper JR. Quantitation of colonic luminal synthesis of butyric acid in piglets. J Pediatr Gastroenterol Nutr 2002;35:324–8.
75. Lifschitz C. Prevention of excessive crying by intestinal microbiota programming. J Pediatr 2013;163:1250–2.
76. Shamir R, St. James-Roberts I, DiLorenzo C, et al. Infant crying, colic, and gastrointestinal discomfort in early childhood: a review of the evidence and most plausible mechanisms. J Pediatr Gastroenterol Nutr 2013;57(Suppl 1):S1–45.
77. Ruhaak LR, Lebrilla CB. Analysis and role of oligosaccharides in milk. BMB Rep 2012;45:442–51.
78. Newburg DS, Grave G. Recent advances in human milk glycobiology. Pediatr Res 2014;75:675–9.
79. Manthey CF, Autran CA, Eckmann L, et al. Human milk oligosaccharides protect against enteropathogenic escherichia coli attachment in vitro and EPEC colonization in suckling mice. J Pediatr Gastroenterol Nutr 2014;58:167–70.
80. Li M, Monaco MH, Wang M, et al. Human milk oligosaccharides shorten rotavirus-induced diarrhea and modulate piglet mucosal immunity and colonic microbiota. ISME J 2014;8:1609–20.
81. Cammarota G, Ianiro G, Gasbarrini A. Fecal microbiota transplantation for the treatment of clostridium difficile infection: a systematic review. J Clin Gastroenterol 2014;48:693–702.
82. Nitzan O, Elias M, Chazan B, et al. Clostridium difficile and inflammatory bowel disease: role in pathogenesis and implications in treatment. World J Gastroenterol 2013;19:7577–85.
83. van Nood E, Speelman P, Nieuwdorp M, et al. Fecal microbiota transplantation: facts and controversies. Curr Opin Gastroenterol 2014;30:34–9.
84. Smits LP, Bouter KE, de Vos WM, et al. Therapeutic potential of fecal microbiota transplantation. Gastroenterology 2013;145:946–53.

Informing and Educating Parents About the Risks and Outcomes of Prematurity

U. Olivia Kim, MD, Mir A. Basir, MD, MS*

KEYWORDS

- Parent • Infant premature • Patient education • Counseling • Ethics
- Decision support techniques

KEY POINTS

- Current process of educating parents is suboptimal mostly because of modifiable factors.
- Proven methods to educate and inform parents are underused.
- Effective parent-clinician communication depends collectively on parents, clinicians, and the health care systems.
- Efforts must focus on improving communication and not on decreasing information provided to parents.

INTRODUCTION

Neonatal-perinatal medicine, although a relatively young subspecialty, has developed rapidly through its many advances in technology and treatment options. In the not too distant past, Patrick Bouvier Kennedy, son of President John F. Kennedy, was born at 34 weeks' gestation with immature lungs and, despite heroic measures, did not survive. Now survival of a 23-week premature infant is not unusual. This has created a sense of innovation and vigor that is exciting to the physicians who have chosen to specialize in this field, but is overwhelming and intimidating to the parents who find themselves as involuntary participants. Despite intensive care, all premature infants do not survive, and in the long-term, survivors are at increased risk of significant morbidities. Hence, the commitment to the care of premature infants gives rise to medical, ethical, and social dilemmas. Families bear the emotional and financial consequences of premature birth, and informed parents have the right to make treatment choices for their child, especially in clinical situations lacking sufficient evidence to direct

Disclosure: The authors having nothing to disclose.
Section of Neonatology, Department of Pediatrics, Children's Corporate Center, Suite 410, 999 N. 92nd Street, Medical College of Wisconsin, Milwaukee, WI 43226, USA
* Corresponding author.
E-mail address: mbasir@mcw.edu

treatment decisions. Hence, it is essential to inform parents regarding expectations of survival and outcome.[1]

In most institutions, this task is left to individual providers, which results in parents receiving information that may be inconsistent, inaccurate, and biased by the practitioner's own values and beliefs.[2] These current inadequacies in informing and educating parents results in "tokenistic parent involvement" and "devalued parental input," as clinicians feel that parents are "not well informed." To improve parental autonomy and encourage clinicians to truly involve parents in the care of their child, there is an urgent need to improve the provision of information to parents. **Table 1** outlines the information-seeking behaviors and informational needs of parents of premature infants.[3] Perhaps because of fear or denial of the impending preterm delivery, most parents initially are passive recipients of information. They neither seek out information nor even ask questions. It is up to the clinician to initiate parental education by supplying relevant information and walking the journey of prematurity with them.

HISTORICAL PERSPECTIVE

In the past, when hospitals did not exist, parents were the primary caregivers for their sick children and made all the decisions regarding their care. With the advent of

Table 1
Parental information-seeking behavior during prenatal period and the neonatal intensive care hospitalization

Variables	Prenatal Period	Early NICU Period	Later NICU Period
Infant status	• Threatened preterm birth	• Acute illness • High mortality period	• Convalescent • Nearing discharge
Parent status	• Anxious, uncertain • Mourning loss of normal pregnancy	• State of shock • Mother hospitalized • Unfamiliar NICU environment	• Familiar NICU environment • Infant is stable • Anxiety ↑at discharge
Parents learning process	• Parents are passive learners • Do not know what is important and what to ask • Learning initiated by others	• Begin self-initiated learning • Still mostly passive learners	• Become active learners • Ask questions • Use of books and Internet
Parents primary concern	• Maintain pregnancy • Infant health issues • Mother's medical issues	• Infant health issues • Infant care • Coping • Mother's recovery	• Infant health issues • Infant care • Coping
Topics parents want more information on	• Infant health issues • What to expect during labor • Guide to information sources	• Infant health issues • Understanding technical information • Coping	• Infant health issues • Infant care • Coping
Primary information resource	• Obstetric physician and nurse • Neonatologist	• NICU physician • NICU nurse	• NICU physician • NICU nurse

Abbreviation: NICU, neonatal intensive care unit.
Adapted from Brazy JE, Anderson BM, Becker PT, et al. How parents of premature infants gather information and obtain support. Neonatal Netw 2001;20(2):41–8.

modern medicine, hospitalization often became necessary. During such hospitalizations, medical professionals provided the required care, and parental involvement was considered unnecessary and even detrimental. In some nurseries, parents were allowed to view their children only through a window until the infant was ready for discharge.[4] The harmful results of the separation between parents and child became evident with an increase in "parenting disorders," including child neglect and abuse. In 1956, the Platt commission investigated these issues and encouraged parental involvement in their child's medical care. Consequently, restrictive hospital policies started to change and parents were welcomed into the hallowed halls of medicine.[5] However, the pendulum swung in 1982, when the Baby Doe law was designed to protect the interests of infants with disabling conditions. Some felt that this law encouraged overtreatment of extremely premature infants without consideration to long-term outcomes and parental concerns.[6] Parent advocates voiced concern that "in delivery-room and nursery crises, families have been at the mercy of an accelerating life-support technology and of their physicians' personal philosophies and motives concerning its use."[6] In response, Dr Jerold Lucey, editor of *Pediatrics*, arranged a conference in 1992 including parents and prominent US neonatologists to discuss these issues, and "The Principles for Family-Centered Neonatal Care" was then published.[7] Three of the 10 principles emphasize the need for open and honest communication on medical and ethical issues between parents and professionals. Currently, family-centered care is embraced in neonatal intensive care units (NICUs) and health care systems nationwide. Parental presence during their child's hospitalization is encouraged and facilitated through participation in daily rounds, bedside infant care, and shared medical decision-making between parents and clinicians.[8] However, medical professionals continue to hold the upper hand in decision-making. If parents choose an option different from that recommended by the physician, the medical professional doubts if the parents are "truly informed." Clearly there is more work to be done.

WE IMPROVE EACH OTHER

It is important to realize that to effectively inform and educate parents, factors related not just to the clinician but also to the parents and the health care systems come into play.[9] Throughout the literature, authors have identified both unique and ubiquitous characteristics within each group that can contribute to successful information transference, **Fig. 1**. The entanglement of many common factors among these 3 stakeholders (clinicians, parents, and health care systems) make it necessary to direct solutions for improving information provision by all involved.

IT'S NOT WHAT YOU SAY BUT HOW YOU SAY IT

Although neonatal counselors may focus on updated facts, statistics, and risks during consultations with parents, it's the delivery of this information that will determine if the parents hear, understand, and accept what is said. It is this part of counseling for prematurity that we wish to focus on so that we might delineate practical ways for medical providers to better convey information to parents. Let's begin by remembering a few fundamental facts. **Box 1** summarizes these "etiquettes."

IT'S NOT JUST THE NEONATOLOGIST WHO PROVIDES PARENTS INFORMATION ON PREMATURITY

First, it is important to recognize that nurses, both in obstetrics and neonatal intensive care, are the resources from which families get most of their information and support

Clinician Factors

- Trained in communication [identifies barriers, individualizes information]

- Motivated to form relationship [uses names, listens, supportive, explains]

- Utilizes tools [translators, information-aids]

- Asks parents [concerns, needs, fears, goals]

- Periodically checks understanding

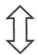 **CLINICIAN-PARENT COMMUNICATION**

Health care System Factors

- Values communication

- Provides communication training

- Invests in information/decision aids

- Provides in house translational services

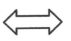

Parent Factors

- Health Literacy

- Baseline knowledge of prematurity

- Motivated [shares beliefs, concerns, preferences, opinions, emotions]

Fig. 1. Factors influencing clinician-parent communication.

during the hospitalization. According to the parents, nurses are the "best source" of information.[3] Second, before delivery, most pregnant women look to their obstetric provider for information and guidance regarding premature birth. Although the obstetric providers have an established relationship with the parents and have the most opportunities to educate and inform parents, studies show that obstetric providers are hesitant to provide information on the outcomes of premature infants. Moreover, obstetric providers are least likely to discuss neurologic outcomes.[10] In our survey, 50% of the obstetric providers reported that they "struggle" to answer parental questions regarding premature infants.[10] Further worsening this scenario, the amount of time parents spend prenatally with the neonatal counselor is extremely limited. Despite recommendations that this information be provided in small increments over several meetings for maximal maternal understanding,[1] studies show that prenatal education on prematurity to parents is often provided in only one encounter: during admission for threatened premature delivery.[2] Under these suboptimal conditions, counseling is broad, rushed, overwhelming, and can even be detrimental. The obstetric team, especially nurses, have an unrealized advantage to make a greater impact on the teaching of parents.

IT'S OKAY TO CHEAT

Some providers feel it's a sign of weakness to refer to a reference source when providing parents information, subsequently they base the information they give to parents on what they recall, which may not be accurate. When neonatal versus obstetric medical professional–provided gestational-age-specific outcome estimates are compared with actual outcome data, both groups underestimate survival and

---

Box 1
The etiquettes of counseling

- A good first impression:
  - ○ Introduce yourself [offer your business card]
  - ○ Sit down and speak in a nonhurried manner
  - ○ Describe your role in their medical care
  - ○ Ask them for their relevant information
    - ■ Use their names whenever possible.
- Let them know the purpose of the meeting:
  - ○ "I'm here to talk to you about your baby and answer any questions you might have."
- Use nontechnical language
- Use supplemental tools to reinforce information:
  - ○ Written information
  - ○ Visual aids (pictures or graphs)
  - ○ Audio recordings
  - ○ Reliable Internet sites
- Tailor the content and rate of information to the parents:
  - ○ Allow parents to ponder the information
  - ○ Frequently check for parental understanding by asking them to briefly state what they have understood.
- Build partnerships:
  - ○ Show empathy and respect

---

overestimate morbidities.[10,11] Consistency of information across providers and confidence in the source providing the information are important for parental learning.[3] Use of educational tools and pocket data cards improve physician recall and can make the information consistent across providers.[12] These cards should be used not to "spit out numbers" at parents but in a manner that engages them. While reviewing the data, the clinician can sit next to the parents and gently point out the statistics. When parents view the information on the card, the benefits of prolonging the pregnancy also become obvious and may motivate them to comply with their obstetrician's recommendations. Parents often ask for a copy of the card as well.

MORE MIGHT BE BETTER: PARENTS WANT MORE DETAILED INFORMATION

Most clinicians recognize that not all parents are cut from the same cloth. Some parents ask many questions and want to know details, whereas others find comfort in generalities. However, published literature overwhelmingly suggests that most parents of premature infants want to be informed about the potential risks and outcomes for their child and seek more information than is currently provided to them.[3,7,13] Despite half a million premature births annually in the United States, issues related to viability, survival, or outcomes of premature infants is not included in routine prenatal education.[14] Parents faced with a preterm birth realize their lack of knowledge and ask that this information be provided as quickly as possible after hospital admission.[15]

One mother wrote, "[He] told me all the issues…I didn't even think that… it was an option to even have a [baby at] 26 weeks…. We were, in all honesty and bluntness, prepared to have a burial for this child. We didn't know what to expect, or severe abnormalities, and we talked about it…through the night."[16] Further complicating this situation is the skewed view of premature infants portrayed by the media. Stories of "miracle babies" disillusion parents and often fill them with unrealistic expectations.[14] Given the decreased capability of parents to learn complex new information under duress and during threatened preterm delivery, some have recommended including basic prematurity information in routine prenatal education, whereas others are of the opinion that this will unnecessarily frighten pregnant women, yet another controversy.[14]

"DON'T FORGET ABOUT US": INFORMATION NEEDS OF PARENTS OF MODERATE AND LATE PREMATURE INFANTS

A large number of births are between 32 and 36 weeks' gestation. A review of 28 studies showed that these children have more school problems, less-advanced cognition, more behavior problems, and higher prevalence of psychiatric problems when compared with their full-term peers.[17] We assessed parental knowledge of both short-term and long-term outcomes for premature infants born at gestational age of less than 34 weeks, and we found no difference in parental knowledge of short-term outcomes, although knowledge of long-term outcomes decreased with advancing gestational age.[18] This may be because long-term outcomes of a moderately premature infant is less of a priority for clinicians, as no urgent decisions need to be made regarding extent of treatment. Despite that fact, other obstetric treatment decisions may be influenced by parental knowledge and preferences. In the United States, preterm labor induction beyond 27 weeks' gestation has increased.[19] In many instances, iatrogenic preterm delivery may be clearly indicated; however, in other instances it may not. In fact most of such preterm deliveries are not based on evidence endorsed by the American College of Obstetrics and Gynecology or published expert opinion.[20] The National Perinatal Association recently recommended that clinicians communicate the risks of late preterm birth to parents, explaining that underdeveloped organ systems, including the brain, may lead to complications.[21] Currently, clinicians are uncertain of how much of this information needs to be shared with parents and some clinicians are of the opinion that providing such information may harm parents.[22] However, this information is important for parents to know to provide informed consent for obstetric procedures. In clinical situations when there is no clear evidence to determine whether to interrupt or let the pregnancy continue, outcome information for the moderate-late preterm infant needs to be shared with the parents to enable them to effectively participate in decision-making before delivery. However, in clinical situations when delivery is clearly beneficial, this information can be shared with the parents during the postnatal period before the infant's discharge. We have found that these parents are just as anxious as parents of extremely premature infants, but they are less aware of the long-term implications of prematurity.[18]

A SPOONFUL OF SUGAR HELPS THE MEDICINE GO DOWN: NEGATIVE PROGNOSTIC INFORMATION AND PARENTAL PARTICIPATION IN END-OF-LIFE DECISION-MAKING

Historically, medical professionals have underestimated the benefits, willingness, and ability of parents to participate in their child's care. This was recently evidenced by medical professional reluctance to include parents in daily attending rounds.[23]

Evaluation of parental attitudes and feelings after the death of their child resulting from withdrawal of mechanical ventilation after joint parent-physician decision-making shows that parents can participate as worthy partners with their physicians in life and death decisions. These parents then seem to adjust to their loss with healthy grieving.[24] We assessed parental anxiety using the State Trait Anxiety Inventory (STAI), a validated tool. Contrary to the opinions of many medical providers, presenting more details on morbidities associated with prematurity (when done properly) actually decreased maternal anxiety and increased their knowledge of long-term problems, including neurologic, behavior, and learning disorders.[25] We should never forget that although many mothers want to be involved in these types of critical decision-making, they instinctively carry a spark of hope that their infant might survive. It is neither our responsibility nor prerogative to extinguish that flame. One mother said, "I don't know what the legalities are, but my feeling at the time was that oh, we needed a lot of positive reinforcement …and what we got was the exact opposite." Let us remember that you don't have to make the parents cry to convince yourself that they understand the gravity of the situation.

"TEACH US SO WE CAN LEARN": HOW PARENTS WANT THE INFORMATION TO BE PRESENTED

When it comes to receiving information, each parent's personal characteristics and their past experiences significantly influence how they receive and respond to information. Some show interest, ask questions, and develop a rapport with the clinicians. With others, the conversation is short due to absence of these cues. Regardless of the social dynamics, all parents deserve to know the risks, concerns, and potential outcomes for their premature infant. Current evidence suggests that parental information-seeking behavior can actually be changed to make parents more active participants. This is supported by the observation that through the course of neonatal hospitalization, as the parents start to understand their child's health issues and become familiar with the neonatal intensive care environment, medical professionals, and medical technology, they become active learners, asking questions and seeking out more information through books and the Internet.[3] After discharge from the NICU, parents stated that they wanted consistent, clear, detailed information and with limited jargon. Moreover, parents wanted information that was specific and individualized for their child. If possible, they also wanted to have this information repeated over several meetings.[26] Delivering information in ways that are relevant and meaningful to the parents is a challenge, and yet this can be achieved if the clinicians spend time to understand parental values, concerns, and goals. Parents also want the underlying tone of the clinician conversation to show support and care.

DIFFERENT STROKES FOR DIFFERENT FOLKS: COMMUNICATING EVIDENCE TO PARENTS

Most parents want to know the chance of survival for their child and many even want to know the gestational-age–specific probabilities of specific complications of prematurity.[27] The American Academy of Pediatrics recommends that this information be provided to the parents, which is easier said than done.[1] Effectively describing statistics to parents can be arduous; however, it is important that clinicians know how to best provide this information because usually the first question posed by parents to clinicians is "what are the chances that my baby will survive?" Clinicians often answer this question in various ways: (1) using generalities, for example, "it is rare for an infant born at this gestational age to survive," (2) giving numerical probabilities such as "1 of

10 infants born at this gestational age will survive," and (3) giving graphic or pictorial representations of the estimates.[28] For example, some have developed decision aids using visual cards to convey numerical evidence.[27] Using generalities is discouraged because there is significant variation in interpretation. For example, patients interpret "rare" as 24% $\pm$ 30%, whereas physicians interpret "rare" as 5% $\pm$ 6%.[29] Even in clinical situations that are similar, no single approach works with all parents. Provision of written handouts with verbal information increased recall of numerical information, including chance of survival and probability of certain neonatal outcomes in pregnant women admitted for threatened preterm delivery.[25] Based on the literature, some suggestions are presented in **Box 2**.

"HELP US TO REMEMBER": PARENTS WANT WRITTEN AND OTHER SUPPLEMENTAL INFORMATION

Although parents state they prefer information to be provided in face-to-face meetings, they find that supplemental sources of information, such as written material, enhances their ability to understand and participate in consultations, especially when the

---

Box 2
Tips, slips, and skills in communicating evidence to parents

- Flexibility in providing evidence:

  One style does not work for all. Assess and change your style according to how parents seem to learn the best.

- No lecturing:

  Encourage active partnership.

- Check comprehension:

  Have parents summarize what they understand.

- When informing about the chance of a certain outcome, present proportion and not probability:

  It is easier to understand "1 out of 10 survive" than "10% survive."

- Use lower denominators:

  "1 out of 10" is easier to comprehend than "10 out of 100."

- Be aware of "framing bias":

  Parents may perceive "1 out of 10 survive," as a positive outcome and "9 out of 10 die," as a negative outcome when actually there is no difference between the two. State the information both ways.

- When comparing 2 treatments, present absolute risk difference and not relative risk:

  Absolute risk is easier to understand and provides estimate of the magnitude of the difference. "Treatment A will reduce the risk of NEC from 2 in 100 to 1 in 100." Whereas, relative risk may be misleading. "Treatment A will reduce the risk of NEC by 50%," as it exaggerates the positive effect when the magnitude of change is small.

- Avoid placing categorical labels to data:

  Designating developmental morbidity as mild/moderate/severe inappropriately adds a value label to the information. Alternately, the test scores may be provided without the labels.

- Supplemental resources:

  Reinforce information with written handouts and audio-recordings of the meeting.

written information is given to them before the meeting with the clinician.[15] At our center, we assessed maternal comprehension after verbal counseling alone and found mothers lacked knowledge of long-term outcomes.[22] Subsequently, in a randomized trial, maternal recognition of long-term outcomes and recall of outcome data was found to be significantly higher in mothers who received written information before face-to-face consultation with a neonatal provider compared with those who were not given supplemental information.[25] Other groups have successfully developed and used similar written guidelines,[30] visual aids,[27,31,32] and audio recordings[33,34] to augment information provision. Interestingly, although these educational tools are well-received by parents, some physicians do not recommend the use of this augmentation because of concerns that the clinical condition could change rapidly and these static sources of information would not be used effectively.

"LET US SEE WHAT YOU SEE": PARENTAL ACCESS TO THEIR CHILD'S MEDICAL RECORD DURING THE NEONATAL HOSPITALIZATION

Parents also report the desire to access information from their child's medical records during the hospitalization. Some were unsure if they were "allowed" to access the medical record, but they reported looking at it anyway. One parent noted, "all the time I look at what happened the night before: his saturation, if they needed to stimulate him, increased his oxygen. I look at his chart every day."[26] The transition to electronic medical records (EMRs) makes it virtually impossible for parents to sneak a look at their child's record on a regular basis. We surveyed 85 parents and 133 medical provider opinions in the NICU regarding direct parental access to their child's EMR.[34] Both medical professionals and parents agreed that direct EMR access may increase parental understanding of their child's care; however, medical professionals were hesitant to allow direct access because of perceived negative repercussions, including increased documentation time, potential harm to parents, and scrutiny. Further study will clarify if this access is akin to Pandora's Box or improved family-centered care.

TURNING THE *TITANIC*: HEALTH CARE SYSTEM CHALLENGES

The American Academy of Pediatrics outlines institutional expectations to inform parents anticipating birth of an extremely premature infant.[1] Health care systems uniquely influence potentially modifiable factors. Most premature infants and their families are cared for in community-based nonacademic hospitals where medical providers and the hospital administration are often unclear about the legal and ethical aspects surrounding prematurity. In a national study including responses from 337 hospitals in 47 states, we evaluated several counselor-independent elements to counseling and found several deficiencies that compromised parental learning. They included (1) lack of hospital-specific outcome data, (2) lack of identified regional or national data for data provision to parents, (3) lack of institutional multidisciplinary consensus guidelines, (4) lack of interpreters for Spanish-speaking parents, and (5) lack of a library of written/audio/video information-aids to supplement verbally provided information.[2] Prominent neonatal clinicians and ethicists have voiced their concern that health care systems have invested human and financial resources in saving premature infants, as this is lucrative; however, hospitals do not invest in the poorly reimbursed services essential for these premature infants and their families to thrive after discharge.[35] Changing the culture of national health care systems in these economic times may be the greatest challenge yet.

SENDING WITHOUT EQUIPPING: COMMUNICATION TRAINING FOR COUNSELORS

There is a lack of specific training in prenatal counseling and communication for neonatal clinicians.[2,36] Such training can optimize presentation of information and help identify and minimize barriers by (1) identifying and playing to the parent's strengths; (2) overcoming the socioeconomic, educational, cultural, and racial differences often present between clinicians and parents; (3) eliciting parental values, preferences, and needs; (4) establishing goals and expectations through shared deliberation with parents; and (5) develop a trusting partnership with parents. Communication and interpersonal skills is now a competency required by the Accreditation Council for Graduate Medical Education for all Neonatal-Perinatal Medicine fellows in training. However, formal and discrete education on how to optimally provide information and develop a healthy partnership with parents remain lacking.

LEAVE YOUR BAGGAGE AT THE DOOR: MINIMIZING BIAS WHEN SHARING OUTCOME DATA WITH PARENTS

In part due to parental advocacy, investigators have systematically gathered outcome data for premature infants, including some infants who have reached young adulthood. However, appropriate interpretation of published data to predict outcome of a particular preterm infant is difficult because of the many differences in the population, families, and institutional practices.[37] Center-specific data overcome some of these variations, but is limited by patient numbers and long-term information availability. Data that perfectly fit the patient are not available in most cases, and the best the clinician can do is to identify these differences while sharing information with parents and adjusting the estimates to personalize the information. Remember that follow-up studies categorize developmental outcomes as mild, moderate, and severe, whereas in reality these outcomes are a continuum. Use of categorical terms adds bias by adding a value label to the information.[38] How information is presented, including the choice of words and body language, may introduce bias. For example, stating "the chance of survival is 80%" or "the chance of mortality is 20%" may lead to different conclusions because of framing bias, even though the meaning is the same.[39] Although it is not possible to remove all bias while sharing information with parents; however, recognizing that bias exists, even in you, is important to strive to achieve neutrality.

THE DEBATE: PROVIDING INFORMATION FOR RESUSCITATIVE DECISION-MAKING FOR EXTREMELY PREMATURE INFANTS

This is perhaps one of the most difficult and controversial aspects of counseling for prematurity. To review the ethical aspects of delivery room resuscitation of extremely premature infants is outside the scope of this review and is not our intent. However, it is discussed in a separate review within this journal. Neonatal clinicians and ethical experts have strong differences in opinion regarding the best course of therapy for the extremely premature infant and how to relay this information to the parents.[40] These antithetic convictions erupted when the Canadian Pediatric Society Fetus and Newborn Committee published their guidelines in "Counseling and Management for Anticipated Extremely Preterm Birth."[41] After reviewing the literature, the Canadian Pediatric Society proposed 15 recommendations that addressed the timing of prenatal counseling, promoted joint decision-making, and offered gestational age–specific advice. However, instruction on how to best counsel, what information to include, and how to personalize the discussion were omitted. Hence, the recommendations were ill-received by many. Many clinical neonatologists publicly rejected the new position statement by claiming it was "a way to avoid responsibility for life-and-death decisions by proposing and following simple and scientifically flawed algorithms."[40] This recent public disagreement demonstrates the strong bias/opinions present among well-intentioned medical professionals and the importance of the information provided to parents. Clinician bias/opinion determine institutional "philosophy" of treatment of extremely premature infants. Resuscitation practices vary significantly in the same city. Currently, there is no mechanism in place to guide parents to hospitals that share the same "philosophy" of care as the parents.

FINAL THOUGHTS: SUMMARY

Experienced clinicians routinely tailor the extent of information provided to accommodate the immediate parental/patient needs, as well as parental preferences and assimilating capacities. However, clinicians must guard against stereotyping parents and justify providing less information to parents from certain backgrounds, to save clinician time or to avoid controversial aspects of treatments.[42] In situations that are novel and unanticipated, like premature delivery, parents usually do not have preexisting preferences. Therefore, education on prematurity is necessary to build a foundation of knowledge for parents to construct their preferences that reflect their family's values and beliefs.[43] Effectively informing and educating parents of premature infants is too important to be left to mere chance. It requires a collective effort by clinicians, parents and health care systems to establish clinical guidelines, train clinicians in patient communication, develop information aids to supplement verbal information, and provide prematurity information during routine prenatal visits. **Fig. 2** outlines this strategy. Ultimately, it is our job to equip parents so that they can advocate for their child. If done successfully, we might find new and worthy allies in the trenches of the NICU.

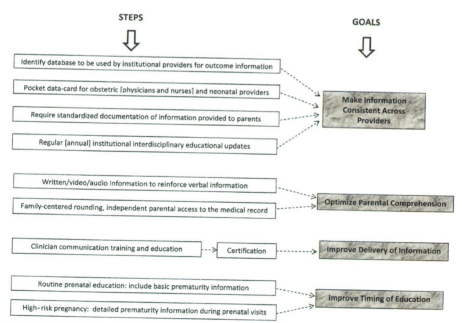

Fig. 2. Steps to improve parental comprehension of clinician provided information.

REFERENCES

1. Batton DG, Committee on Fetus and Newborn. Clinical report—antenatal counseling regarding resuscitation at an extremely low gestational age. Pediatrics 2009;124(1):422–7.
2. Mehrotra A, Lagatta J, Simpson P, et al. Variations among US hospitals in counseling practices regarding prematurely born infants. J Perinatol 2013;33(7):509–13.
3. Brazy JE, Anderson BM, Becker PT, et al. How parents of premature infants gather information and obtain support. Neonatal Netw 2001;20(2):41–8.
4. Fanaroff AA, Kennell JH, Klaus MH. Follow-up of low birth weight infants—the predictive value of maternal visiting patterns. Pediatrics 1972;49(2):287–90.
5. Davies R. Marking the 50th anniversary of the Platt report: from exclusion, to toleration and parental participation in the care of the hospitalized child. J Child Health Care 2010;14:6–23.
6. Harrison H. Parents and handicapped infants. N Engl J Med 1983;309(11):664–5.
7. Harrison H. The principles for family-centered neonatal care. Pediatrics 1993;92(5):643–50.
8. Committee on Hospital Care. Family-centered care and the pediatrician's role. Pediatrics 2003;112(3):691–6.
9. Epstein RM, Street RL. Patient-centered communication in cancer care: promoting healing and reducing suffering. 2007.
10. Powell MR, Kim UO, Weisgerber MC, et al. Readiness of obstetric professionals to inform parents regarding potential outcome of premature infants. J Obstet Gynaecol 2012;32(4):326–31.
11. Haywood JL, Goldenberg RL, Bronstein J, et al. Comparison of perceived and actual rates of survival and freedom from handicap in premature infants. Am J Obstet Gynecol 1994;171(2):432–9.
12. Blanco F, Suresh G, Howard D, et al. Ensuring accurate knowledge of prematurity outcomes for prenatal counseling. Pediatrics 2005;115(4):e478–87.
13. Perlman NB, Freedman JL, Abramovitch R, et al. Informational needs of parents of sick neonates. Pediatrics 1991;88(3):512–8.
14. Catlin A. Thinking outside the box: prenatal care and the call for a prenatal advance directive. J Perinat Neonatal Nurs 2005;19(2):169–76.
15. Grobman WA, Kavanaugh K, Moro T, et al. Providing advice to parents for women at acutely high risk of periviable delivery. Obstet Gynecol 2010;115(5):904–9.
16. Young E, Tsai E, O'Riordan A. A qualitative study of predelivery counseling for extreme prematurity. Paediatr Child Health 2012;17(8):432–6.
17. de Jong M, Verhoeven M, van Baar AL. School outcome, cognitive functioning, and behaviour problems in moderate and late preterm children and adults: a review. Semin Fetal Neonatal Med 2012;17(3):163–9.
18. Govande VP, Brasel KJ, Das UG, et al. Prenatal counseling beyond the threshold of viability. J Perinatol 2013;33(5):358–62.
19. Davidoff MJ, Dias T, Damus K, et al. Changes in the gestational age distribution among US singleton births: impact on rates of late preterm birth, 1992 to 2002. Semin Perinatol 2006;30(1):8–15.
20. Gyamfi-Bannerman C, Fuchs KM, Young OM, et al. Nonspontaneous late preterm birth: etiology and outcomes. Obstet Gynecol 2011;205(5):456.e1–6.
21. Phillips RM, Goldstein M, Hougland K, et al. Multidisciplinary guidelines for the care of late preterm infants. J Perinatol 2013;33(Suppl 2):S5–22.
22. Govande VP, Lagatta J, Basir MA. Reply to Stokes and Watson. J Perinatol 2013;33(10):823–4.

23. McPherson G, Jefferson R, Kissoon N, et al. Toward the inclusion of parents on pediatric critical care unit rounds. Pediatr Crit Care Med 2011;12(6):e255–61.
24. Benfield DG, Leib SA, Vollman JH. Grief response of parents to neonatal death and parent participation in deciding care. Pediatrics 1978;62(2):171–7.
25. Muthusamy AD, Leuthner S, Gaebler-Uhing C, et al. Supplemental written information improves prenatal counseling: a randomized trial. Pediatrics 2012; 129(5):e1269–74.
26. Harvey ME, Nongena P, Gonzalez-Cinca N, et al. Parents' experiences of information and communication in the neonatal unit about brain imaging and neurological prognosis: a qualitative study. Acta Paediatr 2013;102(4):360–5.
27. Guillen U, Suh S, Munson D, et al. Development and pretesting of a decision-aid to use when counseling parents facing imminent extreme premature delivery. J Pediatr 2012;160(3):382–7.
28. Epstein RM, Alper BS, Quill TE. Communicating evidence for participatory decision making. JAMA 2004;291(19):2359–66.
29. Sutherland HJ, Lockwood GA, Tritchler DL, et al. Communicating probabilistic information to cancer patients: is there 'noise' on the line? Soc Sci Med 1991;32(6): 725–31.
30. Kaempf JW, Tomlinson M. Long-term health outcomes of extremely premature infants. Pediatrics 2007;119(2):410–1.
31. Jennings L, Yebadokpo AS, Affo J, et al. Antenatal counseling in maternal and newborn care: use of job aids to improve health worker performance and maternal understanding in Benin. BMC Pregnancy Childbirth 2010;10:75.
32. Kakkilaya V, Groome LJ, Platt D, et al. Use of a visual aid to improve counseling at the threshold of viability. Pediatrics 2011;128(6):e1511–9.
33. Koh TH, Jarvis C. Promoting effective communication in neonatal intensive care units by audiotaping doctor-parent conversations. Int J Clin Pract 1998;52(1):27–9.
34. Chung RK, Kim UO, Shepherd ST. Pandora's box or improved family-centered care: direct parental access to their child's electronic medical record during hospitalization. Abstract presented at the Pediatrics Academic Society, 2014.
35. Lantos J. Cruel calculus: why saving premature babies is better business than helping them thrive. Health Aff (Millwood) 2010;29(11):2114–7.
36. Boss RD, Hutton N, Donohue PK, et al. Neonatologist training to guide family decision making for critically ill infants. Arch Pediatr Adolesc Med 2009;163(9): 783–8.
37. Meadow W, Lagatta J, Andrews B, et al. The mathematics of morality for neonatal resuscitation. Clin Perinatol 2012;39(4):941–56.
38. Batton D. Resuscitation of extremely low gestational age infants: an Advisory Committees Dilemma. Acta Paediatr 2010;99(6):810–1.
39. Haward MF, John LK, Lorenz JM, et al. Effects of description of options on parental perinatal decision-making. Pediatrics 2012;129(5):891–902.
40. Janvier A, Barrington KJ, Aziz K, et al. CPS position statement for prenatal counselling before a premature birth: simple rules for complicated decisions. Paediatr Child Health 2014;19(1):22–4.
41. Jefferies AL, Kirpalani HM, Canadian Paediatric Society Fetus and Newborn, Committee. Counselling and management for anticipated extremely preterm birth. Paediatr Child Health 2012;17(8):443–6.
42. Epstein RM, Korones DN, Quill TE. Withholding information from patients—when less is more. N Engl J Med 2010;362(5):380–1.
43. Epstein RM, Peters E. Beyond information: exploring patients' preferences. JAMA 2009;302(2):195–7.

Ethical Issues in DNA Sequencing in the Neonate

CrossMark

David P. Dimmock, MD*, David P. Bick, MD

KEYWORDS

- Newborn screening • Whole genome sequencing
- Severe combined immunodeficiency polymerase chain reaction

KEY POINTS

- The goal of presymptomatic genetic and genomic testing is to identify newborns with potentially serious or fatal disorders that can be successfully treated, and thereby achieve significant reduction in morbidity and mortality.
- DNA testing is now routinely employed for presymptomatic newborn screening as well as for rapid diagnosis of congenital anomalies.
- The breadth of sequencing now possible raises issues of consent and feasibility of data return.

INTRODUCTION

The goal of presymptomatic genetic and genomic testing is to identify newborns with potentially serious or fatal disorders that can be successfully treated, and thereby achieve significant reduction in morbidity and mortality.

With the recognition of genetic disorders in the newborn there is the potential to offer new lifesaving therapies such as dietary intervention for phenylalanine hydroxylase deficiency (PKU). In other conditions such as hypothyroidism in Down syndrome or hypocalcemia in the 22q11 microdeletion syndrome, the early identification of an untreatable condition allows prompt screening for potential comorbid conditions, thus preventing complications and improving outcomes. The dramatic reduction in the cost of DNA testing has enabled widespread and comprehensive implementation of such technology in neonatal practice. The last 10 years has seen the implementation of routine DNA-based newborn screening for severe combined immunodeficiency (SCID)[1] as well as whole-genome sequencing for the evaluation of symptomatic children.[2] Such implementation has not been without its controversy[3] and is a far cry from the routine practice of many neonatologists. The purpose of this article is to describe

Medical College of Wisconsin, 8701 West Watertown Plank Road, Milwaukee, WI 53226, USA
* Corresponding author.
E-mail address: ddimmock@mcw.edu

Clin Perinatol 41 (2014) 993–1000
http://dx.doi.org/10.1016/j.clp.2014.08.016   **perinatology.theclinics.com**

the currently employed DNA diagnostic tests, noting their key benefits and limitations as applied in the newborn period.

GOALS OF CLINICAL DNA TESTING IN THE NEONATE

The goal of pre-symptomatic genetic and genomic testing is to identify newborns with potentially serious or fatal disorders that can be successfully treated, and thereby achieve significant reduction in morbidity and mortality. The 50-year history of newborn screening demonstrates that the prompt identification of genetic disorders both save lives and is a cost-efficient public health undertaking.[4] Not all genetic disorders have a ready treatment. Nonetheless, changes in care that result from definitive genetic diagnosis improve health surveillance in most cases. Additionally parents report significant comfort in the knowledge of a confirmed genetic disorder.[5]

As knowledge of the causes of genetic disorders increases, detection technologies advance, and better treatment regimens emerge, the complexity of testing and resultant interpretation will increase. In addition, there is an increasing ability to make diagnosis of adult-onset conditions before symptoms arise, including those with limited therapeutic options. This may arise either purposefully or incidentally as a result of screening for other conditions.

KEY BENEFITS OF DNA TESTING
Utility of DNA Testing When a Diagnosis Is Clinically Apparent

In situations in which a clinical diagnosis is apparent from examination alone, there is significant benefit to providing genetic testing to confirm results. For example, in the diagnosis of trisomy 13, in which difficult therapeutic decisions such as withdrawal of therapy are often considered, a definitive molecular result provides an additional level of confidence in the diagnosis. In addition, for several common conditions there are clinical look-alikes such as pseudotrisomy 13, for which the inheritance pattern is different.[6] Similarly, the origin of the extra genetic material in Down syndrome (translocation vs trisomy 21) has significant implications for recurrence risks.

Ability of DNA Diagnosis to End Further Workup or Screening

In certain clinical situations such as a newborn with progressive liver disease several genetic disorders are considered. Historically, to make a definitive diagnosis that would allow for definitive treatment, enzymatic or functional testing of a liver biopsy specimen was needed. In disorders such as symptomatic Arthrogryposis-Renal dysfunction-Cholestasis (ARC) syndrome, in which such procedures carry a risk, DNA-based testing can resolve the diagnosis more safely.[7]

Treatment Dependent on Molecular Results

There is increasing interest in therapeutics that are targeted at the underlying molecular genetic defect. For example, in individuals with a premature termination codon (PTC) (ie, a change in the DNA code that leads the translation machinery to produce a truncated protein that does not function) specific medications have been developed and are in clinical trials that allow the cellular machinery to read through such a termination codon and produce a full-length protein.[8]

Key Benefit of DNA Testing to the Family

Identification of the specific mutation(s) in an affected family member allows for efficient identification of other presymptomatic family members at risk for disease. This allows for screening and preventive therapy in such individuals. Important examples of this include hereditary hemorrhagic telangiectasia (HHT)[9] von Hippel-Lindau (VHL),[10] retinoblastoma[11] and Alagille syndrome.[12]

KEY PROBLEMS WITH DNA TESTING

There have been dramatic advances in the speed of returning results from targeted testing[1] to whole genome sequencing[13] in the newborn period. At the point of care for most institutions, testing remains expensive and poorly reimbursed. Moreover, results are frequently not completed to allow for timely management decisions to be made.

DNA test results may be perceived by consumers, including physicians, as more deterministic than other tests.[14,15] Such conclusions ignore the dramatic success of treatment following early identification of disorders such as phenylketonuria by changing the patient's environment and the variable penetrance of many adult-onset disorders. Nonetheless, the identification of genetic disorders may have the potential to lead to altered perceptions of self- and potential psychological harm.[16] If testing finds an adult-onset disorder that leads to identification of other at-risk family members, these diagnoses potentially affect the ability of these family members to get life and disability insurance.

TESTING MODALITIES
Polymerase Chain Reaction Detection of Nongermline DNA: Newborn Screening for Severe Combined Immunodeficiency—the T-Cell Receptor Excision Circle Assay

In its simplest form, DNA testing can be designed to detect and quantify the amount of a specific DNA sequence. Such detection frequently uses nucleic acid amplification techniques such as polymerase chain reaction (PCR) with subsequent quantification of the number of DNA copies detected. In many instances, a second target is also selected to serve as a control. In the neonatal setting, practitioners are most familiar with the use of such techniques to detect pathogens such as PCR detection of herpes virus[17,18] or HIV. However, such molecular techniques can be used to evaluate for the presence or absence of human genomic DNA sequences.

SCID is a group of disorders caused by more than a dozen single-gene defects. All known gene mutations cause a defect in the development of normal naïve T cells. During normal T-cell development, genomic rearrangement leads to the production of T-cell receptor excision circles (TRECs). One specific TREC has been shown to serve as a reliable surrogate marker for the number of naïve T cells. Quantitative PCR can be employed to quantify TREC number on dried blood spots providing an approximate quantification of naïve T cells. Consequently, individuals with T cell leukopenia have low levels of the TRECs.[19] This is the basis for severe combined immunodeficiency test on dried blood spots successfully employed for newborn screening.[1] Variations on this technique can be used to detect B cell-related immunodeficiency,[20] as well as testing for infectious diseases from newborn screening blood spot cards.[21–24] Although cost-effective,[25] the detection of SCID subjects an apparently healthy child to an expensive and risky procedure.

Pathogenic Variant Screening for High-Risk Infants

Aminoglycoside antibiotics are used relatively frequently in the neonatal intensive care unit (ICU), but they can lead to significant hearing impairment. This risk of hearing loss is largely conferred by mutations in the mitochondrial 12S rRNA gene, the most frequent of which is the mt.1555A>G mutation.[26] Screening for such mutations is possible at birth.[27,28] However, it is currently unclear how to weight knowledge of such risk factors when deviating from well-established therapies that have a demonstrated benefit in preventing mortality.[29] Further adaptive research will be required to evaluate how to integrate such knowledge into routine clinical care.

Germline Chromosome Complement

Birth defects are present in approximately 3% of neonates born in the United States,[30] and genetic factors have been documented as an important cause as part of syndromic or isolated defects.[31,32] Many recognizable syndromes in the newborn period are the result of the duplication or deletion of large regions of genomic material. The most commonly recognized disorders are the trisomies: trisomy 13 (Patau syndrome), trisomy 18 (Edwards syndrome), trisomy 21 (Down syndrome) and monosomy X (Turner syndrome). Such disorders are readily detectable by routine cytogenetic analysis. In these cases, white blood cells are grown in culture, and the chromosomes are stained to make them visible under a microscope.

Approximately 1% of neonates are thought to have syndromic multiple congenital anomalies (MCA). Of these, it is estimated that 40% may be given a clinical diagnosis, mostly as a result of chromosomal abnormalities such as Down syndrome, with the remaining 60% (approximately 25,000 babies each year in the United States) having an unidentified MCA syndrome.[33]

Higher-resolution testing for duplication or deletion of specific smaller regions of chromosomes requires a different molecular technique. Throughout most of the 1990s, this relied upon fluorescent in situ hybridization to interrogate specific known loci.

The widespread use of chromosome array comparative genomic hybridization (CMA) has demonstrated a strong underlying genetic contribution to MCAs.[5] Specifically, 10% to 20% of infants with MCA, previously categorized as undefined with standard cytogenetic technology alone, have clinically defined microdeletion syndromes.[34] In a large cohort evaluating the effects of CMA, the establishment of a microdeletion syndrome led to increased appropriate referrals, appropriate laboratory testing, and increased provider confidence in care. Just as significantly, CMA and subsequent identification of microdeletion improved parental satisfaction and improved ability for families to find a support group of families with a similar disorder.[5]

Genome-wide testing in the form of chromosomal microarray is already in widespread clinical use.[34,35] This test raises several complex issues for patients and families. For example, chromosomal microarray will

- Detect germ line deletions of genes that predispose to later-onset disease and that are not the primary target of investigation; find copy number variants of unknown clinical significance
- In the instance single nucleotide polymorphisms (SNP) based arrays are used, they will detect variants related to pharmacogenomic or cancer risk

Consequently, such tests have the potential to reveal unintended information as well as information directly germane to the clinical question under consideration.[36] That said, microarray has significantly increased the diagnostic yield in newborns,[34] including children with critical congenital heart disease.[37]

Prenatal screening for these conditions has been revolutionized by the availability of next-generation sequencing technologies in the evaluation of cell-free fetal DNA in maternal circulation. DNA from this source contains approximately equal proportions of copy number to chromosome number as the fetal placental cells. The technique allows for low-resolution whole-genome sequencing and alignment of reads to a reference DNA. After subtraction from maternal DNA it is possible to count how many copies of each chromosome there are.[38] Although this is a relatively reliable screening tools in high-risk pregnancies[38] and in lower-risk pregnancies[39] to detect an extra chromosome copy such as trisomy 21, these tests can lead to false positives as a results of confined placental mosaicism,[40] as well as false negatives as a result of fetal mosaicism.[41] Consequently, such prenatal tests should not be relied upon to make a definitive diagnosis without follow-up amniocentesis, chorionic villus sampling, or postnatal chromosome testing.

Early detection and intervention in congenital heart defects is generally seen to improve outcomes and, for ductal-dependent lesions, these may reduce mortality. Furthermore, presymptomatic identification reduces the chance of clinical deterioration before treatment is initiated. This ultimately reduces length of stay in the ICU, while improving mortality and neurologic outcome.[42] Such defects may not be detected by pulse oximetry screening.[42] The published literature suggests that approximately 80% of clinically identified cases of 22q11 microdeletion syndrome have such cardiac defects.[43] Therefore, there has been a drive to extend the reach of newborn screening to detect this chromosomal defect. At this point in time, there remains much to be understood about the frequency of 22q11 microdeletion syndrome.[43]

GENOME-WIDE SEQUENCING

Genome-wide sequencing has recently entered clinical trials for use in neonatal care as an option for patients with rare or uncertain phenotypes.[3] Whole-genome sequencing has been demonstrated to have a superior diagnostic yield to many other forms of genetic testing.[2,3,44,45] However, there are many challenges related to the interpretation of such data.[46] Furthermore, many individuals remain concerned about the risks of such less targeted testing, as it will reveal secondary or incidental findings.[47] There remain many controversies concerning which incidental findings should be returned.[2,3,36,47,48] Consequently, careful application of such technology in potentially vulnerable newborns is recommended.[3,36,41]

SUMMARY/DISCUSSION

DNA testing for disorders and DNA-based screening are rapidly evolving. With new more powerful tests, there is an increasing ability to see a child's potential future if left untreated and change newborns' outcomes. However, there remain significant ethical and structural issues to be considered before routine implementation. These issues include when to deploy screening tests and what threshold must be reached before such testing can be considered for newborn screening. Institutions and providers will have to establish what policies and procedures should be in place for primary results return and who should decide which secondary (incidental) results are to be returned. Despite these concerns, the evolution of DNA testing over the past decade has had significant impact in reducing neonatal morbidity and mortality.

REFERENCES

1. Routes JM, Grossman WJ, Verbsky J, et al. Statewide newborn screening for severe T-cell lymphopenia. JAMA 2009;302:2465–70.
2. Jacob HJ, Abrams K, Bick DP, et al. Genomics in clinical practice: lessons from the front lines. Sci Transl Med 2013;5:194cm5.
3. Kingsmore SF. Incidental swimming with millstones. Sci Transl Med 2013;5:194ed10.

4. Boyle CA, Bocchini JA Jr, Kelly J. Reflections on 50 years of newborn screening. Pediatrics 2014;133:961–3.
5. Coulter ME, Miller DT, Harris DJ, et al. Chromosomal microarray testing influences medical management. Genet Med 2011;13:770–6.
6. Pseudotrisomy 13. In: OMIM. Available at: http://omim.org/entry/264480. Accessed June 1, 2014.
7. Gissen P, Tee L, Johnson CA, et al. Clinical and molecular genetic features of ARC syndrome. Hum Genet 2006;120:396–409.
8. Sermet-Gaudelus I, Boeck KD, Casimir GJ, et al. Ataluren (PTC124) induces cystic fibrosis transmembrane conductance regulator protein expression and activity in children with nonsense mutation cystic fibrosis. Am J Respir Crit Care Med 2010;182:1262–72.
9. McDonald J, Pyeritz RE. Hereditary hemorrhagic telangiectasia. In: Pagon RA, Adam MP, Ardinger HH, et al, editors. Seattle (WA): GeneReviews; 1993.
10. Frantzen C, Links TP, Giles RH. Von Hippel-Lindau disease. In: Pagon RA, Adam MP, Ardinger HH, et al, editors. Seattle (WA): GeneReviews; 1993.
11. Lohmann DR, Gallie BL. Retinoblastoma. In: Pagon RA, Adam MP, Ardinger HH, et al, editors. Seattle (WA): GeneReviews; 1993.
12. Spinner NB, Leonard LD, Krantz ID. Alagille syndrome. In: Pagon RA, Adam MP, Ardinger HH, et al, editors. Seattle (WA): GeneReviews; 1993.
13. Saunders CJ, Miller NA, Soden SE, et al. Rapid whole-genome sequencing for genetic disease diagnosis in neonatal intensive care units. Sci Transl Med 2012;4:154ra135.
14. Dar-Nimrod I, Heine SJ. Genetic essentialism: on the deceptive determinism of DNA. Psychol Bull 2011;137:800–18.
15. Wijdenes-Pijl M, Dondorp WJ, Timmermans DR, et al. Lay perceptions of predictive testing for diabetes based on DNA test results versus family history assessment: a focus group study. BMC Public Health 2011;11:535.
16. Ross LF, Saal HM, David KL, et al. Technical report: ethical and policy issues in genetic testing and screening of children. Genet Med 2013;15:234–45.
17. Kimberlin DW, Lakeman FD, Arvin AM, et al. Application of the polymerase chain reaction to the diagnosis and management of neonatal herpes simplex virus disease. National Institute of Allergy and Infectious Diseases Collaborative Antiviral Study Group. J Infect Dis 1996;174:1162–7.
18. Mitchell PS, Espy MJ, Smith TF, et al. Laboratory diagnosis of central nervous system infections with herpes simplex virus by PCR performed with cerebrospinal fluid specimens. J Clin Microbiol 1997;35:2873–7.
19. Baker MW, Grossman WJ, Laessig RH, et al. Development of a routine newborn screening protocol for severe combined immunodeficiency. J Allergy Clin Immunol 2009;124:522–7.
20. Somech R, Lev A, Simon AJ, et al. Newborn screening for severe T and B cell immunodeficiency in Israel: a pilot study. Isr Med Assoc J 2013;15:404–9.
21. Boppana SB, Ross SA, Novak Z, et al. Dried blood spot real-time polymerase chain reaction assays to screen newborns for congenital cytomegalovirus infection. JAMA 2010;303:1375–82.
22. Choi KY, Schimmenti LA, Jurek AM, et al. Detection of cytomegalovirus DNA in dried blood spots of Minnesota infants who do not pass newborn hearing screening. Pediatr Infect Dis J 2009;28:1095–8.
23. Lewensohn-Fuchs I, Osterwall P, Forsgren M, et al. Detection of herpes simplex virus DNA in dried blood spots making a retrospective diagnosis possible. J Clin Virol 2003;26:39–48.

24. Grosse SD, Dollard S, Ross DS, et al. Newborn screening for congenital cyto-megalovirus: options for hospital-based and public health programs. J Clin Virol 2009;46(Suppl 4):S32–6.
25. Chan K, Davis J, Pai SY, et al. A Markov model to analyze cost-effectiveness of screening for severe combined immunodeficiency (SCID). Mol Genet Metab 2011;104:383–9.
26. Pandya A. Nonsyndromic hearing loss and deafness, mitochondrial. In: Pagon RA, Adam MP, Ardinger HH, et al, editors. Seattle (WA): GeneReviews; 1993.
27. Wang QJ, Zhao YL, Rao SQ, et al. Newborn hearing concurrent gene screening can improve care for hearing loss: a study on 14,913 Chinese newborns. Int J Pediatr Otorhinolaryngol 2011;75:535–42.
28. Chen G, Wang X, Fu S. Prevalence of A1555G mitochondrial mutation in Chinese newborns and the correlation with neonatal hearing screening. Int J Pediatr Otorhinolaryngol 2011;75:532–4.
29. Clark RH, Bloom BT, Spitzer AR, et al. Empiric use of ampicillin and cefotaxime, compared with ampicillin and gentamicin, for neonates at risk for sepsis is associated with an increased risk of neonatal death. Pediatrics 2006;117:67–74.
30. Canfield MA, Honein MA, Yuskiv N, et al. National estimates and race/ethnic-specific variation of selected birth defects in the United States, 1999-2001. Birth Defects Res A Clin Mol Teratol 2006;76:747–56.
31. Turnpenny P, Ellard S. Congenital abnormalities and dysmorphic syndromes. Emery's elements of medical genetics. 12th edition. London: Elsevier Churchill; 2005.
32. Yoon PW, Rasmussen SA, Lynberg MC, et al. The national birth defects prevention study. Public Health Rep 2001;116(Suppl 1):32–40.
33. Rosenthal ET, Biesecker LG, Biesecker BB. Parental attitudes toward a diagnosis in children with unidentified multiple congenital anomaly syndromes. Am J Med Genet 2001;103:106–14.
34. Miller DT, Adam MP, Aradhya S, et al. Consensus statement: chromosomal microarray is a first-tier clinical diagnostic test for individuals with developmental disabilities or congenital anomalies. Am J Hum Genet 2010;86:749–64.
35. Available at: http://www.bcbs.com/blueresources/tec/vols/23/aCHG_genetic_evaluation_patients.pdf. Accessed November 2011.
36. Dimmock D. A personal perspective on returning secondary results of clinical genome sequencing. Genome Med 2012;4:54.
37. Connor JA, Hinton RB, Miller EM, et al. Genetic testing practices in infants with congenital heart disease. Congenit Heart Dis 2014;9:158–67.
38. Chiu RW, Akolekar R, Zheng YW, et al. Non-invasive prenatal assessment of trisomy 21 by multiplexed maternal plasma DNA sequencing: large scale validity study. BMJ 2011;342:c7401.
39. Bianchi DW, Parker RL, Wentworth J, et al. DNA sequencing versus standard prenatal aneuploidy screening. N Engl J Med 2014;370:799–808.
40. Hall AL, Drendel HM, Verbrugge JL, et al. Positive cell-free fetal DNA testing for trisomy 13 reveals confined placental mosaicism. Genet Med 2013;15:729–32.
41. Wang Y, Zhu J, Chen Y, et al. Two cases of placental T21 mosaicism: challenging the detection limits of non-invasive prenatal testing. Prenat Diagn 2013;33:1207–10.
42. Knowles R, Griebsch I, Dezateux C, et al. Newborn screening for congenital heart defects: a systematic review and cost-effectiveness analysis. Health Technol Assess 2005;9:1–152, iii–iv.
43. Bales AM, Zaleski CA, McPherson EW. Newborn screening programs: should 22q11 deletion syndrome be added? Genet Med 2010;12:135–44.

44. Gilissen C, Hehir-Kwa JY, Thung DT, et al. Genome sequencing identifies major causes of severe intellectual disability. Nature 2014;511(7509):344–7.
45. Burke W, Dimmock D. Clinical decisions. Screening an asymptomatic person for genetic risk. N Engl J Med 2014;370:2442–5.
46. MacArthur DG, Manolio TA, Dimmock DP, et al. Guidelines for investigating causality of sequence variants in human disease. Nature 2014;508:469–76.
47. Strong KA, Derse AR, Dimmock DP, et al. In the absence of evidentiary harm, existing societal norms regarding parental authority should prevail. Am J Bioeth 2014;14:24–6.
48. Mayer AN, Dimmock DP, Arca MJ, et al. A timely arrival for genomic medicine. Genet Med 2011;13:195–6.

Screening for and Treatments of Congenital Immunodeficiency Diseases

James Verbsky, MD, PhD[a],*, John Routes, MD[b]

KEYWORDS

- Severe combined immunodeficiency (SCID) • T-cell lymphopenia
- T-cell receptor excision circles (TRECs) • Newborn screening (NBS)
- Hematopoietic stem cell transplantation (HSCT)

KEY POINTS

- Newborn screening (NBS) for severe combined immunodeficiency (SCID) is possible with the T-cell receptor excision circle assay.
- This program has proved effective at diagnosing SCID as well as other disorders associated with T-cell lymphopenia.
- With early diagnosis and infection prophylaxis, infants born with SCID have the best opportunity for successful treatment with stem cell transplant.
- The successful development and implementation of the T-cell receptor excision circles assay for SCID raises the possibility of other immune deficiency screening programs.
- Challenges remain for the NBS program for SCID, such as vulnerable populations that are reluctant to screen, as well as the need for qualified immunologists to care for the children detected.

INTRODUCTION

Newborn screening (NBS) programs are highly successful public health programs designed to detect rare, but treatable, inborn errors of metabolism. A NBS program for severe combined immunodeficiency (SCID) was developed recently and was implemented in several states. This article provides a description of this screening program, summarizes its initial findings, and reviews the pitfalls of this program.

HISTORICAL PERSPECTIVES OF NEWBORN SCREENING

Population-based screening programs began in 1963 with the demonstration that phenylketonuria can be detected in the neonatal period for all newborns, before the

[a] Division of Rheumatology, Department of Pediatrics, Medical College of Wisconsin, Milwaukee, WI, USA; [b] Division of Allergy/Immunology, Department of Pediatrics, Medical College of Wisconsin, Milwaukee, WI, USA
* Corresponding author. Pediatric Rheumatology, Children's Corporate Center, Suite C465, 9000 West Wisconsin Avenue, PO Box 1997, Milwaukee, WI 53201-1997.
E-mail address: jverbsky@mcw.edu

Clin Perinatol 41 (2014) 1001–1015
http://dx.doi.org/10.1016/j.clp.2014.08.017   perinatology.theclinics.com

onset of cognitive symptoms, allowing dietary modification and prevention of long-term disability.[1] The ability to screen for other disorders has increased dramatically, leading to controversies about expanding screening programs. To address these concerns, Wilson and Jungner[2] published a pivotal report that attempted to strike a balance between the desire for early detection and treatment of disease, and the potential harms to patients and society.[2] This report defined the characteristics of disorders that were amenable to NBS, such as disease incidence and severity, the presence of a sensitive test to detect the disorder, as well as a curative treatment (**Box 1**). Although the characteristics outlined by Wilson and Jungner[2] guided the development and implementation of NBS programs and created a platform for understanding of the ethics of screening tests, there is an ongoing need for expansion and reassessment of these criteria as novel medical technologies are developed.[3–5] The Health Resources and Services Administration (HRSA) commissioned the American College of Medical Genetics (ACMG) to develop national NBS standards. This task force ultimately recommended that NBS for 31 conditions be mandated in all states.[5] Despite these national efforts at uniformity for NBS programs, each state administers its own panel of tests.

The primary imperative of NBS remains the identification and early intervention of treatable disorders. These screening programs have been highly successful in preventing the long-term disability associated with inborn errors of metabolism, and congenital hypothyroidism is one of the best examples of this.[6] Congenital hypothyroidism is one of the most common inborn errors of metabolism, occurring in 1 in 2500 infants. Congenital hypothyroidism is characterized by progressive neurologic dysfunction that can lead to mental retardation, which can be prevented by early treatment with hormone replacement. With the implementation of NBS for hypothyroidism, the incidence of mental retardation caused by this disorder has been reduced by more than 90%.[6] NBS for congenital hypothyroidism has proved to be a highly cost-effective when the long-term costs of caring for individuals who develop mental impairment caused by congenital hypothyroidism are considered.

As understanding of the molecular basis of diseases improves, novel methods to detect disorders that are amenable for high-throughput population-based screening are increasingly available and are constantly being evaluated for possible additions

---

Box 1
Wilson and Jungner NBS criteria

1. The condition sought should be an important health problem.

2. There should be an accepted treatment of patients with recognized disease.

3. Facilities for diagnosis and treatment should be available.

4. There should be a recognizable latent or early symptomatic stage.

5. There should be a suitable test or examination.

6. The test should be acceptable to the population.

7. The natural history of the condition, including development from latent to declared disease, should be adequately understood.

8. There should be an agreed policy on whom to treat as patients.

9. The cost of case finding (including diagnosis and treatment of patients diagnosed) should be economically balanced in relation to possible expenditure on medical care.

10. Case finding should be a continuing process and not a once-and-for-all project.

to the NBS panel.[7,8] However, each new test proposed for population-based screening should be evaluated on the principles first proposed by Wilson and Jungner[2] and subsequently amended by HRSA. However, other societal factors, such as the desire to limit government, privacy issues, and issues related to informed consent, make adding additional NBS tests an increasingly difficult process.

SEVERE COMBINED IMMUNODEFICIENCY: A DEADLY DISORDER PREVENTABLE WITH EARLY DETECTION AND TREATMENT

SCID encompasses multiple genetic disorders that result in deficiencies in cellular and humoral immunity caused by a profound deficiency of T cells.[9,10] Most infants with SCID seem physically normal at birth, only coming to attention once they have obtained potentially life-threatening infections. SCID was estimated to occur in 1 in 50,000 to 100,000 live births,[11] but since the implementation of NBS programs the true incidence is probably closer to 1 in 50,000 live births; well within the recommended guidance of incidence of screening.[12]

The clinical course of SCID is well understood, and lifesaving treatments are readily available. Children born with SCID are well at birth and subsequently develop failure to thrive, severe infections, and death without intervention.[11,13] Pneumonias caused by *Pneumocystis jiroveci*, adenovirus, cytomegalovirus (CMV), and respiratory syncytial virus are common. Chronic viral diarrhea leading to villous atrophy, malabsorption, and failure to thrive is also common. SCID may also be diagnosed when a serious infection develops after vaccination with a live, attenuated vaccine, such as disseminated rotavirus after administration of the live oral rotavirus vaccine.[14] In other countries, systemic mycobacterial infection can be seen after vaccination with bacille Calmette-Guérin.[15] Viral and opportunistic infections acquired in the first few months of life can be persistent and fatal even with aggressive treatment.[16] Without screening, the median age of diagnosis of SCID is 6.6 months of life[17] with a mean of 2 months' delay from the onset of symptoms to diagnosis.[13]

T-cell deficiency syndromes may also present early in infancy with autoimmunelike phenomena of rashes, liver dysfunction, hepatosplenomegaly, and diarrhea. These disorders may be caused by a mutation in an SCID-causing gene that codes for a protein with residual function (hypomorphic mutation). In this situation, there is production of a few abnormal autoreactive T cells that traffic into the periphery and mediate a form of autoimmunity known as Omenn syndrome. For example, hypomorphic mutations in *RAG1* or *RAG2* cause Omenn syndrome, whereas null mutations cause SCID.[18–20] Maternally engrafted T cells can also cause a variety of rashes and inflammatory complications similar to Omenn syndrome but frequently less severe.[21]

Hematopoietic stem cell transplantation (HSCT) is the definitive treatment of SCID.[10,17,22,23] Enzyme replacement for adenosine deaminase (ADA) deficiency is also sometimes performed.[24–26] Although still considered investigational, gene therapy is becoming an increasing promising therapeutic option for some forms of SCID.[25,27–29] Patients who receive transplants within the first 3.5 months of life, at a time when the bone marrow is especially receptive for stem cell engraftment and before the development of severe infections, have the best prognosis for survival, with 95% survival compared with 76% survival for those who received transplants later.[10,17] In the past, only children with family histories suggestive of SCID benefited from early diagnosis and transplantation, but with the addition of NBS all children will have this opportunity.

Based on the information previously outlined, it is clear that SCID meets all the criteria for NBS. However, a test was needed that was amenable to population-based screening. SCID is a disorder caused by numerous genetic defects, but all forms of SCID are defined by a deficiency of newly formed (naive) T cells. Several testing modalities have been proposed, including complete blood count (CBC) enumeration of peripheral blood lymphocyte counts. Quantification of peripheral blood lymphocyte counts by CBC is not an ideal test, because it may fail to identify some infants with SCID with normal numbers of B cells and/or NK (natural killer) cells, maternal engraftment of T cells, and/or expansions of rare T-cell clones.[30–34] CBCs are also expensive, and because they cannot be done on NBS screening cards, venipuncture is necessary. These features make this testing modality unsuitable for mass screening.

A novel assay was developed that measures specific intracellular DNA fragments generated during T-cell development, which are markers of naive T cells, known as the T-cell receptor excision circles (TREC) assay. During normal development of T cells in the thymus, the variable (V), diverse (D), and joining (J) segments of the T-cell receptor locus undergo DNA rearrangement (VDJ rearrangement), generating a diverse pool of T-cell receptors (**Fig. 1**). By-products of this process are small, circular pieces of DNA known as TRECs. As T cells divide, the TRECs do not replicate and are thus diluted in an exponential manner. TRECs consequently exist only in naive T cells.[35] This aspect of this assay is important because certain conditions, such as maternal engraftment of T cells or expansion of a few T-cell clones as in Omenn syndrome, can result in a significant number of T cells in an infant with SCID. These T cells have undergone multiple rounds of proliferation that dilute the TRECs. Therefore, in these instances the TREC value is low even though high numbers of T cells may be present. Regardless of the molecular cause or the presence of maternal engraftment, all forms of SCID are characterized by a deficiency in naive T cells, and therefore are detected by the TREC assay.[36–38] The current TREC assay uses quantitative real-time (qRT) polymerase chain reaction (PCR) to quantitate by 1 specific TREC, δRec-ψJα, which is present in approximately 70% of all T cells that express the alpha/beta T-cell receptor.[39] Alpha/beta T cells constitute approximately 85% to 90% of all T cells in peripheral blood, making this an excellent biomarker. If the TREC value is low, the PCR may have not worked because of poor-quality DNA. Therefore, DNA integrity is addressed by performing real-time (RT) PCR on a housekeeping gene (eg, beta-actin, RNaseP).

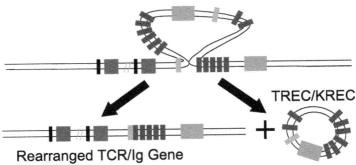

TREC/KREC

Rearranged TCR/Ig Gene

Fig. 1. VDJ rearrangement as the basis of the TREC and KREC assays. T-cell receptor or immunoglobulin molecules generate diversity by rearranging DNA segments bringing variable, diversity, and junctional segments together. As these segments are joined, a circular episomal DNA fragment is produced, known as a TREC or kappa-deleting recombination excision circle (KREC). Ig, immunoglobulin.

In 2005, the TREC assay was adapted for analysis of DNA isolated from dried blood spots on NBS cards.[37] Investigators in Wisconsin further optimized the TREC assay for population-based screening, and showed that the TREC assay was highly sensitive and specific for SCID, reproducible, and amenable to high-throughput population-based testing.[36] In 2008, Wisconsin became the first state to implement mandatory NBS for T-cell deficiency.[40] Massachusetts began screening in February 2009,[41] followed by California, Louisiana, and New York (**Fig. 2**).[42,43] In 2010, based on the Wisconsin experience that showed that the TREC assay successfully detected a baby with SCID, the Secretary's Advisory Committee on Heritable Disorders in Newborns and Children recommended to the Secretary of the Department of Health and Human Services that SCID be added to the Recommended Uniform Screening Panel (www.hrsa.gov/heritabledisorderscommittee/correspondence/feb2010letter.htm).

SCREENING ALGORITHM

All states participating in NBS for SCID have algorithms in place to address a course of action when a screening test is positive. In Wisconsin, the algorithm is designed to ensure adequate follow-up of infants with likely SCID, while limiting the number of false-positive results (**Fig. 3**). All infants undergo screening by the TREC assay, and, if normal, no further intervention is recommended. Any infant with a TREC level less than the cutoff value is retested and DNA integrity is analyzed by quantifying beta-actin levels by qRT-PCR. If the beta-actin level is normal with abnormally low TRECs, an abnormal report is issued and the primary care provider and designated clinical immunologists are contacted for confirmatory testing by flow cytometry. If the beta-actin result is low, the screening test is repeated with a new NBS card. For preterm infants at less than 37 weeks adjusted gestational age (AGA), the screening test is repeated either until normal or until the infant reaches 37 weeks AGA. All full-term and preterm infants with an AGA of 37 weeks with an abnormal TREC assay undergo lymphocyte subset analysis by flow cytometry. Infants with abnormal flow cytometry tests are then referred for evaluation by a clinical immunologist.

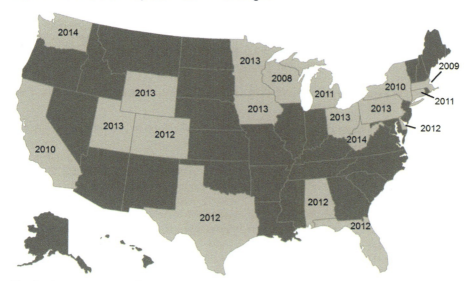

Fig. 2. States screening for SCID and dates screening began. Puerto Rico and Ottawa, Canada, have also implemented NBS for SCID.

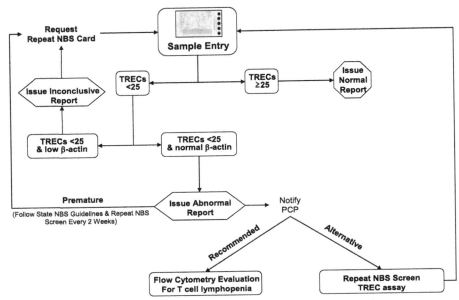

Fig. 3. Algorithm for NBS for SCID in Wisconsin. PCP, primary care provider.

Most states have a similar algorithm, although some states choose to perform flow cytometry regardless of gestational age if the TREC assay is repeated and remains abnormal.[41–43] Initial studies of population-based screening for SCID detected a considerably higher rate of false-positives in preterm infants.[40,44] In Wisconsin, premature infants with abnormal TREC assays are retested every 2 weeks until they reach a corrected gestational age equivalent of 37 weeks, and then they are tested by flow cytometry. This procedure is standard for all abnormal NBS screening tests in premature infants in Wisconsin, significantly reduces the number of false-positive tests, and reduces the cost incurred by limiting the number of infants who have to undergo lymphocyte subset analysis by flow cytometry. Furthermore, a retrospective analysis of preterm infants who died showed that none of these deaths were related to SCID.[44]

RESULTS OF 6 YEARS OF SCREENING FOR SEVERE COMBINED IMMUNODEFICIENCY IN THE UNITED STATES

Numerous reports have been published showing the effectiveness of NBS for SCID using the TREC assay.[40,42,43,45] The results are encouraging and lead to several conclusions. First, the TREC assay is extremely sensitive, with very few false-positive results. During the first 3 years of screening for SCID in Wisconsin, for example, 207,696 infants were screened, and only 0.19% of infants required rescreening because of prematurity or inadequate sample quality.[45] Seventy-two infants were ultimately classified as abnormal and underwent flow cytometric analysis, accounting for only 0.035% of infants screened. Of these, 38 infants were ultimately found to be normal, resulting in a false-positive rate of 0.018% and specificity of 99.98%. Similar rates were reported in other states.[42,43] The high specificity of this assay is important because confirmatory testing by flow cytometry is expensive, and a high false-positive rate would significant increase the cost of screening. Second, the TREC assay is good at detecting T-cell lymphopenia, including both SCID and other defects that result in significant T-cell lymphopenia. In Wisconsin, of the 72 infants who failed the test, 33 had T-cell lymphopenia of varying degrees, resulting in a positive predictive value of the test predicting T-cell lymphopenia of 46%. These results are consistent with other published data.[42,43]

More importantly, results from these studies showed that the TREC assay detects known and unknown causes of SCID or T-cell lymphopenia. Numerous defects known to cause SCID or T-cell lymphopenia have been detected in the first several years of screening (**Box 2**).[42,43,45] Some surprises have occurred, including 1 infant who was identified with a de novo mutation in the *RAC2* gene, which was previously reported to result in an immunodeficiency caused by neutrophil dysfunction.[40,44–46] Furthermore, secondary defects that result in T-cell lymphopenia, such as gastroschisis or chromosomal abnormalities, are also detected (**Box 3**). There have been no known unrecognized cases of SCID in states that offer NBS since the implementation of neonatal screening in 2008 (ie, no known false-negative tests). Although the TREC assay did not detect rare cases of combined immunodeficiencies (discussed later), it has proved to be nearly 100% sensitive in detecting SCID.

The TREC assay is inexpensive, currently costing between $5 and $10 per test.[40,47,48] Furthermore, the cost of transplantation of infants detected by the acquisition of SCID-defining infections is estimated to be 2 to 3 times more than the cost of transplantation of an infant with SCID detected by NBS and who is without infections.[49] These costs must be incorporated into the total cost of caring for infants with SCID to ensure that screening for this condition is cost-effective. Several studies concluded that the cost of the TREC assay is within the range of acceptable costs.[47,48,50,51]

LIMITATIONS OF THE T-CELL RECEPTOR EXCISION CIRCLES ASSAY

With the nationwide implementation of TREC screening, pediatricians need to understand the goals and limitations of this test. Although the TREC screen can detect a wide variety of causes of T-cell lymphopenia, it is not a screening test for all primary immunodeficiencies (PIDs). SCID represents a small proportion of all PIDs, and there are numerous serious but treatable congenital immunodeficiencies that do not result in T-cell or B-cell lymphopenia (eg, chronic granulomatous disease, congenital neutropenia, toll-like receptor defects). In addition, there are combined immunodeficiencies (CID) that do result in clinically significant T-cell defects that may be missed by the

---

Box 2
Genetic defects resulting in SCID or severe T-cell lymphopenia detected by the TREC assay

Interleukin (IL) 7 receptor

ADA

IL2 receptor gamma chain

Jak3

RAG1

RMRP1

22q11 deletion syndrome (DiGeorge)

Rac2 defect

CHARGE (coloboma, heart defect, atresia choanae, retarded growth and development, genital abnormality, and ear abnormality)

Ataxia telangiectasia

Box 3
Secondary causes of T-cell lymphopenia detected by the TREC assay

Jacobsen syndrome

VACTERL (vertebral defects, anal atresia, cardiac defects, tracheo-esophageal fistula, renal anomalies, and limb abnormalities)

Thrombocytopenia absent radii syndrome

Cardiac defects

Trisomy 21/chromosomal defects

Ectrodactyly ectodermal dysplasia syndrome

Gastrointestinal abnormalities (ie, gastroschisis, ileal atresia)

Multiple congenital anomalies

---

assay. Bare lymphocyte syndrome, caused by deficiencies in transcription factors that induce human lymphocyte antigen (HLA) class II expression, results in a severe lack of CD4 cells and significant risk of infections similar to SCID. Bare lymphocyte syndrome is typically missed by the TREC assay because CD8 cells are present in bare lymphocyte syndrome, so the assay can be within the normal range.[52] ZAP-70 defects similarly result in significant CD8 lymphopenia and a CID phenotype, but can have normal TREC levels.[53] ADA deficiency is a common cause of SCID and late-onset ADA deficiency can be missed by the TREC assay.[54] In addition, the TREC assay detects less than 50% of cases of ataxia telangiectasia, which is a CID.[55,56] Several rare disorders, such as Ora1, Stim1, or CD40 ligand deficiency, show an infectious phenotype similar to SCID but have normal numbers of T cells, and it is unknown whether the TREC assay can detect these disorders.[57,58] As time goes on, an increasing number of CID are likely to be missed by the TREC assay. Thus, even in states that screen for SCID, it is important that any infant with abnormal or severe infections be evaluated by a clinical immunologist with expertise in diagnosing these rare disorders.

CAN NEWBORN SCREENING BE EXPANDED TO DETECT MORE IMMUNE DEFICIENCIES?

Although NBS for SCID has proved to be an excellent screening test for the detection of SCID and T-cell lymphopenia, there are still many clinically significant PIDs that are not detected by the TREC assay. NBS for all PIDs is currently not possible, and is not recommended based on the Wilson and Jungner[2] criteria. Many serious PIDs are too rare to justify NBS, because the cost of screening for these disorders is likely to be prohibitive, which shows one advantage of the TREC assay in that it detects any genetic defect that results in low T-cell numbers, and does not evaluate for the specific genetic cause. A similar DNA-based assay is also available that detects deficiencies in B lymphocytes by enumerating kappa-deleting recombination excision circles (KRECs).[59] Similar to T cells, B-cell receptors also undergo rearrangement of their DNA to make immunoglobulin, which acts as the B-cell receptor (see **Fig. 1**). During the rearrangement of genes for the kappa chain of the immunoglobulin molecule, KRECs are generated and indicate successful generation of a mature B cell. Thus, the number of KRECs enumerated by RT-PCR serves as a biomarker of the number of newly formed B cells. The KREC assay is therefore very sensitive in the diagnosis of congenital forms of agammaglobulinemia, such as X-linked agammaglobulinemia, in which very few or no B cells are formed. The KREC assay can also detect CIDs that have low numbers of B cells, such as Nijmegen breakage syndrome, which is missed by the TREC assay.[56] The KREC assay is also useful to help define certain subtypes of SCID: T-B- SCID should show low TRECs and low KRECs; T-B+ SCID should have low TRECs and normal KRECs; and pure B-cell deficiencies should show normal TRECs and low KRECs.[56] The KREC assay is amenable to multiplexing with the TREC assay, which would lower costs considerably because the assays are performed using the same aliquot of eluent from the dried blood spot, which should reduce the cost of these assays if performed together.

With the advent of DNA-based screening, several other disorders can be detected. 22q11.2 deletion syndrome (DiGeorge syndrome) is a prime example. 22q11.2 deletion syndrome is characterized by congenital heart disease, hypoparathyroidism, and variable defects in thymic development and T-cell generation. In infants with severe T-cell lymphopenia, the TREC assay is capable of detecting 22q11.2 deletion syndrome. However, most infants with 22q11.2 deletion syndrome show less profound T-cell lymphopenia and the TREC assay detects less than 10% of all infants with 22q11.2 deletion syndrome.[60] A novel RT-PCR assay has been developed that detects haploinsufficiency of the TBX1 gene, which is present in nearly all cases of 22q11.2 deletion syndrome. This assay is amenable to NBS and would detect nearly all infants with 22q11.2 deletion syndrome.[60] Although infants with 22q11.2 deletion syndrome who are missed by the TREC assay are not at risk for infection-related morbidity/mortality, these infants do have significant health problems as well as long-term issues with learning disabilities and mental disorders.[61] Although anticipatory care can markedly improve the long-term outcomes of these infants, there is considerable debate on whether 22q11.2 deletion syndrome should be included in NBS.

CLINICAL COMPLEXITIES IN NEWBORN SCREENING FOR SEVERE COMBINED IMMUNODEFICIENCY

Before the initiation of NBS the clinical diagnosis of SCID was frequently based on a constellation of findings of severe, persistent, and/or opportunistic infections in the context of severe T-cell lymphopenia and abnormal T-cell function. A family history is also useful for diagnosis. However, some patients with laboratory and clinical evidence of SCID lack a genetic diagnosis, and HSCT should be recommended in these cases. With the advent of NBS for SCID, clinicians are currently faced with the dilemma of identifying infants who have significant T-cell lymphopenia but who do not have SCID-defining infections. Although they have marked T-cell lymphopenia, some of the identified infants have T-cell counts that are higher than those of typical infants with SCID, which is currently defined as fewer than 200 T cells/mm^3. Furthermore, when infants with severe T-cell lymphopenia are detected, they are frequently treated with intravenous immunoglobulin and other prophylactic medications that prevent or delay the acquisition of SCID-defining infections. The intermediate immunologic phenotype and lack of SCID-defining infections leads to a difficult clinical dilemma of deciding on a potentially dangerous treatment (ie, HSCT) of an otherwise healthy infant. Furthermore, it is anticipated that new genetic causes of T-cell lymphopenia will be discovered by NBS. Because the natural history of these disorders will not have been defined, the optimal treatment will be unknown.

In Wisconsin, we detected several infants with severe T-cell lymphopenia but with more than 200 T cells/mm^3. In one case, an infant with an abnormal TREC assay and T-cell lymphopenia had an older sister born before NBS for SCID who had invasive opportunistic infections, failure to thrive, and autoimmune enteropathy.[45] She lacked TRECs and had a low T-cell count (<1500 cells/mm^3) with greatly expanded and activated CD8 cells. This constellation of clinical and immunologic findings indicated a serious combined immunodeficiency (CID) and HSCT was performed. The brother detected by NBS has not been transplanted and has been treated with immunoglobulin replacement and prophylactic antibiotics. He is currently thriving without infections or other complications. This case highlights that, without a genetic diagnosis, the optimal treatment and long-term prognosis of infants with idiopathic CIDs is unclear and presently needs to be individualized on case-by-case basis.

Another issue that is critical to successful implementation of NBS for SCID is how to educate vulnerable populations, including the Amish, Mennonite, and Navajo, that may be reluctant to screen their children and that have high rates of SCID. Furthermore, if NBS for SCID is performed and detects an infant with SCID, the parents may opt against treatment. In this situation, courts have consistently ruled that lifesaving treatments must be initiated and an HSCT is likely to be performed in the affected infant. Although this is expected to lead to a beneficial outcome in a particular infant, legal intervention may lead to increased opposition to any NBS in the community at large. These complex societal problems need to be addressed if NBS is to be implemented successfully in high-risk populations.

Another important problem is the lack of clinical immunologists properly trained in the diagnosis of infants with SCID. Moreover, because the treatment of SCID is HSCT, centers where patients are evaluated should also have an active pediatric HSCT service, and, ideally, one that is accustomed to transplantation for PIDs. HSCT center experience and volume are important, because patients who receive HLA-mismatched transplants seem to have better outcomes at large centers compared with small centers. In states lacking this expertise, how would infants get the proper evaluation and treatment? Would there be a statewide referral to centers of excellence or would parents and doctors struggle to make the proper consultation? Will the decision to send affected infants to centers of excellence be influenced by the particular insurance carrier? Would the ability of infants covered under title XIX be eligible for referral? These important issues are not currently being addressed at the governmental level and need urgent attention as the TREC assay is increasingly implemented nationwide.

PRACTICAL ASPECTS OF NEWBORN SCREENING FOR SEVERE COMBINED IMMUNODEFICIENCY

The TREC assay is also useful to predict the degree of T-cell lymphopenia. Numerous defects that result in moderate T-cell lymphopenia are detected by the TREC assay, such as 22q11.2 syndrome, chromosomal abnormalities, and lymphatic defects, but in these instances the TRECs are typically low but not absent.[45] In all of the cases of SCID in 5 years of screening in Wisconsin, the TREC assay was 0, whereas in secondary causes of T-cell lymphopenia and in cases of moderate T-cell lymphopenia the TREC assay was low but detectable.[45] This observation can be useful when recommending intervention in a newly detected infant.

Once an infant is detected with SCID, it is critical to prevent the acquisition of any infections that can affect the success of HSCT. We have developed guidelines for supportive care and infectious disease prophylaxis based in part on national consensus guidelines, including isolation parameters and pharmacologic therapy, which are started in any infant suspected of SCID (**Table 1**).[62] Infants suspected of SCID but without infectious symptoms are cared for at home as long as the infant lives close to a hospital that is well versed in taking care of sick children, the home environment is not worrisome, and the parents are comfortable. No sick contacts or public exposures are allowed. Strict hand washing is recommended. One potential infectious

Table 1	
Recommended supportive care anticipatory guidelines for infants with suspected SCID	
Guideline	**Reason**
Avoid public places, daycare Limited contact with young children Strict hand washing	Prevent transmission of community-acquired diseases
No breast feeding	Prevent transmission of CMV
Boil ingestible water	Prevent cryptosporidium infection
Avoid all live and live, attenuated vaccines (MMR, varicella, rotavirus, influenza)	Prevent infection with vaccine-related viruses
Blood products: leukodepletion and irradiation essential; CMV negative when available	Prevent transmission of CMV and graft-versus-host disease

Abbreviation: MMR, measles, mumps, and rubella.

agent that is difficult to prevent is CMV; a virus that is transmitted by oral secretions and breast milk. The acquisition of CMV can negatively affect the success of HSCT. We have recommended no breast feeding or contact with secretions (masks) while the infant undergoes evaluation. Mothers are screened for CMV and, if negative, breast feeding and some contact precautions are lifted. The pretransplant evaluation includes a panel of PCR tests to evaluate for viral disease, in particular CMV, and surveillance PCR assays are repeated monthly or bimonthly. Infants who test positive for viral infection are hospitalized and antiviral therapy implemented. Infants are screened for antibodies to human immunodeficiency virus (HIV)–1, which would indicate maternal HIV infection. Infants identified as possible SCID undergo a prophylaxis regimen designed to prevent bacterial, fungal, and viral infections (see **Table 1**). Infants with SCID do not receive any live vaccinations, and we withhold other routine immunizations as well because these children are on antibody replacement. We instruct family members and close contacts to be up to date on immunizations against influenza and pertussis. Although transmission of varicella, measles, and rotavirus through vaccination is highly unlikely,[63] we do not recommend that close contacts or family members be vaccinated with live viral vaccines unless there is a community outbreak or there are other special circumstances.

SUMMARY

All forms of SCID are characterized by reduced numbers of naive T cells, making the TREC assay, which enumerates naive T-cell numbers from dried blood spots, an ideal tool for NBS of this disorder. NBS for SCID using the TREC assay seems to be cost-effective and is extremely sensitive in detecting infants with SCID. Published results in states that have implemented NBS for SCID indicate that early detection of SCID markedly improves the prognosis. Although the TREC assay is highly effective at detecting SCID, it does not detect all combined immunodeficiencies. Therefore, clinicians must aggressively evaluate infants with failure to thrive and opportunistic infections for PIDs, even in states that screen for SCID. NBS for SCID has highlighted several important limitations to this screening program, including difficulties in screening at-risk populations, the limitations of this assay in detected other immunodeficiencies, the best treatment plan of infants with severe T-cell lymphopenia but no genetic diagnosis, and the lack of expertise to properly diagnose and treat affected infants in certain geographic locations. The long-term success of NBS for SCID depends on addressing these and other problems as they arise. However, the success of this program has created the opportunity to generate other screening programs to detect infants with serious immune deficiencies before the acquisition of life-threatening infections.

REFERENCES

1. Guthrie R, Susi A. A simple phenylalanine method for detecting phenylketonuria in large populations of newborn infants. Pediatrics 1963;32:338–43.
2. Wilson JM, Jungner G. Principles and practice of screening for disease. Geneva (Switzerland): WHO; 1968.
3. Fleischman AR, Lin BK, Howse JL. A commentary on the President's Council on Bioethics report: the changing moral focus of newborn screening. Genet Med 2009;11:507–9.
4. Andermann A, Blancquaert I, Beauchamp S, et al. Revisiting Wilson and Jungner in the genomic age: a review of screening criteria over the past 40 years. Bull World Health Organ 2008;86:317–9.
5. Newborn screening: toward a uniform screening panel and system. Genet Med 2006;8(Suppl 1):1S–252S.
6. Rose SR, Brown RS, Foley T, et al. Update of newborn screening and therapy for congenital hypothyroidism. Pediatrics 2006;117:2290–303.
7. Kharrazi M, Hyde T, Young S, et al. Use of screening dried blood spots for estimation of prevalence, risk factors, and birth outcomes of congenital cytomegalovirus infection. J Pediatr 2010;157:191–7.
8. Bales AM, Zaleski CA, McPherson EW. Patient and family experiences and opinions on adding 22q11 deletion syndrome to the newborn screen. J Genet Couns 2010;19:526–34.
9. Buckley RH. The multiple causes of human SCID. J Clin Invest 2004;114:1409–11.
10. Buckley RH, Schiff SE, Schiff RI, et al. Hematopoietic stem-cell transplantation for the treatment of severe combined immunodeficiency. N Engl J Med 1999;340:508–16.
11. Fischer A, Notarangelo LD. Combined immunodeficiencies. In: Stiehm ER, Ochs HD, Winkelstein JA, editors. Immunologic disorders in infants and children. Philadelphia: Elsevier; 2004. p. 3–16.
12. Kaye CI, Accurso F, La FS, et al. Newborn screening fact sheets. Pediatrics 2006;118:e934–63.
13. Stephan JL, Vlekova V, Le Deist F, et al. Severe combined immunodeficiency: a retrospective single-center study of clinical presentation and outcome in 117 patients. J Pediatr 1993;123:564–72.
14. Werther RL, Crawford NW, Boniface K, et al. Rotavirus vaccine induced diarrhea in a child with severe combined immune deficiency. J Allergy Clin Immunol 2009;124:600.
15. Marciano BE, Huang CY, Joshi G, et al. BCG vaccination in patients with severe combined immunodeficiency: complications, risks, and vaccination policies. J Allergy Clin Immunol 2014;133:1134–41.
16. Buckley RH. Molecular defects in human severe combined immunodeficiency and approaches to immune reconstitution. Annu Rev Immunol 2004;22:625–55.
17. Myers LA, Patel DD, Puck JM, et al. Hematopoietic stem cell transplantation for severe combined immunodeficiency in the neonatal period leads to superior thymic output and improved survival. Blood 2002;99:872–8.

18. Villa A, Notarangelo LD, Roifman CM. Omenn syndrome: inflammation in leaky severe combined immunodeficiency. J Allergy Clin Immunol 2008;122:1082–6.
19. Villa A, Santagata S, Bozzi F, et al. Omenn syndrome: a disorder of Rag1 and Rag2 genes. J Clin Immunol 1999;19:87–97.
20. Honig M, Schwarz K. Omenn syndrome: a lack of tolerance on the background of deficient lymphocyte development and maturation. Curr Opin Rheumatol 2006;18:383–8.
21. Denianke KS, Frieden IJ, Cowan MJ, et al. Cutaneous manifestations of maternal engraftment in patients with severe combined immunodeficiency: a clinicopathologic study. Bone Marrow Transplant 2001;28:227–33.
22. Buckley RH. A historical review of bone marrow transplantation for immunodeficiencies. J Allergy Clin Immunol 2004;113:793–800.
23. Buckley RH. Transplantation of hematopoietic stem cells in human severe combined immunodeficiency: longterm outcomes. Immunol Res 2011;49:25–43.
24. Brigida I, Sauer AV, Ferrua F, et al. B-cell development and functions and therapeutic options in adenosine deaminase-deficient patients. J Allergy Clin Immunol 2014;133:799–806.
25. Aiuti A, Cattaneo F, Galimberti S, et al. Gene therapy for immunodeficiency due to adenosine deaminase deficiency. N Engl J Med 2009;360:447–58.
26. Chan B, Wara D, Bastian J, et al. Long-term efficacy of enzyme replacement therapy for adenosine deaminase (ADA)-deficient severe combined immunodeficiency (SCID). Clin Immunol 2005;117:133–43.
27. Aiuti A, Slavin S, Aker M, et al. Correction of ADA-SCID by stem cell gene therapy combined with nonmyeloablative conditioning. Science 2002;296:2410–3.
28. Hacein-Bey-Abina S, Le Deist F, Carlier F, et al. Sustained correction of X-linked severe combined immunodeficiency by ex vivo gene therapy. N Engl J Med 2002;346:1185–93.
29. Hacein-Bey-Abina S, Von Kalle C, Schmidt M, et al. A serious adverse event after successful gene therapy for X-linked severe combined immunodeficiency. N Engl J Med 2003;348:255–6.
30. Lev A, Simon AJ, Ben-Ari J, et al. Co-existence of clonal expanded autologous and transplacental-acquired maternal T cells in recombination activating gene-deficient severe combined immunodeficiency. Clin Exp Immunol 2014;176:380–6.
31. Gil J, Busto EM, Garcillan B, et al. A leaky mutation in *CD3D* differentially affects $\alpha\beta$ and $\gamma\delta$ T cells and leads to a T$\alpha\beta$−T$\gamma\delta$+B+NK+ human SCID. J Clin Invest 2011;121:3872–6.
32. Villa A, Sobacchi C, Notarangelo LD. V(D)J recombination defects in lymphocytes due to RAG mutations: severe immunodeficiency with a spectrum of clinical presentations. Blood 2001;97:81–8.
33. Mella P, Imberti L, Brugnoni D, et al. Development of autologous T lymphocytes in two males with X-linked severe combined immune deficiency: molecular and cellular characterization. Clin Immunol 2000;95:39–50.
34. Brugnoni D, Notarangelo LD, Sottini A, et al. Development of autologous, oligoclonal, poorly functioning T lymphocytes in a patient with autosomal recessive severe combined immunodeficiency caused by defects of the Jak3 tyrosine kinase. Blood 1998;91:949–55.
35. Douek DC, Vescio RA, Betts MR, et al. Assessment of thymic output in adults after haematopoietic stem-cell transplantation and prediction of T-cell reconstitution. Lancet 2000;355:1875–81.

36. Baker MW, Grossman WJ, Laessig RH, et al. Development of a routine newborn screening protocol for severe combined immunodeficiency. J Allergy Clin Immunol 2009;124:522–7.

37. Chan K, Puck JM. Development of population-based newborn screening for severe combined immunodeficiency. J Allergy Clin Immunol 2005;115:391–8.

38. Morinishi Y, Imai K, Nakagawa N, et al. Identification of severe combined immunodeficiency by T-cell receptor excision circles quantification using neonatal Guthrie cards. J Pediatr 2009;155:829–33.

39. Verschuren MC, Wolvers-Tettero IL, Breit TM, et al. Preferential rearrangements of the T cell receptor-delta-deleting elements in human T cells. J Immunol 1997; 158:1208–16.

40. Routes JM, Grossman WJ, Verbsky J, et al. Statewide newborn screening for severe T-cell lymphopenia. JAMA 2009;302:2465–70.

41. Comeau AM, Hale JE, Pai SY, et al. Guidelines for implementation of population-based newborn screening for severe combined immunodeficiency. J Inherit Metab Dis 2010;33:S273–81.

42. Vogel BH, Bonagura V, Weinberg GA, et al. Newborn screening for SCID in New York State: experience from the first two years. J Clin Immunol 2014;34: 289–303.

43. Kwan A, Church JA, Cowan MJ, et al. Newborn screening for severe combined immunodeficiency and T-cell lymphopenia in California: results of the first 2 years. J Allergy Clin Immunol 2013;132:140–50.

44. Accetta DJ, Brokopp CD, Baker MW, et al. Cause of death in neonates with inconclusive or abnormal T-cell receptor excision circle assays on newborn screening. J Clin Immunol 2011;31:962–7.

45. Verbsky JW, Baker MW, Grossman WJ, et al. Newborn screening for severe combined immunodeficiency; the Wisconsin experience (2008-2011). J Clin Immunol 2012;32:82–8.

46. Ambruso DR, Knall C, Abell AN, et al. Human neutrophil immunodeficiency syndrome is associated with an inhibitory Rac2 mutation. Proc Natl Acad Sci U S A 2000;97:4654–9.

47. Audrain M, Thomas C, Mirallie S, et al. Evaluation of the T-cell receptor excision circle assay performances for severe combined immunodeficiency neonatal screening on Guthrie cards in a French single centre study. Clin Immunol 2014;150:137–9.

48. Chan K, Davis J, Pai SY, et al. A Markov model to analyze cost-effectiveness of screening for severe combined immunodeficiency (SCID). Mol Genet Metab 2011;104:383–9.

49. Lipstein EA, Vorono S, Browning MF, et al. Systematic evidence review of newborn screening and treatment of severe combined immunodeficiency. Pediatrics 2010;125:e1226–35.

50. McGhee SA, Stiehm ER, McCabe ER. Potential costs and benefits of newborn screening for severe combined immunodeficiency. J Pediatr 2005;147:603–8.

51. Modell V, Knaus M, Modell F. An analysis and decision tool to measure cost benefit of newborn screening for severe combined immunodeficiency (SCID) and related T-cell lymphopenia. Immunol Res 2014;60(1):145–52.

52. Lev A, Simon AJ, Broides A, et al. Thymic function in MHC class II-deficient patients. J Allergy Clin Immunol 2013;131:831–9.

53. Grazioli S, Bennett M, Hildebrand KJ, et al. Limitation of TREC-based newborn screening for ZAP70 severe combined immunodeficiency. Clin Immunol 2014; 153:209–10.

54. la Marca G, Canessa C, Giocaliere E, et al. Tandem mass spectrometry, but not T-cell receptor excision circle analysis, identifies newborns with late-onset adenosine deaminase deficiency. J Allergy Clin Immunol 2013;131:1604–10.
55. Mallott J, Kwan A, Church J, et al. Newborn screening for SCID identifies patients with ataxia telangiectasia. J Clin Immunol 2013;33:540–9.
56. Borte S, von DU, Fasth A, et al. Neonatal screening for severe primary immunodeficiency diseases using high-throughput triplex real-time PCR. Blood 2012; 119:2552–5.
57. Picard C, McCarl CA, Papolos A, et al. STIM1 mutation associated with a syndrome of immunodeficiency and autoimmunity. N Engl J Med 2009;360: 1971–80.
58. Feske S, Gwack Y, Prakriya M, et al. A mutation in Orai1 causes immune deficiency by abrogating CRAC channel function. Nature 2006;441:179–85.
59. van Zelm MC, Szczepanski T, van der Burg M, et al. Replication history of B lymphocytes reveals homeostatic proliferation and extensive antigen-induced B cell expansion. J Exp Med 2007;204:645–55.
60. Tomita-Mitchell A, Mahnke DK, Larson JM, et al. Multiplexed quantitative real-time PCR to detect 22q11.2 deletion in patients with congenital heart disease. Physiol Genomics 2010;42A:52–60.
61. Bales AM, Zaleski CA, McPherson EW. Newborn screening programs: should 22q11 deletion syndrome be added? Genet Med 2010;12:135–44.
62. Verbsky J, Thakar M, Routes J. The Wisconsin approach to newborn screening for severe combined immunodeficiency. J Allergy Clin Immunol 2012;129: 622–7.
63. Lindegren ML, Kobrynski L, Rasmussen SA, et al. Applying public health strategies to primary immunodeficiency diseases: a potential approach to genetic disorders. MMWR Recomm Rep 2004;53:1–29.

Pulse Oximetry in Very Low Birth Weight Infants

Richard A. Polin, MD*, David A. Bateman, MD, Rakesh Sahni, MD

KEYWORDS

- Oxygen saturation • Neonatal • Resuscitation • Intensive care

KEY POINTS

- During neonatal care, pulse oximetry is readily used to target oxygen saturation (Spo_2) during delivery room resuscitation, in situations associated with an increased risk of hypoxemia, in prevention of hyperoxia, and for screening of congenital heart disease.
- The optimal Spo_2 for very low birth weight infants remains a moving target, because uncertainty still exists as to the most appropriate range.
- Randomized clinical trials have demonstrated that 21% oxygen is as effective as 100% oxygen for resuscitation of term and late preterm infants and is associated with lower mortality.
- Although controversial, for resuscitation of infants less than 32 weeks it is recommended to choose initial inspired oxygen between 30% and 90% and titrate it to achieve the recommended Spo_2 value ranges.
- In the management of preterm infants receiving supplemental oxygen a single target Spo_2 range that minimizes mortality and severe ROP remains undetermined; however, data from clinical trials suggest that use of a higher oxygen saturation target range than previously recommended (eg, 90%–95%) is prudent.

INTRODUCTION

The development of pulse oximetry is arguably one of the most important advances in clinical monitoring during the past three decades. Its introduction in clinical practice has led to a revolutionary advancement in patient assessment and monitoring because it allows for a simple, noninvasive, and reasonably accurate estimation of arterial oxygen saturation. Pulse oximeters have become available for widespread application in neonatal care, and oxygen saturation has even been proposed as the "fifth vital sign."[1] In neonatal care, pulse oximetry is readily used to target oxygen saturation (Spo_2) during delivery room resuscitation, in situations associated with an increased risk of hypoxemia (eg, during intubation), in prevention of hyperoxia, and

Division of Neonatal-Perinatal Medicine, Department of Pediatrics, College of Physicians and Surgeons, Columbia University, 3959 Broadway MSCHN 1201, New York, NY 10032–3702, USA
* Corresponding author.
E-mail address: rap32@cumc.columbia.edu

Clin Perinatol 41 (2014) 1017–1032
http://dx.doi.org/10.1016/j.clp.2014.08.018   **perinatology.theclinics.com**
0095-5108/14/$ – see front matter © 2014 Elsevier Inc. All rights reserved.

for screening of congenital heart disease. Accumulating evidence from large, blinded, randomized, controlled trials in neonates now shows that relatively small differences in Spo$_2$ target ranges can have a surprisingly strong influence on important clinical outcomes.[2–6] The optimal Spo$_2$ for very low birth weight (VLBW) infants remains a moving target, because uncertainty still exists as to the most appropriate range. This article describes the historical perspective, physiologic principles, and the use of pulse oximetry in targeting different oxygen ranges at various time-points throughout the neonatal period (at delivery, early weeks, later period) in VLBW infants.

HISTORICAL PERSPECTIVE

The theoretic background for noninvasive assessment of blood oxygenation was set in the early 1900s when it was observed that spectral changes of light absorbance in vivo are related to tissue perfusion.[7] In the 1930s and 1940s, photo cells permitted German, English, and American physiologists to build ear oximeters with red and infrared light, requiring calibration. In 1940, Squire[8] reported on a blood-oxygen meter for use on the hand that computed saturation based on changes of red and infrared light transmission caused by pneumatic tissue compression. In 1942, Millikan[9] coined the word "oximeter" for a portable ear device that read energy absorption in the red and infrared light spectra. Subsequently, Wood[10] used this approach to compute absolute saturation continuously from the ratios of optical density changes with pressure in an ear oximeter by interrupting tissue perfusion. However, all these early oximeters relied either on compression and reperfusion of the measuring site or on the arterialization of capillary blood through heating and thus were inconveniently large, difficult to use, and, most importantly, inaccurate.[7–11] A true revolution in the development of noninvasive oximetry occurred with the work of the Japanese electrical engineer Aoyagi,[12] who was interested in measuring cardiac output noninvasively by dye dilution method using commercially available ear oximetry. He balanced the red and infrared signals to cancel the pulse noise, which prevented measuring the dye washout accurately. He discovered that changes of oxygen saturation voided his pulse cancellation and realized that these pulsatile changes could be used to compute saturation from the ratio of ratios of pulse changes in the red and infrared. His ideas and equations led to the development of the first pulse oximeter in late 1974. Over the next two decades, after the explosive development of technologies in light emission and signal processing, pulse oximeters underwent astonishing improvements and became available for widespread application throughout medical practice.[11–13]

PHYSIOLOGIC PRINCIPLES OF PULSE OXIMETRY OPERATION

Conceptually, it is most useful to view the pulse oximeter waveform as measuring the change in blood volume during a cardiac cycle in the region being studied. Pulse oximetry is based on two physical principles: the presence of a pulsatile signal generated by arterial blood (AC component), which is relatively independent of nonpulsatile arterial blood, venous and capillary blood, and other tissues (DC component); and oxyhemoglobin (O$_2$Hb) and reduced hemoglobin (Hb) have different absorption spectra.[14] Currently available oximeters use sensors placed around a hand or foot with two light-emitting diodes that emit red and infrared light, most commonly at wavelengths of 660 and 940 nm, respectively. Light is detected on the other side using a photo diode. These two wavelengths are used because O$_2$Hb and Hb have different absorption spectra at these particular wavelengths. In the red region, O$_2$Hb absorbs less light than Hb, whereas the reverse occurs in the infrared region. Therefore, any change in light absorption should be attributed to the variations of the arterial blood volume related to the cardiac cycle.[12,15–17] By obtaining the ratio of light absorption in the red and infrared spectra and then calculating the ratio of these two ratios (ratio of absorption ratios), the Spo_2 can be calculated as follows[12]:

$$Spo_2 = f(AC_{red}/DC_{red})/(AC_{infrared}/DC_{infrared})$$

where, f is the calibration constant that is manufacturer specific.

In addition to the digital readout of Spo_2, most pulse oximeters display a photoplethysmogram resulting from surges in arterial blood volume and subsequent increased light absorption that occur with each heartbeat. The peaks in the photoplethysmographic waveform coincide with each heartbeat and are used to generate a pulse rate, and the waveform display can also help clinicians distinguish an artifactual signal from the true signal.

OXYGEN SATURATION TARGETS DURING RESUSCITATION

Michal Sedziwoj (1566–1636), a Polish scientist and alchemist, is credited with the discovery of oxygen. By heating saltpeter, he concluded that air contained a life-giving substance (later shown to be oxygen). More than 170 years later Mayow, Scheele, and Priestly reached a similar conclusion, but none of them realized that the "life-giving" substance was oxygen. Ultimately it was Lavoisier who named the gas "oxygine" and recognized it as an element.[18] Francois Chaussier (1746–1828) began using oxygen for neonatal resuscitation in 1780 and its use quickly spread throughout Europe. After William Little's description of brain damage following asphyxia, the use of oxygen achieved even greater popularity. The development of the Apgar score further emphasized the importance of an infant's "pink color" in determining the adequacy of resuscitation. As late as 2000, the American Heart Association (AHA) and the International Liaison Committee on Resuscitation (ILCOR) recommended 100% oxygen for resuscitation.[19] However, over the past 15 years Saugstad and others have questioned the safety of 100% oxygen for neonatal resuscitation.[20–26] Recent studies indicate that use of high concentrations of oxygen increases free radial production and inflammatory gene expression.[27,28] Randomized clinical trials in humans have demonstrated that 21% oxygen is as effective as 100% oxygen for resuscitation of term and late preterm infants and is associated with lower mortality.[21–26,29–31] Other benefits of using 21% oxygen for resuscitation (eg, reduced time to first breath or cry and improved Apgar scores) are controversial.[21,23,26,29,30,32–34]

The clinical assessment of skin color is an imprecise way to detect cyanosis.[35] Furthermore, in healthy newborn infants, cyanosis is commonly observed in the minutes after birth, because the fetal oxyhemoglobin saturation values range between 40% and 50%.[36] Continuous pulse oximetry in the delivery room is considered standard of care and recommended by ILCOR/AHA for the following situations: when resuscitation is anticipated, when positive pressure ventilation is used for more than a few breaths, when supplementary oxygen is needed, or when cyanosis is persistent.[20] The pulse oximeter probe should be attached to a preductal site (right upper extremity). Studies suggest that data acquisition is quickest if the probe is attached to the infant before the probe is attached to the machine.[37] ILCOR guidelines recommend that a pulse oximeter be attached within 60 seconds of birth; however, a recent study by McCarthy and colleagues[38] suggested that goal is difficult to achieve even in a highly skilled tertiary facility.

In term and preterm infants who do not require any resuscitation (including oxygen), oxygen saturation values increase slowly following delivery and achieve values greater than 90% by 5 to 8 minutes of life.[39] Values in infants delivered vaginally rise more quickly than those delivered by cesarean section.[39,40] Dawson and colleagues[41] published normative values for oxygen saturation (10th–97th percentile) in a large number of term and preterm infants (**Fig. 1**). ILCOR and the AHA recommend an oxygen saturation value in the interquartile range of preductal saturations measured in healthy term babies following vaginal birth at sea level (**Fig. 2**).[37] However, other countries have chosen different saturation targets and there are no data to decide which target is correct.[42] Preterm infants receiving continuous positive airway pressure (CPAP) achieve reference oxygen values more quickly than spontaneously breathing preterm infants.[43] Oxygen saturation targets may be achieved by initiating resuscitation with air or blended oxygen. In term newborn infants, resuscitation should generally be initiated with room air; however, if the infant is still bradycardic (<60/minute) or saturation values do not increase as expected, the concentration of oxygen should be increased to 100%.[37] Given that cerebral blood flow is restored more quickly with 100% oxygen in animals with circulatory collapse we recommend that infants who are severely bradycardic or asystolic should receive 100% oxygen until the heart rate is restored.[44]

The choice of an inspired oxygen concentration for resuscitation of infants less than 32 weeks is controversial.[37,45–47] ILCOR recommends choosing initial inspired oxygen between 30% and 90% and titrating it to achieve the recommended saturation value ranges (see **Fig. 2**).[37] There have been several randomized clinical trials in preterm infants resuscitated with varying concentrations of oxygen. In each of the studies, the initial inspired oxygen concentration was titrated to achieve a predetermined target saturation value. Wang and colleagues[48] randomized 41 preterm infants (23–32 weeks gestation) to resuscitation with 21% or 100% oxygen. Saturation values remained significantly lower in infants resuscitated with room air than those receiving 100% oxygen. Furthermore, target saturation values could not be achieved by 3 minutes of life in the low inspired oxygen concentration group.[48] It is noteworthy that there were no significant differences in heart rate by 2 minutes of life. This suggests that cardiac output (and cerebral blood flow) were restored even though the saturation values

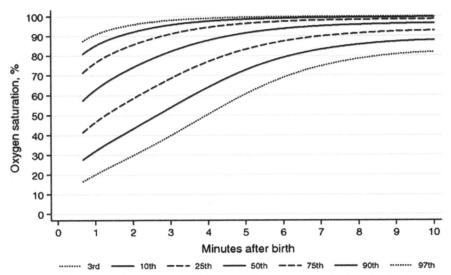

Fig. 1. The 3rd, 10th, 25th, 50th, 75th, 90th, and 97th SpO_2 percentiles for all infants with no medical intervention after birth. (*From* Dawson JA, Kamlin CO, Vento M, et al. Defining the reference range for oxygen saturation for infants after birth. Pediatrics 2010;125:e1344.)

Newborn Resuscitation

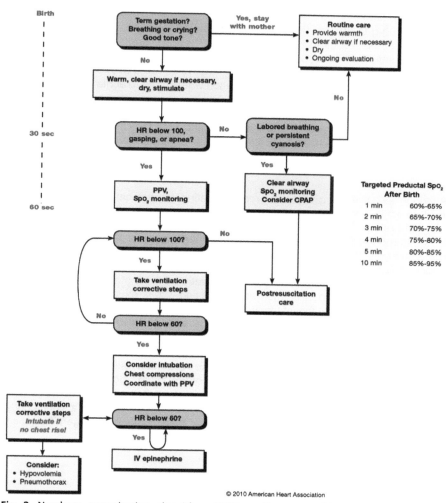

© 2010 American Heart Association

Fig. 2. Newborn resuscitation algorithm. CPAP, continuous positive airway pressure; HR, heart rate; IV, intravenous; PPV, positive pressure ventilation. (*From* Kattwinkel J, Perlman JM, Aziz K, et al. Part 15: neonatal resuscitation: 2010 American Heart Association Guidelines for Cardiopulmonary Resuscitation and Emergency Cardiovascular Care. Circulation 2010;122:S910; with permission.)

remained depressed. Escrig and colleagues[45] randomized 42 infants less than or equal to 28-weeks gestation to resuscitation with 30% or 90% oxygen. The target saturation value was 85%. In contrast to the prior study, there were no differences in oxygen saturation values at any time point. However, the probability of being ventilated with room air was significantly greater at 10 and 20 minutes of life in infants initially resuscitated with 30% oxygen.

Although the benefits of room-air resuscitation on mortality are clear, few studies have assessed the effect of oxygen on the risk of bronchopulmonary dysplasia

(BPD) or long-term neurodevelopmental outcomes. Two studies have addressed whether use of low or high inspired oxygen concentrations for resuscitation results in different pulmonary outcomes. Vento and colleagues[49] randomized 78 infants less than 1000 g to 30% or 90% oxygen. The low-oxygen group had less evidence of oxidative stress, required fewer days of oxygen and mechanical ventilation, and had a lower incidence of BPD. More recently Kapadia and colleagues[47] randomized 88 preterm infants 24- to 34-weeks gestation to 21% or 100% oxygen. Similar to previous studies, the inspired oxygen concentration was titrated to achieve the saturation values described in the 2010 AHA guidelines. The low oxygen group had less evidence of oxidative stress, fewer ventilator days, and a lower incidence of BPD. There has been a single meta-analysis of neurodevelopmental outcomes in infants ventilated with 21% or 100% oxygen. At 12 to 24 months of age, there were no differences in outcomes.[31] However, 27% of the patients were lost to follow-up, there was considerable heterogeneity between the trials, and all of the studies were quasi randomized and unblinded.[50]

Although ILCOR/AHA guidelines precisely define oxygen saturation targets, it is difficult to achieve them. Goos and colleagues[51] demonstrated that during the resuscitation of preterm infants less than 30-weeks gestation there were large deviations from the European Resuscitation Council guidelines in the first 10 minutes after birth. To determine which oxygen resuscitation strategy was most effective at achieving and maintaining oxygen saturations of 85% to 92%, Rabi and coworkers[52] randomized infants less than 32-weeks gestation to resuscitation with a static concentration of 100% oxygen or an oxygen titration strategy using 100% oxygen or 21% oxygen. At 8 and 10 minutes of life, the infants who were assigned to the oxygen titration strategy beginning with 100% oxygen spent a greater proportion of time in the targeted saturation range than the infants receiving a static concentration of 100% oxygen. Most recently, Gandhi and colleagues[53] investigated whether using a Transitional Oxygen Targeting System, which plots real-time saturation values, was better than standard saturation targeting at maintaining preterm infants between the 10th and 50th percentile oxygen saturation curves described by Dawson and colleagues.[41] Saturation values were maintained within the specified target range for a significantly longer time in preterm infants resuscitated using the Transitional Oxygen Targeting System display.

OXYGEN SATURATION TARGETS DURING NEONATAL INTENSIVE CARE

The motivation for establishing a rational set of target limits for oxygen saturation in preterm infants receiving supplemental oxygen, and the persistent difficulty in doing so, cannot be understood outside the context of the epidemiology and pathogenesis of retinopathy of prematurity (ROP). That most neonatologists understand the story of this relationship as a "modern parable" or "cautionary tale," replete with villains, heroes, unexpected plot twists, and avoidable tragedies, is because of the efforts of William Silverman (1917–2005), who used it to advocate evidence-based medical practice based on randomized controlled trials.[54,55]

In 1942, Wilson and coworkers[56] recognized that periodic breathing observed in preterm infants could be abolished with oxygen. Wilson was cautious about advocating the therapeutic use of oxygen, but other investigators were more enthusiastic.[57] As oxygen use proliferated, an epidemic of blindness in preterm infants caused by retrolental fibroplasia (RLF) arose in the world's developed countries, becoming within a single decade the most common cause of blindness in children.[54,58] In the early 1950s, comparative observations in Britain and Australia noted a difference in rates of RLF between nurseries that used oxygen liberally and those that did not.[59,60] Early observations about the role of oxygen in the pathogenesis of RLF were augmented by clinical observations and laboratory models.[61,62]

A randomized controlled trial begun in 1953 tested whether the incidence of RLF could be altered by exposure to restricted versus unrestricted levels of oxygen.[63] This trial, enrolling all infants with birth weight less than 1500 g in 18 hospitals, found that the incidence of cicatrical RLF was 3.5 times greater with unrestricted use than with use based on clinical need. The incidence of "active RLF" was twice as high. There was no difference in mortality noted. A smaller randomized trial performed at Bellevue Hospital found a 22% incidence of cicatrical RLF among preterm infants continuously exposed to "high" oxygen concentration (mean Fio_2, 69% [standard deviation, 6.5%]) but none in infants in the "low" oxygen group (mean Fio_2, 38% [standard deviation, 7.7%]).[64]

During the next decade, the incidence of RLF declined sharply as oxygen use was curtailed. However, the restricted use of oxygen came with an unexpected cost. In 1960, a review of a series of autopsied preterm infants noted that deaths from hyaline membrane disease increased 2.5-fold during a 4-year period of restricted oxygen use (1954–1958) compared with a similar period (1944–1948) of routine oxygen use.[65] These observations were later confirmed epidemiologically.[66,67] Reviewing data in the United Kingdom, Cross[67] estimated that each case of blindness prevented resulted in an excess of 16 deaths. The studies described previously were performed in an era when neither the technology to measure delivered oxygen (Fio_2) nor blood levels of oxygen (Pao_2, Sao_2) were routinely available.[68,69] Most of the devices related to oxygen that are now used became commercially available in the 1970s to 1980s.[7,11,12,68,69] Therefore, infants in the 1960s nursed in a restricted oxygen environment likely experienced repeated episodes of cyanosis (and therefore low saturation values). Some of the increased mortality was almost certainly related to the severe restriction of oxygen that would not be tolerated in any modern neonatal intensive care unit (NICU).

In 1987, Bancalari and colleagues[70] performed a prospective observational study to determine whether continuous $TcPo_2$ monitoring reduced the risk of ROP in infants with birth weight less than or equal to 1300 g. Although they noted a reduction in ROP in infants with birth weight greater than or equal to 1000 g, they found no reduction in ROP in infants less than 1000 g, who had the greatest exposure to oxygen and were at highest risk for the disease. The investigators cautioned that, "...by continuously adjusting the Fio_2 in an attempt to keep the $TcPo_2$ within a specified range, oscillations in $TcPo_2$ are frequently amplified, thereby achieving an effect exactly the opposite of what is desired."[70] In a second report based on this cohort, the investigators found that the adjusted odds ratio for each 12-hour period in which $TcPo_2$ exceeded 80 mm Hg was 1.9 (95% confidence interval, 1.2–3.0).[71]

Without a detailed understanding of the relationship between oxygen exposure and the pathogenesis of ROP on a cellular level, rational limits on the use of oxygen that minimized ROP in preterm infants could not be achieved. During 1990s, the relationship between premature birth, retinal oxygen status, insulin-like growth factor, vascular endothelial growth factor, and vascular growth and proliferation was gradually elucidated.[43,57,72–74] This mechanism provided the rationale for the STOP-ROP trial, published in 2000.[75] The investigators reasoned that although hyperoxia might be responsible for intense vascular proliferation early in the disease, supplemental oxygen might actually downregulate neovascularization after ROP had become established. A total of 649 extremely low birth weight infants with prethreshold ROP and receiving supplemental oxygen were randomized to receive oxygen at a conventional

Spo$_2$ target range (89%–94%) or at a higher range (96%–99%). Although some measures of ROP severity improved in the high saturation group, there was no difference between groups in the rates of the primary outcome or progression to threshold ROP. Death rates were similar in both groups but worse pulmonary status was noted in infants randomized to the high-saturation group.

In Australia, another large multicentered trial, the Benefits of Oxygen Saturation Targeting (BOOST) trial, explored the possible benefit of higher levels of oxygen saturation.[76] This trial enrolled 350 infants with gestational age less than 30 weeks, randomized to a standard Spo$_2$ range (91%–94%) or a high Spo$_2$ range (95%–98%). The study found no differences in growth or neurodevelopmental outcome at 12 months corrected age and no difference in rates of death or ROP. However, it noted higher rates of BPD (supplemental oxygen need at 36-weeks postmenstrual age) and need for oxygen after hospital discharge in the high-saturation group. From these two randomized clinical trials, it became apparent that Spo$_2$ levels greater than or equal to 95% offered no benefit to small preterm infants.

By early part of this millennium, it was clear that the incidence of ROP was not decreasing, despite new monitoring technology and better understanding of ROP pathogenesis.[77] Several observations suggested that lower target Spo$_2$ range might decrease incidence of severe ROP and BPD in VLBW infants without causing harm.[78–81] In a single NICU that set guidelines for a target Spo$_2$ range of 85% to 93% and imposed a strictly enforced protocol, the incidence of severe ROP (stage 3–4) decreased from 12.5% to 2.5% in a 5-year period (1997–2001).[78] During the same period, survival rates improved in this NICU. The severe ROP rate for infants in Vermont Oxford Network stayed about the same. These observations led to the widespread adoption of lower target saturation ranges and a subsequent decline in the incidence of severe ROP (**Fig. 3**). However, without guidance of a strong evidence base, advisory bodies were uncertain what saturation range to recommend. In the United States, the AAP suggested that a target Spo$_2$ range from 85% to 95% was

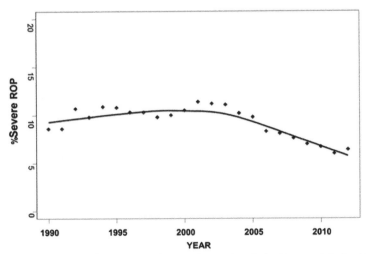

Fig. 3. Median incidence of severe ROP in member units of the Vermont-Oxford Network, 1990–2012. (*From* Vermont Oxford Network database of very low birth weight infants. Burlington (VT): Vermont Oxford Network; 2014. Nightingale Internet Reporting System. Accessed May 15, 2014; with permission.)

desirable.[48] In Europe, consensus guidelines suggested 85% to 93%.[82] Both statements lamented the absence of data needed to support any recommendation.

The absence of solid evidence on which to base rational oxygen use led to calls for randomized controlled trials.[55,83,84] By the mid-2000s, three large, double-blind, randomized clinical trials with similar design were launched in Europe, Australia, New Zealand, the United States, and Canada.[3,4,6] These trials focused on infants less than 28-weeks gestational age. Common design features included two standardized target saturation groups: low (Spo_2 = 85%–89%) and high (Spo_2 = 91%–95%). Blinding in all three studies was attained using an altered pulse oximeter algorithm offset to read 88% to 92% for the specified target range. Composite outcomes were death or severe ROP, and death or neurodevelopmental disability 18 to 24 months. Death was included in these measures because it is a competing outcome.

The first of these trials, the SUPPORT trial,[3] was a multicenter randomized trial involving 23 centers in the United States. It used a 2 × 2 factorial design, also testing two delivery room practices: initial CPAP without surfactant versus intubation and mechanical ventilation with surfactant. The trial enrolled 1316 infants 24- to 27-weeks gestational age who were randomized to one of the two Spo_2 target ranges noted previously, with blinding attained using the altered pulse oximeter. Results of the trial showed no difference in the composite primary outcome: death before hospital discharge or severe ROP (28% vs 32%; low vs high). However, the incidence of each of the component outcomes differed significantly: severe ROP was greatly reduced in the low-Spo_2 group (8.6% vs 17.9%), but the rate of death increased in the low-saturation group (19.9% vs 16.2%). No difference in rates of BPD or necrotizing enterocolitis (NEC) was noted.

In a follow-up study of infants who participated in the SUPPORT trial, investigators found no difference in the composite outcome of death or neurodevelopmental impairment at 18- to 22-months corrected age among those assigned to a lower or higher target range of oxygen saturation.[5] A significantly elevated mortality rate persisted in the low-Spo_2 group.

Interim results of the second trial, BOOST II,[6] conducted in Australia, New Zealand, and United Kingdom, appeared in 2013. The report was based on the enrollment of 2448 infants less than 28-weeks gestational age. Halfway through the study, an error was discovered in the pulse oximeter algorithm that caused poor separation between the intended target saturation groups. Following introduction of a corrected algorithm, a higher death rate was noted in the low-Spo_2 target group (23% vs 16%). A decreased rate of severe ROP (11% vs 14%) and a higher rate of NEC (10% vs 8%) were also noted in the low-Spo_2 target group. The BOOST II trial was halted before completion by the study's safety committee. A report on the primary composite outcome (death or severe neurodevelopmental delay at 18–24 months) has not yet been published. **Fig. 4** shows the significantly elevated hazard ratio for death in the low- versus high-Spo_2 target groups obtained after the pulse oximeter algorithm was revised.[6]

The third study with similar design, the Canadian Oxygen Trial,[4] found no difference in the composite primary outcome (death or neurodevelopmental impairment at 18 months), no difference in rates among the outcome components, and no difference in incidence of severe ROP. It did find a significantly longer duration of in-hospital oxygen need in the high-saturation group.

A retrospective meta-analysis that included results available for the three trials in late 2013 showed no difference between the low- and high-saturation groups in rates of death or severe neurosensory disability at 18 to 24 months with either the original or the revised algorithm.[30] Among secondary outcomes, the analysis found higher

Revised Algorithm

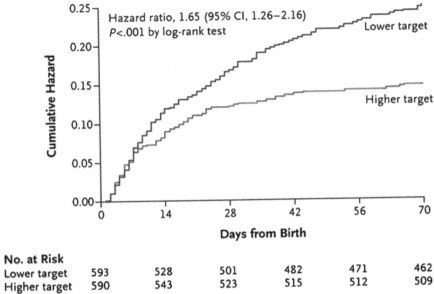

Fig. 4. Cumulative hazard estimates for death before hospital discharge in the two oxygen saturation target groups for the revised oximeter algorithm, BOOST II trial. CI, confidence interval. (*From* Stenson BJ, Tarnow-Mordi WO, Darlow BA, et al. Oxygen saturation and outcomes in preterm infants. N Engl J Med 2013;368:2012; with permission.)

risk ratios (95% confidence interval) for mortality (1.41 [1.14–1.74]) and NEC (1.25 [1.05–1.49]) and a lower risk ratio for severe ROP (0.74 [0.59–0.92]) for low- versus the high-saturation groups. Risk ratios were similar for BPD, intra-ventricular hemorrhage (grades 2–4), and patent ductus arteriosus. A prospective meta-analysis based on individual patient data will be conducted when BOOST II follow-up results become available.[85]

In summary, despite the efforts of three major international randomized trials, a single target saturation range that minimized mortality and severe ROP remained undetermined. However, data from these trials suggest that use of a higher oxygen saturation target range than previously recommended (eg, 90%–95%) is prudent in the management of preterm infants receiving supplemental oxygen.[86] The three randomized clinical trials leave many unanswered questions that may be fruitful areas of investigation. Recent studies have demonstrated the difficulty of maintaining the SpO_2 of VLBW infants receiving supplemental oxygen within any target range.[2,87] In a study by Lim and colleagues,[87] a group of 45 infants less than 37-week gestational age on CPAP spent only about 30% of time with SpO_2 within the specified target range (89%–93%). The influence of these excursions on the incidence of ROP, mortality, and other outcomes is unknown.

Ethical Storm over the SUPPORT Trial Consent Form

In early 2013, the Office for Human Research Protection (OHRP) investigated allegations brought by the advocacy group Citizens United. At issue was whether the consent form used in the SUPPORT trial misled parents about the risks of participating in the study.

OHRP concluded that parents were indeed misled.[88] The University of Alabama at Birmingham (UAB), one of the SUPPORT study sites, was cited for "failure to describe the reasonably foreseeable risks of blindness, neurologic damage and death." The letter contained a lengthy review of prior studies dating back to the 1950s, a review of SUPPORT outcome data, and extracts of the consent form used by UAB. It concluded, "Accordingly, we determine that the informed consent document for this trial failed to adequately inform parents of the reasonably foreseeable risks and discomforts of research participation." Although the determination itself was confined to a criticism of the consent form used by UAB, it was clear that OHRP believed that increased mortality was a "reasonably foreseeable risk" of study participation and the conduct of the study could be considered unethical. That the investigators had acted unethically was asserted by the report and editorial in the *NY Times*.[89]

In the weeks that followed the letter of determination, the conduct of the SUPPORT trial and the OHRP determination were vigorously defended.[90–94] One defense of SUPPORT came from the National Institutes of Health,[91] which had approved and funded the SUPPORT trial. Although acknowledging the deficiencies in UAB's consent form and unequivocally supporting the role of the OHRP, the authors suggested that the OHRP ruling "has had the effect of damaging the reputation of the investigators and, even worse, casting a pall over the conduct of clinical research to answer important questions in daily practice." Given the strong views expressed by opposing parties and the absence of clear standards, OHRP retreated from its original determination.[88] The issue remains under deliberation.

TECHNOLOGIC ADVANCES

Pulse oximetry has been proved to be an extremely useful tool in assessment and monitoring of VLBW infants as they receive neonatal care. However, its widespread use over the last three decades has also revealed some of its inherent limitations. Accurate determination of Spo_2 requires a high-quality arterial signal and is limited by errors resulting from motion, low perfusion, and dyshemoglobinemias. The theoretic model of conventional pulse oximetry assumes that the arterial blood is the only light-absorbing pulsatile component. However, this assumption has been challenged by Spo_2 readings during motion that fall below 85%. That should not be the case if these desaturations were merely the result of uncharacterized noise. The newest generations of pulse oximeters use improved algorithms of signal extraction technology, which assume that nonarterial absorbers also generate a pulsatile signal when motion occurs and that the ratio of absorption ratios should be considered a composite of arterial and nonarterial pulsatile signals, ultimately resulting in more accurate Spo_2 readings especially under critical conditions. These novel conceptual models are also applicable to situations of low signal-to-noise ratio, such as low-perfusion states.[95,96]

Until recently, pulse oximeters have also been limited because they use two wavelengths of light to display Spo_2, assuming that the only light absorbers in the blood are O_2Hb and Hb. This assumption is frequently violated, resulting in serious Spo_2 errors. The new multiwavelength Rainbow Technology pulse oximeters developed by Masimo Corporation (Irvine, CA) have permitted the noninvasive measurement of carboxyhemoglobin, methemoglobin, and total Hb.[97] Reflectance pulse oximeters that are based on absorption analysis of reflected rather than transmitted light have recently been introduced into neonatal clinical practice.[98] With the success of pulse oximetry and recent advances in digital signal processing, there is increasing research interest in the circulatory information derived from the photoplethysmographic waveform. New plethysmograph-derived parameters, such as perfusion index and pleth variability index, have the potential to estimate tissue perfusion and intravascular volume noninvasively.[16] Combined with improved understanding of the underlying physiology of the waveform it is easy to predict the emergence of multifunction pulse oximeters. The incorporation of these technologic advances into evidence-based clinical algorithms will improve the efficiency of this methodology in routine neonatal care. Clinical research is needed to define the utility of these technologies, and to identify new monitoring opportunities.

REFERENCES

1. Mower WR, Sachs C, Nicklin EL, et al. Pulse oximetry as a fifth pediatric vital sign. Pediatrics 1997;99:681–6.
2. Di Fiore JM, Walsh M, Wrage L, et al. Low oxygen saturation target range is associated with increased incidence of intermittent hypoxemia. J Pediatr 2012;161:1047–52.
3. Carlo WA, Finer NN, Walsh MC, et al. Target ranges of oxygen saturation in extremely preterm infants. N Engl J Med 2010;362:1959–69.
4. Schmidt B, Whyte RK, Asztalos EV, et al. Effects of targeting higher vs. lower arterial oxygen saturations on death or disability in extremely preterm infants: a randomized clinical trial. JAMA 2013;309:2111–20.
5. Vaucher YE, Peralta-Carcelen M, Finer NN, et al. Neurodevelopmental outcomes in the early CPAP and pulse oximetry trial. N Engl J Med 2012;367:2495–504.
6. Stenson BJ, Tarnow-Mordi WO, Darlow BA, et al. Oxygen saturation and outcomes in preterm infants. N Engl J Med 2013;368:2094–104.
7. Severinghaus JW, Astrup PB. History of blood gas analysis. VI. Oximetry. J Clin Monit 1986;2:270–88.
8. Squire J. Instrument for measuring quantity of blood and its degree of oxygenation in web of the hand. Clin Sci 1940;4:331–9.
9. Millikan GA. The oximeter, an instrument for measuring continuously the oxygen saturation of arterial blood in man. Rev Sci Instrum 1942;13:434–44.
10. Wood H. Oximetry. In: Glasser O, editor. Medical Physics, Vol. 2. Chicago (IL): Year Book Publishers; 1950. p. 664–80.
11. Severinghaus JW. Takuo Aoyagi: discovery of pulse oximetry. Anesth Analg 2007;105:S1–4 [Tables of contents].
12. Aoyagi T. Pulse oximetry: its invention, theory, and future. J Anesth 2003;17: 259–66.
13. Poets CF, Southall DP. Noninvasive monitoring of oxygenation in infants and children: practical considerations and areas of concern. Pediatrics 1994;93:737–46.
14. Jubran A. Pulse oximetry. In: Tobin MJ, editor. Principles and practice of intensive care monitoring. New York: McGraw Hill, Inc; 1998. p. 261–87.
15. Hanning CD, Alexander-Williams JM. Pulse oximetry: a practical review. BMJ 1995;311:367–70.
16. Sahni R. Noninvasive monitoring by photoplethysmography. Clin Perinatol 2012; 39:573–83.
17. Zonios G, Shankar U, Iyer VK. Pulse oximetry theory and calibration for low saturations. IEEE Trans Biomed Eng 2004;51:818–22.
18. Obladen M. History of neonatal resuscitation. Part 2: oxygen and other drugs. Neonatology 2009;95:91–6.
19. Niermeyer S, Kattwinkel J, Van Reempts P, et al. International guidelines for neonatal resuscitation: an excerpt from the Guidelines 2000 for Cardiopulmonary

Resuscitation and Emergency Cardiovascular Care: International Consensus on Science. Contributors and Reviewers for the Neonatal Resuscitation Guidelines. Pediatrics 2000;106:E29.

20. Perlman JM, Wyllie J, Kattwinkel J, et al. Part 11: neonatal resuscitation: 2010 International Consensus on Cardiopulmonary Resuscitation and Emergency Cardiovascular Care Science With Treatment Recommendations. Circulation 2010;122:S516–38.
21. Saugstad OD. To oxygenate or not to oxygenate–that is the question. Am J Physiol Heart Circ Physiol 2008;295:H1371–2.
22. Saugstad OD. Why are we still using oxygen to resuscitate term infants? J Perinatol 2010;30(Suppl):S46–50.
23. Saugstad OD. Resuscitation of newborn infants: from oxygen to room air. Lancet 2010;376:1970–1.
24. Saugstad OD, Ramji S, Irani SF, et al. Resuscitation of newborn infants with 21% or 100% oxygen: follow-up at 18 to 24 months. Pediatrics 2003;112:296–300.
25. Saugstad OD, Ramji S, Soll RF, et al. Resuscitation of newborn infants with 21% or 100% oxygen: an updated systematic review and meta-analysis. Neonatology 2008;94:176–82.
26. Saugstad OD, Ramji S, Vento M. Oxygen for newborn resuscitation: how much is enough? Pediatrics 2006;118:789–92.
27. Solberg R, Longini M, Proietti F, et al. Resuscitation with supplementary oxygen induces oxidative injury in the cerebral cortex. Free Radic Biol Med 2012;53:1061–7.
28. Wollen EJ, Sejersted Y, Wright MS, et al. Transcriptome profiling of the newborn mouse brain after hypoxia-reoxygenation: hyperoxic reoxygenation induces inflammatory and energy failure responsive genes. Pediatr Res 2014;75:517–26.
29. Saugstad OD. Hyperoxia in the term newborn: more evidence is still needed for optimal oxygen therapy. Acta Paediatr Suppl 2012;101:34–8.
30. Saugstad OD, Aune D. Optimal oxygenation of extremely low birth weight infants: a meta-analysis and systematic review of the oxygen saturation target studies. Neonatology 2014;105:55–63.
31. Saugstad OD, Vento M, Ramji S, et al. Neurodevelopmental outcome of infants resuscitated with air or 100% oxygen: a systematic review and meta-analysis. Neonatology 2012;102:98–103.
32. Bajaj N, Udani RH, Nanavati RN. Room air vs. 100 per cent oxygen for neonatal resuscitation: a controlled clinical trial. J Trop Pediatr 2005;51:206–11.
33. Ramji S, Rasaily R, Mishra PK, et al. Resuscitation of asphyxiated newborns with room air or 100% oxygen at birth: a multicentric clinical trial. Indian Pediatr 2003;40:510–7.
34. Saugstad OD. The oxygen paradox in the newborn: keep oxygen at normal levels. J Pediatr 2013;163:934–5.
35. O'Donnell CP, Kamlin CO, Davis PG, et al. Clinical assessment of infant colour at delivery. Arch Dis Child Fetal Neonatal Ed 2007;92:F465–7.
36. Berger TM. Neonatal resuscitation: foetal physiology and pathophysiological aspects. Eur J Anaesthesiol 2012;29:362–70.
37. Kattwinkel J, Perlman JM, Aziz K, et al. Part 15: neonatal resuscitation: 2010 American Heart Association guidelines for cardiopulmonary resuscitation and emergency cardiovascular care. Circulation 2010;122:S909–19.
38. McCarthy LK, Morley CJ, Davis PG, et al. Timing of interventions in the delivery room: does reality compare with neonatal resuscitation guidelines? J Pediatr 2013;163:1553–7.e1.

39. Rabi Y, Yee W, Chen SY, et al. Oxygen saturation trends immediately after birth. J Pediatr 2006;148:590–4.

40. Rabi Y, Dawson JA. Oxygen therapy and oximetry in the delivery room. Semin Fetal Neonatal Med 2013;18:330–5.

41. Dawson JA, Kamlin CO, Vento M, et al. Defining the reference range for oxygen saturation for infants after birth. Pediatrics 2010;125:e1340–7.

42. Wyllie J. Recent changes to UK newborn resuscitation guidelines. Arch Dis Child Fetal Neonatal Ed 2012;97:F4–7.

43. Vento M, Cubells E, Escobar JJ, et al. Oxygen saturation after birth in preterm infants treated with continuous positive airway pressure and air: assessment of gender differences and comparison wit published normograms. Arch Dis Child Fetal Neonatal Ed 2013;98:F228–32.

44. Matsiukevich D, Randis TM, Utkina-Sosunova I, et al. The state of systemic circulation, collapsed or preserved defines the need for hyperoxic or normoxic resuscitation in neonatal mice with hypoxia-ischemia. Resuscitation 2010;81:224–9.

45. Escrig R, Arruza L, Izquierdo I, et al. Achievement of targeted saturation values in extremely low gestational age neonates resuscitated with low or high oxygen concentrations: a prospective, randomized trial. Pediatrics 2008;121:875–81.

46. Finer N, Saugstad O, Vento M, et al. Use of oxygen for resuscitation of the extremely low birth weight infant. Pediatrics 2010;125:389–91.

47. Kapadia VS, Chalak LF, Sparks JE, et al. Resuscitation of preterm neonates with limited versus high oxygen strategy. Pediatrics 2013;132:e1488–96.

48. Wang CL, Anderson C, Leone TA, et al. Resuscitation of preterm neonates by using room air or 100% oxygen. Pediatrics 2008;121(6):1083–9.

49. Vento M, Moro M, Escrig R, et al. Preterm resuscitation with low oxygen causes less oxidative stress, inflammation, and chronic lung disease. Pediatrics 2009; 124:e439–49.

50. Shah PS. Meta-analysis of neurodevelopmental outcome after room air versus 100% oxygen resuscitation: generating more questions than answers? Commentary on O.D. Saugstad et al.: neurodevelopmental outcome of infants resuscitated with air or 100% oxygen: a systematic review and meta-analysis (Neonatology 2012;102:98-103). Neonatology 2012;102(2):104–6.

51. Goos TG, Rook D, van der Eijk AC, et al. Observing the resuscitation of very preterm infants: are we able to follow the oxygen saturation targets? Resuscitation 2013;84:1108–13.

52. Rabi Y, Singhal N, Nettel-Aguirre A. Room-air versus oxygen administration for resuscitation of preterm infants: the ROAR study. Pediatrics 2011;128:e374–81.

53. Gandhi B, Rich W, Finer N. Achieving targeted pulse oximetry values in preterm infants in the delivery room. J Pediatr 2013;163:412–5.

54. Silverman WA. Retrolental fibroplasia: a modern parable. New York: Grune & Stratton; 1980.

55. Silverman WA. A cautionary tale about supplemental oxygen: the albatross of neonatal medicine. Pediatrics 2004;113:394–6.

56. Wilson JL, Long S, Howard PJ. Respiration of premature infants: response to variations of oxygen and to increased carbon dioxide in inspired air. Am J Dis Child 1942;63:1080–5.

57. Hellstrom A, Perruzzi C, Ju M, et al. Low IGF-I suppresses VEGF-survival signaling in retinal endothelial cells: direct correlation with clinical retinopathy of prematurity. Proc Natl Acad Sci U S A 2001;98:5804–8.

58. Appelbaum A. Retrolental fibroplasia—blindness in infants of low weight at birth. Calif Med 1952;77:259–65.

59. Campbell K. Intensive oxygen therapy as a possible cause of retrolental fibroplasia; a clinical approach. Med J Aust 1951;2:48–50.
60. Crosse VM. The problem of retrolental fibroplasia in the City of Birmingham. Trans Ophthalmol Soc U K 1951;71:609612.
61. Patz A, Eastham A, Higginbotham DH, et al. Oxygen studies in retrolental fibroplasia. II. The production of the microscopic changes of retrolental fibroplasia in experimental animals. Am J Ophthalmol 1953;36:1511–22.
62. Patz A, Hoeck LE, De La Cruz E. Studies on the effect of high oxygen administration in retrolental fibroplasia. I. Nursery observations. Am J Ophthalmol 1952; 35:1248–53.
63. Kinsey VE. Retrolental fibroplasia; cooperative study of retrolental fibroplasia and the use of oxygen. AMA Arch Ophthalmol 1956;56:481–543.
64. Lanman JT, Guy LP, Dancis J. Retrolental fibroplasia and oxygen therapy. J Am Med Assoc 1954;155:223–6.
65. Avery ME. Recent increase in mortality from hyaline membrane disease. J Pediatr 1960;57:553–9.
66. Bolton DP, Cross KW. Further observation on cost of preventing retrolental fibroplasia. Lancet 1974;303:445–8.
67. Cross KW. Cost of preventing retrolental fibroplasia? Lancet 1973;2:954–6.
68. Severinghaus JW. The invention and development of blood gas analysis apparatus. Anesthesiology 2002;97:253–6.
69. Severinghaus JW, Astrup PB. History of blood gas analysis. V. Oxygen measurement. J Clin Monit 1986;2:174–89.
70. Bancalari E, Flynn J, Goldberg RN, et al. Influence of transcutaneous oxygen monitoring on the incidence of retinopathy of prematurity. Pediatrics 1987;79:663–9.
71. Flynn JT, Bancalari E, Snyder ES, et al. A cohort study of transcutaneous oxygen tension and the incidence and severity of retinopathy of prematurity. N Engl J Med 1992;326:1050–4.
72. Pierce EA, Foley ED, Smith LE. Regulation of vascular endothelial growth factor by oxygen in a model of retinopathy of prematurity. Arch Ophthalmol 1996;114: 1219–28.
73. Shweiki D, Itin A, Soffer D, et al. Vascular endothelial growth factor induced by hypoxia may mediate hypoxia-initiated angiogenesis. Nature 1992;359:843–5.
74. Smith LE. Pathogenesis of retinopathy of prematurity. Semin Neonatol 2003;8: 469–73.
75. Group TS-RMS. Supplemental therapeutic oxygen for prethreshold retinopathy of prematurity (STOP-ROP), a randomized, controlled trial. I: primary outcomes. Pediatrics 2000;105:295–310.
76. Askie LM, Henderson-Smart DJ, Irwig L, et al. Oxygen-saturation targets and outcomes in extremely preterm infants. N Engl J Med 2003;349:959–67.
77. Lad EM, Hernandez-Boussard T, Morton JM, et al. Incidence of retinopathy of prematurity in the United States: 1997 through 2005. Am J Ophthalmol 2009; 148:451–8.
78. Chow LC, Wright KW, Sola A. Can changes in clinical practice decrease the incidence of severe retinopathy of prematurity in very low birth weight infants? Pediatrics 2003;111:339–45.
79. Sjöstedt S, Rooth G. Low oxygen tension in the management of newborn infants. Arch Dis Child 1957;32:397–400.
80. Tin W, Milligan DW, Pennefather P, et al. Pulse oximetry, severe retinopathy, and outcome at one year in babies of less than 28 weeks gestation. Arch Dis Child Fetal Neonatal Ed 2001;84:F106–10.

81. Tin WG, Gupta S. Optimum oxygen therapy in preterm babies. Arch Dis Child Fetal Neonatal Ed 2007;92:F143–7.

82. Sweet DG, Carnielli V, Greisen G, et al. European consensus guidelines on the management of neonatal respiratory distress syndrome in preterm infants: 2010 update. Neonatology 2010;97:402–17.

83. Cole CH, Wright KW, Tarnow-Mordi W, et al. Resolving our uncertainty about oxygen therapy. Pediatrics 2003;112:1415–9.

84. Tin W. Oxygen therapy: 50 years of uncertainty. Pediatrics 2002;110:615–6.

85. Askie LM, Brocklehurst P, Darlow BA, et al. NeOProM: Neonatal Oxygenation Prospective Meta-analysis Collaboration study protocol. BMC Pediatr 2011;11:6.

86. Polin RA, Bateman D. Oxygen-saturation targets in preterm infants. N Engl J Med 2013;368:2141–2.

87. Lim K, Wheeler KI, Gale TJ, et al. Oxygen saturation targeting in preterm infants receiving continuous positive airway pressure. J Pediatr 2014;164:730–6.e1.

88. Office for Human Research Protections. Human Research Protections under Federalwide Assurance (FWA) 5960: The Surfactant, Positive Pressure, and Oxygenation Randomized Trial (SUPPORT) June 4, 2013. Available at: www.hhs.gov/ohrp/detrm_letrs/YR13/june13a.pdf.

89. Editorial Board. An ethical breakdown. New York Times 2013;A26.

90. Lantos JD. Learning the right lessons from the SUPPORT study controversy. Arch Dis Child Fetal Neonatal Ed 2014;99:F4–5.

91. Drazen JM, Solomon CG, Greene MF. Informed consent and SUPPORT. N Engl J Med 2013;368:1929–31.

92. Hudson KL, Guttmacher AE, Collins FS. In support of SUPPORT — A view from the NIH. N Engl J Med 2013;368:2349–51.

93. Macklin R, Shepherd L, Dreger A, et al. The OHRP and SUPPORT — Another view. N Engl J Med 2013;369:e3.

94. Wilfond BS, Magnus D, Antommaria AH, et al. The OHRP and SUPPORT. N Engl J Med 2013;368:e36.

95. Cannesson M, Talke P. Recent advances in pulse oximetry. F100 Med Rep 2009; 1:66.

96. Graybeal JM, Petterson MT. Adaptive filtering and alternative calculations revolutionizes pulse oximetry sensitivity and specificity during motion and low perfusion. Conf Proc IEEE Eng Med Biol Soc 2004;7:5363–6.

97. Aoyagi T, Fuse M, Kobayashi N, et al. Multiwavelength pulse oximetry: theory for the future. Anesth Analg 2007;105:S53–8 [Tables of contents].

98. Agashe GS, Coakley J, Mannheimer PD. Forehead pulse oximetry: headband use helps alleviate false low readings likely related to venous pulsation artifact. Anesthesiology 2006;105:1111–6.

Index

Note: Page numbers of article titles are in **boldface** type.

A

Analgesia in newborns, fentanyl, 902–903
 for invasive procedures, 908–909
 for mechanical ventilation, 908, 911
 morphine, 901–902
 nonopioid, 904–907
 opioid, 902–903
 postoperative, 908
Anti-vascular endothelial growth factor antagonist therapy, bevacizumab, 937
 evidence that inhibition of epithelial growth factor inhibits intravitreal angiogensis,
  932, 934–935
 FDA approved agents, 937
 guidelines for, 938–939
 size and dose considerations for adult and preterm infant, 937–938

B

Borderline viability, best interest of infant in, arguments against, 805
  parental decision-making authority in, 805
 constrained parental autonomy in decision-making and, 806
 controversies in caring for the extremely premature infant, **799–814**
 counseling debate in, parental values *versus* physician or health care team, 807–808
  parent participation in decision-making, 807
  probability and utility in decision-making, 807
 debate about cost in, direct and indirect, 808
  rationing of care in, 809
 doctor knows best in, 805
 guidelines are discriminatory and lack ethical and scientific basis, ageism within
  and at border of gray zone, 803–804
  response to ageism, 804–805
 mandatory trial of assessment and treatment, accuracy of assessment of
  gestational age after birth, 801–802
  assessment of vigorousness adds prognostic information and therefore
   decreases uncertainty, 802
  testing early treatment responses provides facts to help determine long-term
   prognosis, 802
  treatment withdrawal is ethically equivalent to withholding in parents perspective,
   802–803
 preterm birth care as emergency situation, 803
 resuscitation guidelines in, argument against, trial of assessment and treatment
  for all, 800–801
  gestational age-based, 799–800

Clin Perinatol 41 (2014) 1033–1043
http://dx.doi.org/10.1016/S0095-5108(14)00105-5
0095-5108/14/$ – see front matter © 2014 Elsevier Inc. All rights reserved.

United States Postal Service

Statement of Ownership, Management, and Circulation
(All Periodicals Publications Except Requester Publications)

1. Publication Title
Clinics in Perinatology

2. Publication Number
0 0 1 - 7 4 4

3. Filing Date
9/14/14

4. Issue Frequency
Mar, Jun, Sep, Dec

5. Number of Issues Published Annually
4

6. Annual Subscription Price
$285.00

7. Complete Mailing Address of Known Office of Publication (Not printer) (Street, city, county, state, and ZIP+4®)
Elsevier Inc.
360 Park Avenue South
New York, NY 10010-1710

Contact Person
Stephen R. Bushing

Telephone (Include area code)
215-239-3688

8. Complete Mailing Address of Headquarters or General Business Office of Publisher (Not printer)
Elsevier Inc., 360 Park Avenue South, New York, NY 10010-1710

9. Full Names and Complete Mailing Addresses of Publisher, Editor, and Managing Editor (Do not leave blank)

Publisher (Name and complete mailing address)
Linda Belfus, Elsevier, Inc., 1600 John F. Kennedy Blvd. Suite 1800, Philadelphia, PA 19103-2899

Editor (Name and complete mailing address)
Kerry Holland, Elsevier, Inc., 1600 John F. Kennedy Blvd. Suite 1800, Philadelphia, PA 19103-2899

Managing Editor (Name and complete mailing address)
Adrianne Brigido, Elsevier, Inc., 1600 John F. Kennedy Blvd. Suite 1800, Philadelphia, PA 19103-2899

10. Owner (Do not leave blank. If the publication is owned by a corporation, give the name and address of the corporation immediately followed by the names and addresses of all stockholders owning or holding 1 percent or more of the total amount of stock. If not owned by a corporation, give the names and addresses of the individual owners. If owned by a partnership or other unincorporated firm, give its name and address as well as those of each individual owner. If the publication is published by a nonprofit organization, give its name and address.)

Full Name	Complete Mailing Address
Wholly owned subsidiary of	1600 John F. Kennedy Blvd, Ste. 1800
Reed/Elsevier, US holdings	Philadelphia, PA 19103-2899

11. Known Bondholders, Mortgagees, and Other Security Holders Owning or Holding 1 Percent or More of Total Amount of Bonds, Mortgages, or Other Securities. If none, check box ☐ None

Full Name	Complete Mailing Address
N/A	

12. Tax Status (For completion by nonprofit organizations authorized to mail at nonprofit rates) (Check one)
The purpose, function, and nonprofit status of this organization and the exempt status for federal income tax purposes:
☐ Has Not Changed During Preceding 12 Months
☐ Has Changed During Preceding 12 Months (Publisher must submit explanation of change with this statement)

PS Form 3526, August 2012 (Page 1 of 3) (Instructions Page 3)) PSN 7530-01-000-9931 PRIVACY NOTICE: See our Privacy policy in www.usps.com

---

13. Publication Title
Clinics in Perinatology

14. Issue Date for Circulation Data Below
June 2014

15. Extent and Nature of Circulation

		Average No. Copies Each Issue During Preceding 12 Months	No. Copies of Single Issue Published Nearest to Filing Date
a. Total Number of Copies (Net press run)		1,715	1,669
b. Paid Circulation (By Mail and Outside the Mail)	(1) Mailed Outside-County Paid Subscriptions Stated on PS Form 3541. (Include paid distribution above nominal rate, advertiser's proof copies, and exchange copies)	1,119	1,047
	(2) Mailed In-County Paid Subscriptions Stated on PS Form 3541 (Include paid distribution above nominal rate, advertiser's proof copies, and exchange copies)		
	(3) Paid Distribution Outside the Mails Including Sales Through Dealers and Carriers, Street Vendors, Counter Sales, and Other Paid Distribution Outside USPS®	291	259
	(4) Paid Distribution by Other Classes Mailed Through the USPS (e.g. First-Class Mail®)		
c. Total Paid Distribution (Sum of 15b (1), (2), (3), and (4))	▶	1,410	1,306
d. Free or Nominal Rate Distribution (By Mail and Outside the Mail)	(1) Free or Nominal Rate Outside-County Copies Included on PS Form 3541	65	98
	(2) Free or Nominal Rate In-County Copies Included on PS Form 3541		
	(3) Free or Nominal Rate Copies Mailed at Other Classes Through the USPS (e.g. First-Class Mail)		
	(4) Free or Nominal Rate Distribution Outside the Mail (Carriers or other means)		
e. Total Free or Nominal Rate Distribution (Sum of 15d (1), (2), (3) and (4))	▶	65	98
f. Total Distribution (Sum of 15c and 15e)	▶	1,475	1,404
g. Copies not Distributed (See instructions to publishers #4 (page #3))	▶	240	265
h. Total (Sum of 15f and g)	▶	1,715	1,669
i. Percent Paid (15c divided by 15f times 100)	▶	95.59%	93.02%

16. Total circulation includes electronic copies. Report circulation on PS Form 3526-X worksheet.

17. Publication of Statement of Ownership
If the publication is a general publication, publication of this statement is required. Will be printed in the December 2014 issue of this publication.

18. Signature and Title of Editor, Publisher, Business Manager, or Owner
Stephen R. Bushing – Inventory Distribution Coordinator

Stephen R. Bushing

Date: September 14, 2014

I certify that all information furnished on this form is true and complete. I understand that anyone who furnishes false or misleading information on this form or who omits material or information requested on the form may be subject to criminal sanctions (including fines and imprisonment) and/or civil sanctions (including civil penalties).

PS Form 3526, August 2012 (Page 2 of 3)

Moving?

Make sure your subscription moves with you!

To notify us of your new address, find your **Clinics Account Number** (located on your mailing label above your name), and contact customer service at:

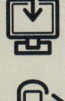

Email: journalscustomerservice-usa@elsevier.com

800-654-2452 (subscribers in the U.S. & Canada)
314-447-8871 (subscribers outside of the U.S. & Canada)

Fax number: 314-447-8029

Elsevier Health Sciences Division
Subscription Customer Service
3251 Riverport Lane
Maryland Heights, MO 63043

*To ensure uninterrupted delivery of your subscription, please notify us at least 4 weeks in advance of move.

Printed and bound by CPI Group (UK) Ltd, Croydon, CR0 4YY

08/06/2025

01896870-0007